Additional Praise for
Take a Load off Your Heart

"I was skeptical: Why one more cardiac self-help book? But then I started reading—till the very end. I could not put it down: well-written, little med-speak and entirely up-to-date and accurate. This is something I can recommend to all my patients."
—V.F. Froelicher, M.D.,
Professor of Medicine, Stanford University

"Whether you're trying to prevent that first heart attack or reduce your risk of a second one, *Take a Load off Your Heart* is the book to read. It tells you what you need to know about exercise, nutrition and handling stress—all in terms you can understand and apply in your daily life."
—Redford Williams, M.D., Director,
Behavioral Research, Duke University Medical Center

"Joe Piscatella and Dr. Barry Franklin have made an important contribution to the heart health of the nation. This eminently readable book combines medical information and suggestions for self-help."
—Nanette K. Wenger, M.D., Professor of Medicine (Cardiology),
Emory University School of Medicine

"*Take a Load off Your Heart* is superb—an outstanding book by two of the foremost experts on lifestyle modification and heart disease prevention. It is must reading for anyone who wants to prevent a heart attack or avoid another if they have already had one."
—Neil F. Gordon, M.D., Ph.D., M.P.H.,
President and CEO, INTERVENT USA

"A must-read for anyone who wants a science-based, comprehensive and sensible approach for reducing their risk of heart disease. It offers the gold-standard dietary recommendations, as well as the new discoveries in nutrition to promote health, all in 'how to' examples that readers will value."
—Penny Kris-Etherton, Ph.D., R.D.,
Distinguished Professor of Nutrition, Penn State University

"This easy-to-read book takes the mystery out of heart disease and translates the latest science into a remarkable 'how-to' manual of prevention. Reliable, current and practical advice for anyone who has a beating heart!"
—Gary J. Balady, M.D., Director of Preventive Cardiology, Boston Medical Center, Boston University School of Medicine

"A comprehensive guide for anyone concerned about heart disease. *Take a Load off Your Heart* is filled with practical advice and cutting-edge information. Read it today!"
—Wayne M. Sotile, Ph.D., author of *Thriving with Heart Disease: A Unique Program for You and Your Family/Living Happier, Healthier, Longer*

"A sensible, clear and comprehensive approach to improving heart health. It highlights the latest findings in cardiovascular research and provides useful tools for putting our current prevention and treatment guidelines into practice."
—Ronald M. Krauss, M.D., Children's Hospital, Oakland Research Institute

"A well-written treasure trove of information. Utilized properly, this book can add a significant dimension to our overall educational effort to positively influence and improve the cardiovascular health of our society."
—Gerald F. Fletcher, M.D., Mayo Clinic Jacksonville

"This is an excellent, easily readable book, which is loaded with information and should be of great value to all who want to take the best possible steps to prevent heart disease."
—Sidney C. Smith, Jr., M.D., Professor of Medicine, Director, Center for Cardiovascular Science and Medicine, University of North Carolina School of Medicine

"Take a short cut to a long life with a few hours of entertaining reading."
—Gerald C. Timmis, M.D., Medical Director, Clinical Research, William Beaumont Hospital

Take a Load off Your Heart

TAKE A LOAD OFF YOUR HEART

109 Things You Can Actually Do to
Prevent, Halt or Reverse Heart Disease

By Joseph C. Piscatella
and Barry A. Franklin, Ph.D.

Workman Publishing • New York

Library of Congress Cataloging-in-Publication Data

Piscatella, Joseph C.
    Take a load off your heart : 109 things you can actually do to prevent, halt or reverse heart disease / by Joseph C. Piscatella and Barry A. Franklin.
        p. cm.
    ISBN 0-7611-2676-7 (alk. paper)
        1. Coronary heart disease—Prevention. 2. Stress management. I. Franklin, Barry A. II. Title.

RC685.C6 P573 2003
616.1'2305—dc21

                                                                2002033852

Cover design by Paul Gamarello. Book design by Michael Fusco.
Cover illustration by Larry Limnidis/The*eye*spot

> The material in this book is provided for information only and should not be construed as medical advice or instruction. Always consult with your physician or other appropriate health professionals before making any changes in diet, physical activity and/or drug therapy.

Workman books are available at special discounts when purchased in bulk for premiums and sales promotions as well as for fund-raising or educational use. Special editions or book excerpts can also be created to specification. For details, contact the Special Sales Director at the address below.

Workman Publishing Company, Inc.
708 Broadway
New York, NY 10003-9555
www.workman.com

Printed in the U.S.A.
First printing: January 2003
10 9 8 7 6 5 4 3 2

To my wife, Bernie, my most constructive critic, ardent supporter and best friend. The journey with her has been a gift from God. —J.C.P.

To my wife, Linda, for her love, patience, understanding, encouragement and support. She has helped, in so many ways, to turn my dreams into reality. —B.A.F.

Acknowledgments

I t takes a team of dedicated people to put a book together. In particular, we are grateful to the medical professionals who gave of their time and expertise, providing information and insight and offering valuable suggestions. These include William C. Roberts, M.D., Beverly Utt, R.D., M.P.H., and Suzette Kroll, R.D.

The book would not be possible without our respective staff support, particularly Lou Imhof at the Institute for Fitness & Health; Brenda White and Dee LaPointe at William Beaumont Hospital; and Dave Harvey, Donna Selenich and Sue Tomaszycki, who helped with the graphics.

And finally, the dedication and expertise at Workman Publishing have been instrumental. Our thanks to Peter Workman for his faith in our work, to Susan Bolotin and Lynn Strong for their masterful editorial touch, and to the entire Workman team—especially Megan Nicolay, Meghan Rowe Phillips, Jenny Mandel, Kim Shannon, Paul Gamarello and Michael Fusco—for their dedicated support.

Contents

Appendix I: Prescriptions, Procedures and Programs 313

Appendix II: Sources and Web Sites

Before We Start . . .

W E KNOW FROM OUR OWN EXPERIENCE that when questions of health are pressing, many of us want quick answers even before we know exactly what to ask. Since the two of us have counseled literally thousands of patients, we've gotten pretty good at guessing what's on people's minds.

What does a heart attack feel like?

Everyone—not just cardiac patients—needs to know the answer to this one. Among the most common symptoms are pain, pressure or a sense of fullness under the breastbone that lasts two minutes or more. Men often say the pain feels like "having an elephant on my chest"; women typically experience a milder chest pain. The sensation may radiate to the shoulders, neck, jaw, back or arms. (Or it may not.) Women generally experience the radiating pain throughout the neck, jaw, shoulders, arms, back or abdomen; in general, their symptoms are more subtle. Men tend to have sharp pain in their arms and shoulders. Dizziness, sweating, nausea and shortness of breath may also occur.

Should I call 911 even if I don't have all these symptoms?

Not all symptoms may be present. If you think you might be having a heart attack, seek medical help immediately.

Is there anything I should do while I'm waiting for EMS to arrive?

Chew and swallow one regular uncoated adult aspirin (325 mg). It has been estimated that this recommendation alone, if widely adopted, would save an additional 5,000 to 10,000 lives in the United States each year!

What if I'm wrong? I'd feel like an idiot if I got to the hospital and they told me I had indigestion!

This is no time for foolish pride. Balloon angioplasty and new clot-busting drugs can literally halt heart attacks in progress—or at least minimize the damage—if administered soon after the onset of symptoms. Unfortunately, most heart attack victims wait several hours before seeking medical attention. By that time, irreversible heart muscle damage—or even death—can occur.

Is there a particular time of day—or day of the week—when the risk of heart attack is greatest?

You bet. Between six A.M. and noon is the riskiest time of day, perhaps because morning increases in hormone levels, blood pressure and artery stiffness heighten the possibility of clot formation. And more heart attacks happen on Monday than on other days of the week—a phenomenon scientists refer to as "Blue Monday." Why Monday? Many believe that the stress of a frenetic work environment, especially after a relaxing weekend, may be the cause.

———

How big a problem is heart disease in the United States?

Very. Cardiovascular disease afflicts an estimated 100 million Americans, or about half the adult population. And one person dies from cardiovascular disease every 34 seconds. This means that by seven A.M. on any day of the week, 741 people have already died from heart disease. By noon the figure has risen to 1, 271; by midafternoon, some 1,558 have died. By the time the 11 o'clock news has ended, the death toll stands at 2,488.

But what are my own odds of dying from heart disease?

Let's try to say this another way. Your odds of contracting AIDS are one in a million. Your chance of being murdered is one in 10,000. But your risk of dying from cardiovascular disease is one in two.

*I always thought heart disease was a "man's problem,"
but over the past year three female friends of mine
have been diagnosed with serious heart trouble.
Are they the exception?*

The truth is that heart disease is an equal opportunity affliction. It has been diagnosed in almost as many women (6.75 million) as men (6.93 million), but it's the leading cause of death among American women. According to Dr. Nanette Wenger of Emory University Medical School, "Over 250,000 women die of heart disease each year, more than the next 14 causes of death combined." In fact, says Dr. Wenger, "More women than men now die annually of heart disease. While women tend to fear cancer, particularly breast cancer, twice as many females die each year of heart and blood vessel disease as of all forms of cancer combined."

Heart disease is a problem for both sexes, but gender differences do exist. Men may develop the first signs of heart disease at ages 35 to 40. Men aged 30 to 49 are 6.5 times more likely to have a heart attack than women in that age group. The condition doesn't usually affect women until a decade or more later. Between ages 45 to 64, one out of nine women has heart disease. Over age 65, the ratio is one out of three—about the same as men.

*Are there any differences between men's and women's
chances of surviving a heart attack?*

Women stand a greater chance of dying within a year of their first heart attack. Moreover, there is evidence that women are traditionally less likely to get state-of-the art diagnostic cardiac studies and treatments. And when they do get treatment, their disease is generally more advanced than that of their male counterparts. Women are also more likely to die during heart surgery. These findings have led to major funding for the Women's Health Initiative, commissioned by the National Institutes of Health.

I have heart disease, and I'm concerned about my children and grandchildren. At what age should doctors look for a problem?

According to the American Heart Association, screening patients for heart disease risk should start as early as age 20. In particular, people 40 or older, or anyone who has two or more risk factors, should know their chances of developing heart disease. The Framingham Risk Score allows one to estimate his or her risk of having a heart attack in the next decade. (Go to the NHLBI Web site <www.nhlbi.nih.gov> for estimating risk using the Framingham Heart Study predictions.)

What is angina?

There are often no warning signs in the early stages of coronary heart disease. But as the coronary arteries become gradually narrowed and compromised, many people experience angina, or angina pectoris, which in Latin means "pain in the chest." And it is indeed a temporary chest pain caused by the heart muscle receiving insufficient oxygen to maintain its workload. Generally interpreted as a certain indicator of significant coronary artery blockage, angina affects over five million Americans.

Can you tell me more about what it feels like?

Typically, angina comes on as a sharp, sudden pain often described as a feeling of tightness behind the breastbone, heaviness, squeezing, numbness, burning or pressure. It may be confused with heartburn. And the pain may radiate into the arms (generally, the left arm), neck, jaw, back and shoulder. Men usually experience angina more intensely than women.

Is all angina the same?

No. Stable angina, which most often occurs during or soon after physical exertion, eating a heavy meal, going out in very cold or hot weather or as a reaction to emotional stress, will usually force you to stop what you're doing until the pain subsides. Unstable angina, which is often a symptom of an impending heart attack, produces escalating pain at less predictable times, even when you're sleeping. Angina is a progressive condition. The pain may become more frequent, more intense, or both.

How long does an angina attack last?

It can vary from 30 seconds to several minutes, but most attacks last only a few minutes. Your doctor will most likely prescribe one of many appropriate drugs and encourage you to stop smoking and to eat a low-fat diet.

But I'm on angina medication and I still get pain.

If rest in combination with drugs (many experts consider three consecutive nitroglycerin tablets a rule of thumb) doesn't bring relief, seek medical assistance NOW. This would suggest an impending heart attack.

———

What is a heart attack?

A heart attack, also called a myocardial infarction (MI), takes place when blood flow to a portion of the heart is completely stopped. Caused by an abrupt blockage in a coronary artery, usually resulting from the rupture of unstable plaque and a blood clot that seals off the artery, a heart attack produces permanent damage to the cardiac muscle.

How do doctors know if a heart attack is mild or severe?

The percentage of blood that is pumped out of the left ventricle with each beat of the heart is called the ejection fraction. Under normal circumstances, a little more than half the volume of blood is pumped out, so a normal ejection fraction ranges from 55% to 65%. A mild heart attack could result in an ejection fraction of 45%. A major heart attack may cause the ejection fraction to drop to 25% or even lower.

––––––––

What is cardiac arrest?

Almost everyone has heard of someone who suddenly collapsed and died of a heart problem without having had any known risks or warning signs. Most likely that person experienced sudden cardiac death, or cardiac arrest. About 225,000 Americans die of SCD each year.

Is it the same as a heart attack?

No. SCD is related to problems with the heart's electrical conduction system. The most common cause is ventricular fibrillation, a condition that may result in the heart beating chaotically. This causes an inadequate blood supply to all the organs, including the heart and brain. In some cases, however, a heart attack can lead to these chaotic electrical rhythms, which can cause SCD.

Is there anything that can be done for someone in cardiac arrest?

Move quickly! Immediate CPR can save a life. A doctor, nurse or trained paramedic can use defibrillator paddles to electrically shock the heart back to a normal rhythm. These days, you'll even find easy-to-operate defibrillators in major airports, shopping malls and sports stadiums. If defibrillation occurs within the first minute of collapse, the survival rate can be as high as 90%.

Surely there must be some warning!

Some survivors have mentioned lightheadedness, palpitations, or extremely fast or irregular heart rhythms. If you feel those symptoms, you should see your doctor for an evaluation.

––––––––

Three months ago, our neighbor had a thallium exercise stress test that showed normal blood flow to his heart. The doctors told him he was fine. Yesterday, he had a heart attack! Why wasn't this detected?

No medical test can accurately predict future heart attacks 100% of the time. A stress test is often able to detect major coronary blockages (i.e., greater than 70% obstruction) that result in severe deprivation of blood flow to areas of the heart muscle during exercise. But a patient may have several blockages between 30% and 60% and still achieve normal results from a thallium stress test if no single lesion results in enough diminishment of blood flow to register. Recent studies have shown that it is often these more modest lesions that rupture suddenly, causing a heart attack.

Is it true that creases on the earlobes may indicate heart disease?

Maybe. One study followed people under age 65, both with and without known heart disease, over an eight-year period. Those with diagonal carlobe creases had a much higher rate of cardiac problems and procedures. The researchers suggested that the heart and earlobes may be supplied by similar kinds of blocked blood vessels. On the other hand, empiric experience has shown that many people with known heart disease do not have this telltale characteristic.

Can air pollution trigger heart attacks and other cardiac problems?

High levels of air pollution have been linked to heart attacks. The particles found in air pollution can cause vasoconstriction, transiently elevating blood pressure and triggering heart rhythm irregularities; moreover, pollution can increase the likelihood of blood clotting. Although these individual effects may be modest, collectively they can cause serious problems, especially in diseased or damaged hearts. It's unfortunate that we can't do much to decrease the risk from air pollution, other than supporting environmental regulations to reduce it.

Is there a relationship between snoring and heart disease?

We do know that people who snore have a greater risk of dying of heart disease than their nonsnoring counterparts. No one knows why, although snorers are also likely to have hypertension and heart rhythm abnormalities.

My husband became furious at his boss, and within 30 minutes he developed severe chest pain. He was taken by ambulance to the hospital, where doctors confirmed he was having a heart attack. Was this just a coincidence?

Probably not. Recently, researchers at Harvard reported that severe anger can double or even triple the risk of a heart attack, especially within two hours of the episode. Clearly, your husband had underlying heart disease. The argument, however, probably triggered the event.

Can reducing my fat intake prevent a worsening of my heart disease?

Quite possibly. One landmark study showed that heart patients who consumed 23% or less of their total calories from fat showed little or no progression in their heart disease. While it is critical to cut fat (which helps to reduce calories) for weight control, reducing saturated fat and trans fat is more directly connected to lowering cholesterol.

How many meals should I eat a day?

Although some authorities believe that eating three meals a day is the best diet plan, recent studies (in animals and humans) suggest it is better to eat five or six small nutritious meals a day. Two possible explanations: 1) eating large quantities of food at a single sitting may increase the depositing of fat, or lipogenesis, and 2) heavy meals may lead to reduced physical activity. If you feel lethargic after you eat, it's unlikely you're going to get up and burn off any of those calories.

If I do regular exercise, do I also need to change my diet if I want to improve my blood lipid profile?

Yes. Exercise alone results in only *modest* changes in blood lipids and lipoproteins. If you really want to improve your blood cholesterol, HDL and LDL, you must improve your dietary habits.

Can exercise trigger a cardiac event?

Although considerable evidence suggests that regular exercise may help protect against heart disease, unconventionally vigorous physical exertion and other stressors such as emotional upsets can also trigger cardiovascular complications. Consequently, cardiac patients should stop exercising and seek medical help if any of the following symptoms persist despite rest and medication:
- Chest pain or pressure
- Rapid or irregular heartbeat
- Extreme shortness of breath
- Dizziness

Indeed, Dr. Paul Thompson, director of Preventive Cardiology at Hartford Hospital in Connecticut, tells his patients that "any discomfort from your earlobes to your belly button that comes on with exercise and goes away with rest could be angina." If it persists, get help.

Can brisk walking reverse some of the deleterious effects commonly attributed to aging?

Yes. After age 20, aerobic fitness typically declines by approximately 1% per year. A three-month exercise program can lead to a 15% to 20% increase in your heart-lung fitness (or MET capacity), which transforms to a 15-to-20-year functional rejuvenation. The moral of the story? Ponce de León sailed in search of the Fountain of Youth. He should have stayed on land and walked.

I understand that having a potbelly is bad for my heart. Should I be doing sit-ups? If so, how many?

Researchers at the University of Massachusetts had volunteers do 5,004 sit-ups over a 27-day test period. At the end of the study, their muscles were toned, but their stomach fat was no more reduced than the fat on their backs or buttocks. Spot reduction simply does not work.

Well, what should I do?

Engage in large-muscle, rhythmic aerobic exercise on a regular basis and increase activities in daily living (e.g., walking, stair climbing and gardening). A likely reason that spot reducing *appears* to work is that if the intensity of the exercise is sufficiently strenuous and its duration long enough, fat from the entire body—including the target area—will be reduced.

My husband recently had a heart attack, and now he wants to take up scuba diving. This sounds like a bad idea to me, but he says I'm being a worrywart. Who's right?

Death rates from scuba diving are similar to those associated with skydiving and professional car racing, in part because it places a considerable strain on the heart—much more so than regular swimming. So, we're siding with you on this one.

Does regular exercise make the heart more efficient?

Definitely. On average, a regular endurance exercise program will decrease a person's heart rate by more than three million beats per year. That's efficiency!

If the object of an exercise program is to increase heart rate to a certain level and hold it there for 30 minutes or more, why can't I just sit in the steam room or sauna to raise my heart rate?

Ah, if that were only true. But contrary to popular belief, it is not an increased heart rate per se that causes the body to become physically fit. The actual training stimulus is increased body metabolism or oxygen consumption. If you become extremely anxious, for example, your heart rate may transiently skyrocket, yet you're not really getting the equivalent of a workout. If it worked that way, high-strung, nervous types would be the most physically fit people in the world!

Because of my beta-blocker therapy, my resting heart rate is in the fifties and my exercise heart rate is generally in the low eighties. Can I still improve my aerobic fitness with such low training heart rates?

Absolutely! Numerous studies have shown that patients taking beta-blockers can still achieve substantial improvements in aerobic fitness with a regular exercise program despite a reduced training heart rate.

Again, an increase in heart rate alone does not cause your body to become physically fit. The key to improved aerobic fitness is the rise in total body oxygen consumption, which still occurs in exercisers who are taking cardiac medications, including beta-blockers.

How much exercise would I have to do to halt or even reverse coronary heart disease?

The optimal amount of exercise for such cardioprotective benefits remains controversial. However, one major study, which included a low-fat, low-cholesterol diet, showed that burning a minimum of 1,600 calories per week may halt the progression of heart disease, while expending 2,200 calories per week may even lead to a slight regression in heart disease. For many people, this would translate into walking 15 and 20 miles per week, respectively. Further support for this recommendation comes from the American Heart Association, which suggests that the maximum benefits of exercise can be achieved with five to six hours per week of physical activity.

Is sexual activity strenuous enough to cause a heart attack or even sudden cardiac death?

This question is a favorite among middle-aged and older patients with a history of heart problems, so here's the latest news: researchers from Harvard Medical School and the Harvard School of Public Health have concluded that sexual activity is a probable contributor to heart attacks in fewer than 1% of patients. (Another interesting finding was that the risk of a heart attack during or immediately after sexual activity was lower in patients who regularly engaged in vigorous physical exertion.)

In truth, sexual activity is just not that strenuous for most of us. One of the earliest studies of heart disease and sexual activity found that the average maximal heart rate during sexual intercourse was 117 beats per minute and that systolic blood pressure generally increased by only 30 to 40 millimeters of mercury. Achieving similar increases in heart rate and blood pressure during an exercise stress test would require an energy output equivalent to walking on level ground at a pace of three to four miles per hour.

In addition, even if your heart rate rises to fairly high levels during sexual activity, this increase does not necessarily mean that you're expending huge amounts of energy. Emotional stress—and excitement—can also increase nervous system activity and elevate the heart rate.

But is there anything I should be doing to make sex "safer"?

Well, for one thing, you should exercise regularly. In the late 1970s, Dr. Richard Stein reported that heart patients showed a decrease in peak heart rate during sexual intercourse (from 127 to 120 beats per minute) following a 16-week stationary bicycle exercise program. Many of the patients who participated in the program also reported decreased anxiety, increased self-confidence and reduced anginal symptoms. In another study of heart attack survivors, researchers reported that both frequency and quality of sexual activity improved as a result of a physical fitness program.

Is it possible that my medication is having an effect on my sex life?

Yes. Medications people take after heart attacks or coronary interventions to reduce the workload on the heart or control arrhythmias (irregular heartbeats), as well as drugs commonly prescribed to relieve anxiety or depression, can have adverse side effects, most notably impotence in men and diminished sex drive in both men and women. On the other hand, some medications, such as beta-blockers and nitroglycerin, may enhance sexual activity by alleviating angina during exertion. Indeed, some patients may be advised to take such drugs prophylactically, that is, before sexual activity.

Can I take Viagra?

Since the approval by the Food and Drug Administration for the treatment of erectile dysfunction, millions of prescriptions (legal and illegal) for sildenafil citrate (Viagra) have been filled. Reported adverse cardiovascular complications associated with the use of sildenafil include infrequent heart attacks, threatening heart rhythm irregularities, plummeting blood pressure and, in rare instances, death, especially in patients with heart disease who were simultaneously taking nitrates. Yet, according to a recent study of a relatively small group of carefully selected men with erectile dysfunction and known or probable heart disease, sildenafil administered one hour before maximal exercise testing was well tolerated and did not worsen the cardiovascular and electrocardiographic responses to exercise. If you're considering Viagra, check with your doctor.

So let's cut to the chase. Can I have sex?

In general, you can resume sexual activity within a few weeks of a heart attack or coronary artery bypass surgery and within a few days of a balloon angioplasty procedure. As we've said, having sex is comparable to walking at a pace of about three to four miles per hour, so anyone who can do that without abnormal signs or symptoms can probably have sex. Here are some specific concerns:

■ If you're taking an antianginal medication such as nitroglycerin, you might want to ask your doctor about taking it prior to sex. In addition, you should avoid sexual activity after heavy meals and drinking alcohol, when excessively fatigued or in too hot or too cold an environment. (One Japanese study showed that 80% of deaths during sexual intercourse occurred in hotel rooms during extramarital affairs, and most of the victims had been eating and drinking heavily.)

■ If you want to have better sex with less anxiety, you should exercise regularly, eat a low-fat diet, lose weight if necessary, not smoke and not drink more than a moderate amount of alcohol.

■ Experiment to see if you prefer the on-top or on-the-bottom position. While the cardiovascular response is the same, the on-the-bottom spot may slightly reduce cardiac cost, eliminating isometric support of the body weight by the arms.

■ As mentioned above, some medications, by easing the symptoms of angina, may decrease anxiety and enhance sexual activity. On the other hand, men whose cardiovascular medications cause problems such as impotence should never abruptly discontinue taking these drugs without their physician's approval, especially if they're taking beta-blockers such as propranolol (Inderal), atenolol

(Tenormin), metoprolol (Lopressor) or nadolol (Corgard). Often a change in or gradual tapering of medication can solve the problem, or various other treatments for impotence may be prescribed.

————

Are there safe cigarettes?

According to one landmark study, men who smoked cigarettes with reduced levels of tar and nicotine did not have a lower risk of heart attack than those who smoked regular brands—perhaps because they inhaled more deeply than smokers of other types of cigarettes. We know it's not easy, but if you smoke, you must stop.

But I'm afraid I'll gain weight if I stop smoking.

It's very likely that you will. Smoking 24 cigarettes over a 24-hour period increases daily caloric expenditure by about 10%. If you don't want to gain weight, you'll have to reduce your caloric intake, increase your exercise, or both.

————

I recently had a heart attack. When can I return to work?

For young and middle-aged cardiac patients, returning to work is a particularly important objective. More than a decade ago, researchers at Stanford University demonstrated that an occupational work evaluation (treadmill testing and counseling) could accelerate return-to-work rates among heart attack patients by reassuring them, their spouses and physicians that the demands of their job could be safely tolerated.

Today, heart attack victims can often return to their jobs, at least on a part-time basis, within four to six weeks, especially if the work does not involve strenuous physical labor. Patients who have undergone coronary artery bypass surgery may take a bit longer, whereas those undergoing balloon angioplasty generally return within a week. Economic conditions, the patient's state of mind, employer stereotypes and the availability of pension benefits can often make going back to work seem less appealing, but we agree with the late Sterling B. Brinkley of the Department of Health, Education and Welfare, who so aptly summarized our point of view: "Work is an essential ingredient for quality of living. We have seen too many people quit too soon, sitting on porches, watching cars go by. I have also been impressed by the numbers who die within a year or two after retirement. I have wondered if the stimulus of work did not, in fact, give life itself."

Do white-collar workers have any advantage over blue-collar workers when it comes to death from heart disease?

Blue-collar workers are 43% more likely to die of heart disease than white-collar workers, even after differences in risk have been considered. But it remains unclear whether other influences—diet, medical care or cultural factors—play an even greater role than the jobs they do.

Where do heart surgeons get the blood vessels they use for bypass grafts?

Bypass grafts for people with clogged coronary arteries may be constructed with an "extra" vein removed from the leg (a saphenous vein) or with an artery that lies inside the chest wall (an internal mammary artery). Research indicates that artery grafts have a far better long-term patency rate (the percentage of grafts that remain open).

My husband recently had a heart attack. In addition to supporting his efforts at lifestyle change, what can I do?

Learn basic cardiopulmonary resuscitation (CPR). Reversal of sudden cardiac death can be brought about not only by trained physicians, nurses and paramedics, but by any of us, anywhere, using no tools but our hands, our lungs and our brains. To enroll in a CPR course, contact your local office of the American Heart Association, the American Red Cross, a hospital or a local high school that offers community courses. It may be the most valuable course you'll ever take.

My father had a heart attack last summer, but now he insists that he can shovel snow this winter because he's a regular exerciser. Do you agree?

No, we don't agree. Snow shoveling puts a tremendous workload on the heart, and cold temperatures can add to the stress. Several years ago, Dr. Barry Franklin and associates at William Beaumont Hospital in Royal Oak, Michigan, studied the physical demands of snow shoveling on healthy but inactive men. After only 10 minutes, the blood pressure and heart rate of the subjects rose to dangerously high levels, equaling or exceeding the maximum responses of the same subjects during exhaustive treadmill testing. Among people with heart disease, such high numbers can lead to inadequate oxygen supply to the heart muscle, anginal chest pain and potentially fatal heart rhythm disturbances. Furthermore, the marked increases in heart rate and blood pressure that accompany snow shoveling may cause greater than usual flows that dislodge plaque and other fragments from blood vessel walls. The result: a heart attack. Using a snowblower is not necessarily the solution, since pushing one can put considerable demands on the heart, especially in sedentary individuals.

It may be best for middle-aged and older persons at risk for heart disease to hire a snowplow service to clear the driveway. We'd certainly recommend this approach in your father's case. As a reminder for him, we'd suggest that you make a copy of this label and paste it on your snow shovel:

WARNING
use of this instrument
for snow removal may be
hazardous to your health!

A friend who just had coronary artery bypass surgery seems to be very forgetful these days. Is it my imagination, or is there a connection?

Memory problems are a relatively common side effect of coronary bypass surgery. Fortunately, for almost all patients, the lapses usually disappear within a few months.

Folk wisdom says, "Laughter is the best medicine." Is there any truth to the notion?

Laughter is actually very strong medicine. Dr. William Fry, Jr., professor emeritus at Stanford University and a pioneer in laughter research, believes that even the physical act of laughing is good for you. But the most astonishing evidence of the healing power of laughter comes from a 1997 study of 48 heart attack patients. Half watched comedic films for 30 minutes every day; the other half served as controls. After a year, patients in the control group had a greater number of recurrent heart attacks. Indeed, other researchers suggest that laughter is a powerful antidote to stress, reducing hormone levels that can trigger dangerous heart rhythms, blood clotting, or both.

A coworker recently suffered a heart attack. His doctor told him he had already had a heart attack sometime earlier but was unaware of it. Is that possible?

Yes. More than a quarter of all heart attacks go unrecognized. In other words, they occur without severe chest pain and other ominous symptoms. Oftentimes (and more frequently among women than men), mild chest discomfort may be denied or simply considered "heartburn."

What is acute congestive heart failure? It sounds scary.

Generally not as ominous as it sounds, congestive heart failure can occur after a heart attack or whenever the pumping capacity of the heart is significantly compromised. Symptoms include unusual fatigue (especially after mild exertion), shortness of breath, sudden weight gain and swelling in the ankles. Contact your doctor if you have any of these symptoms. On the other hand, chronic congestive heart failure is the most frequent diagnosis in the growing geriatric population. It occurs when the left ventricle has been permanently weakened, decreasing the heart's ability to pump blood properly. Because of the associated poor prognosis, young and middle-aged individuals with this condition are sometimes considered as candidates for a heart transplant.

Why is congestive heart failure more common after a heart attack?

When heart muscle dies and is replaced by scar tissue, which does not have the ability to contract and expand, the heart loses some of its effectiveness as a pump. This is particularly true if scarring has occurred in the left ventricle, the principal pumping chamber of the heart. If the left ventricle is no longer able to pump enough blood to the body but the right venticle continues to pump normally, the difference may cause blood to back up in the lungs and in the large leg veins. This disrupts the circulatory flow and causes distention of the tissues and a leaking of fluid into the abdomen and extremities.

Is that why people with chronic congestive heart failure often have swelling in their ankles and feet?

Yes, and it also explains why they frequently gain weight from fluid buildup, called edema. If the fluid backs up into the lungs, that can cause pulmonary edema—and extreme shortness of breath. If that happens to you, you may have to adjust your sleep position.

Wow, this is pretty depressing.

It's not fun, and certainly the best idea is to avoid having congestive heart failure. But your doctor has lots of ways to make you more comfortable. Commonly prescribed medications include digoxin, diuretics, ACE inhibitors and beta-blockers. In some cases, angioplasty or bypass surgery may be beneficial for patients with congestive heart failure. Moreover, moderate-intensity exercise using interval training (a work-rest approach) is increasingly recommended for those with congestive heart failure.

I've had angina for 12 years. Unfortunately, both angioplasty and coronary artery bypass surgery failed to give me any lasting relief. Now my doctor has recommended EECP. What do you know about this new treatment?

Enhanced external counterpulsation (EECP) is a promising, noninvasive outpatient treatment that may be helpful in relieving or eliminating your symptoms. Patients typically attend one-hour treatment sessions once a day, five days a week for seven weeks. While you lie on a padded table in a treatment room, a nurse or therapist will wrap a set of inflatable cuffs around your calves, thighs and buttocks. The system compresses your lower limbs and, through heartbeat-synchronized inflation and deflation, rhythmically increases blood flow toward your heart (e.g., like exercise). Studies suggest that the treatment can reduce anginal symptoms, possibly by stimulating "collateral circulation," the opening of new, natural pathways around narrowed or blocked coronary arteries.

What is your opinion of chelation therapy? A local clinic provides this treatment option, but it's costly and my health insurance doesn't cover it.

Chelation therapy purports to clean out blocked arteries without surgery. The process involves introducing an amino acid called ethylenediamine tetra-acetic acid (EDTA) into the veins. Normally used to treat mercury or lead poisoning, since it causes heavy metals to be excreted in the urine, this chemical is believed to help reduce damage to artery walls and remove calcium, a key component of plaque, from the bloodstream. Supposedly, it causes potentially harmful heavy-metal molecules (such as calcium, lead, zinc, iron) to be bound with other chemicals and eliminated from the body. A single treatment takes about two hours and costs about $75 to $110 (usually not covered by insurance). A normal treatment schedule calls for 25 to 40 treatments. About 2,500 doctors in the United States offer chelation therapy.

The American Heart Association and the American College of Cardiology recognize chelation therapy in the treatment of heavy-metal poisoning but do not endorse it as an effective method for treating heart disease; in fact, they cite possible adverse side effects such as kidney damage, decreased bone density and heart rhythm irregularities. A just-published study of 84 patients, 41 of whom had undergone an extended series of chelation treatments, concluded that there was no benefit when compared with placebo. Moreover, a review of the topic published in *Circulation* in 1997 found that only four of 50 studies surveyed met the criteria for sound science—and none of those four studies showed that chelation therapy worked in treating heart disease. In support of this conclusion, a more recent study conducted by doctors from the University of Calgary found no benefit from the therapy. Says Dr. D. George Wyse, one of the authors of the study, "My advice to patients is there is no evidence that chelation works."

People say you can avoid heart trouble by taking an aspirin once a day. Is this true?

The answer largely depends on your specific medical history. If you're healthy and without major risk factors for heart disease, the negatives associated with regular aspirin use (stomach bleeding and an increased incidence of stroke) probably outweigh the positives (decreased incidence of cardiac events). However, if you have one or more major risk factors for heart disease, especially if you're over 40 years of age and you're a cigarette smoker and/or you have an elevated blood cholesterol, aspirin may be helpful. In fact, the newest guidelines of the American Heart Association suggest low-dose aspirin for patients with a 10% or higher risk of developing heart disease within 10 years, using the Framingham Risk Score.

■ The Harvard Nurses' Health Study showed a 30% reduction in heart attacks among women aged 50 and older who took aspirin daily, compared with a similar group of women who did not.

■ A study of 4,500 Italian men and women aged 50 and older found that one aspirin per day cut the risk of dying from heart attack or stroke by 50%. This group was followed for 3.6 years before the trial was stopped prematurely due to the clear benefit of aspirin.

■ The ongoing Harvard Physicians' Health Study involved more than 22,000 male doctors, all of whom were in apparently good health. Half the group took a buffered, or coated, aspirin every day; the other half received a look-alike placebo. For those taking aspirin, the risk of heart attack was cut by 47%. In this case, the beneficial effect of aspirin was so apparent that the doctors who monitored the trial felt ethically compelled to recommend that it be stopped and that those volunteers getting the placebo be informed so they, too, could take aspirin.

Recently, the U.S. Preventive Services Task Force reported that aspirin therapy clearly decreased the risk of initial heart attacks in persons "at risk" for heart disease. The downside? Aspirin also increased the risk of stomach bleeding and the incidence of strokes. The Task Force concluded that the benefits outweighed the risks, but only in patients at high risk for developing heart disease. This conclusion was echoed in a just-published paper by the American Heart Association on guidelines for primary prevention of heart disease and stroke.

The bottom line is that aspirin therapy is generally underutilized in this country, especially in emergency settings and in preventing recurrent heart problems. But it's not for everyone. If you're not taking aspirin regularly and think you should be, or if you're taking it and wondering if you shouldn't be, check with your doctor.

I've heard that alcohol can worsen heart disease, but I've also heard that alcohol can prevent it. Which is it?

Drinking alcohol in excessive amounts over many years can lead to alcoholic cardiomyopathy, a weakening of the heart muscle. (Fortunately, complete abstinence from alcohol may often resolve the condition.) In addition, drinking too much can lead not only to cirrhosis of the liver, weight gain and an increased risk for mouth and throat cancer, but can also raise the level of serum triglycerides, which is thought to be a risk factor for heart disease.

On the other hand, a moderate amount of alcohol—about one drink per day—may decrease the risk of heart attack and stroke. Still, we do not recommend that anyone *start* drinking alcohol to prevent heart disease. The risks are too great.

Well, I already drink. Can I keep on drinking?

If you do drink, you should limit your alcohol consumption to no more than one drink per day. Whether white or red wine is more protective than beer or liquor remains unclear.

Although I have a "normal" blood pressure, my doctor says I have a heart rhythm abnormality that puts me at risk for a stroke. The whole thing has me confused.

Patients with a heart rhythm disturbance called atrial fibrillation (AF) are clearly at increased risk for a stroke. The good news is that a procedure called cardioversion (during which a synchronized direct current shocks the heart) can often normalize atrial fibrillation. In addition, your doctor may prescribe an anticoagulant such as Coumadin to decrease the likelihood of blood clot formation.

Is a stroke related to a heart attack?

Atherosclerosis, the underlying condition that leads to coronary heart disease, can also cause stroke. In the case of stroke, however, blockages stop blood flow to the brain, not to the heart.

Is stroke common?

A stroke occurs every minute in America. Each year over 500,000 people suffer a stroke and 144,000 of them die.

What are the warning signs of stroke?

Feeling sudden weakness in an arm, hand or leg, or not feeling one side of the face or body are common precursors of stroke. Other symptoms include:

- Suddenly not being able to see out of one eye
- Suddenly having difficulty talking
- Not being able to understand what someone is saying
- Feeling dizzy or losing balance
- Having the worst headache of your life

If you have one or more stroke symptoms for more than a few minutes, call 911.

———

I had a heart attack five years ago. What's my risk of future cardiac problems?

Doctors rarely talk explicitly to their heart patients about the risk of future cardiac events. Consequently, their patients assume the worst when, in fact, most do just fine.

Years ago, researchers at Stanford University asked a group of patients soon after their heart attacks to rate their likelihood of having another major cardiac problem (fatal or nonfatal) over the next year. Almost uniformly, the interviewees vastly overestimated their subsequent cardiac risk—suggesting that they anticipated an unfavorable prognosis. Yet the annual rate of death in these same patients was actually 1.5%, and only 2% had recurrent nonfatal heart attacks!

Today, increasing numbers of heart patients are entering their seventies, eighties and nineties, oftentimes outliving their counterparts without heart disease. In our experience, these tend to be patients who take care of themselves and, perhaps equally important, develop the *mind-set* necessary to deal with the challenges of heart disease. There is considerable evidence in the psychosocial literature to suggest we get what we expect and attract what we fear. Invariably, those patients who not only survive but thrive *believe* they can achieve longevity and a high quality of life.

Introduction

It's not your father's heart disease anymore.

FOR MANY YEARS, doctors focused on cholesterol as the single most important risk factor for coronary heart disease. The connection was simple: the more cholesterol you had in your bloodstream, the more likely you were to suffer a heart attack. Sure, smoking mattered, as did high blood pressure. But as Dr. Robert Levy, former director of the National Heart, Lung and Blood Institute, once stated, elevated cholesterol was the "chief factor of a heart attack."

Soon after the connection was made, interest in managing blood cholesterol bordered on obsession. Virtually overnight "low-cholesterol" foods appeared in grocery stores, cooking shows featured heart-healthy recipes and "What's your number?" became a popular topic at cocktail parties. And although the recommendation was a kind of one-size-fits-all approach (get your cholesterol under 200 by eating a low-fat diet, exercising regularly and taking medication if necessary), it seemed to work. Average American cholesterol levels fell in the 1980s and '90s. So did heart attack rates.

But the advice didn't work for everyone. Diagnosed with high cholesterol, a friend changed his lifestyle dramatically. He cut down on red meat and fast foods, ate more fruits and vegetables, and began exercising regularly. His total cholesterol dropped from 220 to about 180 . . . just before he had a massive heart attack.

He was not alone. About half of all heart attacks in the United States occur in people who do not have high cholesterol. Indeed, Dr. Thomas Yannios, author of *The Heart Disease Breakthrough*, reports that about 80% of people who get heart disease have the same total cholesterol levels as those who don't.

A New Perspective

Cutting-edge science calls for new thinking about heart disease and its treatment. The most recent findings suggest that cholesterol, while important, is only part of the story, one of multiple factors that in combination can cause a heart attack. Other markers—such as the degree to which the artery wall is injured and inflamed, and how easily your blood clots—are now seen as critical.

In addition, there is a new perspective on achieving lifestyle behaviors to manage heart disease. We pretty much all know that a balanced diet and sufficient exercise are essential for achieving cardiac health. But such knowledge has not led to healthy action. Why? Are we lazy or just plain stupid? Again, new research has the answer. It's chronic stress that keeps many people from shaping a diet and exercise plan. People under stress tend to eat unwisely and to skip exercise. But once stress is managed, healthy dietary and exercise actions are more likely to follow.

These changes in medical thinking lie behind my decision to write this book, but it's a decision consistent with my mission as a writer over the past two decades: to teach people how to apply the most up-to-date science to their everyday lives, all with the goal of achieving better cardiac health. If my readers are heart patients, I want them to have the tools to stabilize and reverse their disease; if they are without heart disease, I want them to have a manual for prevention. That's the "why" of the book. The "how" takes a little more explanation.

Looking Back

The seeds of this book were planted on July 16, 1977, the day I was diagnosed with advanced coronary disease. Four days later I had bypass surgery. *I was 32 years old!* My mother had often told me, "Life is what happens while you're making plans," but still, this was more than a little bit of a surprise. While I was aware that our family had a tendency toward high cholesterol and heart disease, I had never thought about my own risk.

My obliviousness is fairly typical. As Dr. William B. Kannel, former director of the long-running Framingham Heart Study in Massachusetts, says, "If you don't know that you're free of heart disease, don't assume that you are." His studies found that 16% of the time, people with heart disease experience sudden cardiac death as "the first, last and only symptom" of their problem.

So, in a way, I was lucky.

Here's my story. For about a month I had noticed a shortness of breath and pressure in my chest while warming up to play tennis. After about 10 minutes, these feelings would go away. The pain was not sharp—more like an uncomfortable fullness behind my breastbone. It was certainly not of sufficient concern to stop the match. I recall telling myself, "It's probably a touch of bronchitis."

After waiting a few weeks to see if the feeling would clear up on its own, I made an appointment with our family doctor. He had given me a complete physical exam just four months earlier. There had been no problems then, and I didn't expect him to find any now. Just a quick look at my lungs, a prescription, and I'd be on my way home.

I was wrong. The doctor was concerned about the "uncomfortable fullness" and the irregular results of a resting electrocardiogram, and he sent me that very day to a cardiologist. One test led to another, culminating in a cardiac catheterization to x-ray my coronary arteries. The diagnosis changed my life forever: "Joe, you have coronary heart disease, a buildup of cholesterol-filled blockages in the coronary arteries," he said. "This disease affects blood flow to the heart. In your case it's severe, with about 95% of the left main coronary artery obstructed. Your heart isn't getting enough oxygen to keep up with the workload, which is why you had chest pain playing tennis. You are a coronary fatality statistic waiting to happen."

I heard his words, but I had difficulty personalizing the diagnosis. Like most people, I knew that heart disease was a major health issue, perhaps the greatest in the western world. But my appreciation was an arm's length away. What did blocked arteries or heart attacks have to do with me, a 32-year-old guy in the prime of my life?

I would soon learn that heart disease was no longer just facts, figures and other people's families. We were now talking about *my* heart, *my* health, and the impact on *my* family. Looking back on the moment my doctor recommended immediate coronary bypass surgery, I recall the words of the famous Spanish matador, El Cordobés, who once said that his interest in the bullfight increased in direct ratio to the closeness of the bull's horns. My interest was suddenly very great indeed.

After the six-hour operation, in which a piece of vein taken from my leg was used to create a new coronary artery that went around the blockage, I was euphoric, thinking myself "cured." But a postoperative consultation with my cardiologist was sobering. "Let's be straight on what was accomplished," he said. "The surgery reduced the immediate risk of a life-threatening heart attack, and it took away the pain. But you still have coronary heart disease. You had it the day before surgery, you had it the day after surgery and you have it now. The immediate problem has been solved, but the underlying condition remains. You need to assess the risk factors that got you to this point and change those things that can be changed. The way you choose to live is the key to your cardiac future. Things like what you eat and how you exercise will dictate whether or not the disease progresses. It's in your own hands, Joe."

The time following surgery was very traumatic for my family. My wife, Bernie, and I had been married less than 10 years. Our children, Anne and Joe, were six and four. Instead of the "normal" concerns of a young family—picking the best school for the kids, choosing a vacation spot, scheduling soccer carpools—our focus was on living with heart disease. And there was some question even about that.

In an effort to get educated, I met with a lipids specialist at a major university near my home. He talked to me about cholesterol and blood pressure, diet and medications, and a course of action. His information was helpful, but he'd failed to address the question that was most important to me: "Will I live?" I asked him. "Will I have a normal life span or not?"

Perhaps he was having a bad day, possibly he was being brutally honest, or maybe he just had a terrible bedside manner, but this was his never-to-be-forgotten answer: "You probably won't live to see age 40," he said. "I'd be very surprised if you're at your kids' high school graduation."

I left his office shocked and angry. But I was also scared. His "opinion" created so much stress for me that I could hardly function. For about a month I moped around home, depressed, anxious and unable to focus on anything. I had always been actively engaged with life; now I had become a passive observer—except when it came to my heart. In that regard I was ever vigilant, always on guard for something terrible about to happen. One day, on a short walk down the road to our mailbox, I felt a pain in my side and was gripped by panic. It turned out to be nothing more than a muscle cramp, but I believed death was imminent. Afterwards, I realized I had become immobilized by stress and fear.

Bernie put the situation into perspective: "Joe, you can't change the cards you were dealt, but you can play those cards as best you can." She was supported by my doctor, who told me, "When General Patton was asked how he would respond to an enemy attack, he replied with one word: 'counterattack.' When the enemy is heart disease, the strategy is the same. Heart disease is not a death sentence. The key to long-term success is to learn about the disease, reduce your risk factors with healthy lifestyle changes, take your medications, get regular checkups and heed warning symptoms immediately."

I knew they were right. I couldn't change my genetic heritage. Besides, as I soon learned, lifestyle habits can offset and counteract "bad genes." Ten percent of the population will get up in the morning, run five miles and still have a heart attack because of bad genes.

Ten percent will have cream for breakfast, avoid exercise and yet never have a heart attack because they are protected by good genes. But for the remaining 80%, lifestyle habits are the greatest determinant of cardiac health. Dr. William C. Roberts, editor of the *American Journal of Cardiology*, put it this way: "For every person with coronary heart disease because of family genes, there are 499 people who have it because of lifestyle decisions."

Hope and optimism became my allies, education my friend. I made a commitment to learn all that I could about the disease and about the mitigating effect of lifestyle habits, and to do everything possible to overcome my genetic baggage. The starting point was learning what I could control. It was pretty clear that certain lifestyle habits—eating well, exercising regularly, not smoking and managing stress better—were key to my long-term health. But I needed to make a plan, and I didn't know what to do. I was confused.

Confused about diet. What was a healthy diet, anyway? Information and advice changed so rapidly that I called them studies du jour. One day eggs were considered breakfast-table suicide; the next day a new study said they were acceptable. Some experts touted margarine as better, others sided with butter. One day low fat was in, high protein (really, high fat) was out. The next day it was reversed. The dueling science left me bewildered.

Confused about exercise. Some experts counseled slow and steady exercise. Others advised kicking up the pace to "go for the burn" and warned of "no pain, no gain." As a heart patient, could I lift weights? Some doctors said yes, some said no. Not knowing who was right made me fearful.

Confused about smoking. I didn't smoke, but I lived for 18 years with parents who did. In college, my roommates smoked; at my office, many coworkers smoked. "You've actually been smoking from two to seven cigarettes a day for a number of years," a pulmonary doctor told me. "You just never bought a pack yourself." How could I avoid being harmed by cigarette smoke in the future?

Confused about stress. Not much was known in those days about the role of stress, but intuitively I knew that getting all worked up, frequently over minor things, could not be good for my health. I was already feeling "out of time" before I had heart disease. How could I keep the disease from increasing my stress, which in turn would exacerbate my disease?

My need for accurate information and usable advice culminated in my first book, *Don't Eat Your Heart Out.* Over the last two decades, I've continued to pay close attention to the progress in cardiac medicine and treatment. And with the help of dedicated health professionals and the support of my family, I've sorted out how the lifestyle pieces fit together for better cardiac health. More important, I've developed a methodology for putting information into action to achieve long-term lifestyle habits. Called the Piscatella Protocol, this approach involves making changes through a sequence of events that creates adherence. The protocol also utilizes a number of practical tips for heart-healthy living, which I call Heart Savers.

The creation of the Piscatella Protocol was not an academic exercise. It was a course of action for living long and well despite having heart disease. And it has worked:

■ Critical markers such as weight, cholesterol and blood pressure show that I'm in better health now than I was in 1977.

■ Tests show not only that my heart disease has been stabilized, but also that I actually have less disease today than in 1977, a condition called coronary regression.

■ In July of 2002, I celebrated my 25th anniversary of bypass surgery by hiking on Mt. Rainier. And that lipids specialist? He's still practicing. Every time I have a birthday I send *him* a card to let him know I'm still around. I've also derived great satisfaction from keeping him apprised of the many graduation ceremonies I've attended—high school, college, graduate school and law school.

Speaking of those kids whose graduations I was never supposed to see, they're now adults and neither of them demonstrates high cholesterol or other cardiac risk factors. The life skills I learned for rehabilitation, they use for prevention. To a certain extent, that has allowed them to offset any genetic predisposition to heart disease.

Looking Forward

This book, a manual for preventing, stabilizing and reversing heart disease, is my sixth but perhaps my most important. What was known about heart disease and heart-healthy living in 1977 and what is known today are worlds apart. In addition, I've had 25 years of experience in making lifestyle changes, enough time to sort out what is effective and what is not, what is a fad and what is trusted information, what works on paper but breaks down in practical application. Such experience is invaluable. As *Cuckoo's Egg* author Clifford Stoll has written, "Data is not information any more than 50 tons of cement is a skyscraper."

But just to be sure I had the data *and* practical information I needed, I asked Barry A. Franklin, Ph.D., a highly respected national authority on cardiac rehabilitation—and a good friend—to collaborate on the project. (He's the one on the left in the picture that accompanies our "Speaking from Experience" sidebars.) Since 1985, Barry has served as the director on the cardiac rehabilitation program and exercise laboratories at William Beaumont Hospital in Royal Oak, Michigan. He is an expert on cardiac science, the former editor in chief of the *Journal of Cardiopulmonary Rehabilitation* and past president of both the American Association of Cardiovascular and Pulmonary Rehabilitation and the American College of Sports Medicine. His experience running one of the largest and most successful cardiac rehabilitation programs in the country has given him a valuable insight into the human process of making healthy lifestyle changes.

Former New York governor Mario Cuomo has said that his mother gave him two principles for success: 1) Figure out exactly what it is you want to do, and 2) Do it. The Piscatella Protocol operates on those principles. It turns information into action, telling you how to bring about healthy habits once and for all.

■ *Step 1: Assess your cardiac risk.* The 10 critical markers in this section will give you a global view of your cardiac risk. Some markers, such as LDL cholesterol, blood pressure and smoking, are well established. Others, such as homocysteine, C-reactive protein, clotting and personality/behavior are only now emerging.

Each marker is independently important to your cardiac risk. That's why, wherever possible, numeric values have been included as a means of estimating your own risk. For instance, the recommended HDL cholesterol level is 40 or above. If your HDL is 60, this marker does not constitute a risk; however, if your HDL is only 31, you know it's a risk and you need to take action. By comparing your markers to established norms, you'll have a more accurate picture of where you stand. You can assess some markers using self-scoring testing; for others, you'll need to include them in a blood test as part of your annual physical exam.

■ *Step 2: Manage daily stress.* Unfortunately, we can't remove stress from our lives. Stress is a natural by-product of change, and change is constant. There is birth; there is death. The market goes up; the market comes down. But we can learn to handle stress more effectively. People who cope well with stress are in a better position to institute and maintain healthy exercise and eating habits. Read the section on stress and use the Heart Savers to put stress management techniques into practice.

■ *Step 3: Make exercise a habit.* We suggest exercise before dietary change because regular, moderate exercise is easier to achieve. Building up to a 45-minute walk four times a week is easier than giving up your morning doughnut. Making exercise a regular part of your life causes an improvement in outlook. That's because exercise is positive; it's *doing* something. Dietary change, on the other hand, is often seen as negative; it's about what you *can't* have. By starting and sticking with an exercise program, you create a platform of success—one that carries over to healthy eating. In addition, exercise has a positive impact on stress management. Read the section on effective exercise and use the Heart Savers to make it a regular part of your life.

■ *Step 4: Balance your diet*. It's important not to base your dietary decisions on pop science or the latest fad. This step lays out accepted, credible science for heart-healthy eating. It's also important to recognize that eating is a quality-of-life issue. That's why my recommendations are not extremely high or extremely low in fat; instead, they call for balance and moderation.

There are a number of simple actions you can take to improve your diet, control weight and reduce cardiac risk. The diet section will provide you with the principles of the smartest way to eat; the Heart Savers will give you the ability to put those principles into action.

In addition, there is a section on critical drug therapy, from aspirin to beta-blockers, which can enhance lifestyle improvements to benefit cardiac health.

Our intent is to provide straight information based on the latest science tempered by experience and common sense. The result, we hope, is usable advice that will help those with heart disease stabilize and reverse their disease, and those without heart disease to prevent it. Barry and I have written *Take a Load off Your Heart* with the sincere hope that it can make a difference. It will, if you let it.

Joseph C. Piscatella
Institute for Fitness & Health
Gig Harbor, Washington

Step 1
Assess Your Risk

10 Critical Cardiac Markers

MOST HEALTH PROFESSIONALS ONCE AGREED that heart disease was basically a problem of blocked pipes. The plumbing analogy is easy to understand, which may explain its popularity among doctors. As one cardiologist put it, "I describe heart disease to my patients as akin to rust accumulating over the years in an old water pipe. Pretty soon the pipe is blocked and there's no water at the tap. When the coronary arteries get blocked by cholesterol buildup, or plaque, there's no blood for the heart. Then the person suffers a heart attack. It's a concept patients can easily grasp."

Unfortunately, it's not a full and accurate description of how heart disease progresses or how a heart attack takes place. "We now know that the 'rusty pipe' theory is far too simple a notion," says Dr. Ronald Krauss, chairman of the American Heart Association's Council on Nutrition, Physical Activity and Metabolism. "Elevated cholesterol *is* important, but it's only part of the story." New studies suggest that coronary artery injury, inflammation and blood clotting rank right up there with cholesterol as cardiac risks.

Arterial injury is part of the human condition. Each time the heart beats, it pumps 5% of the body's blood back to itself via the coronary arteries. And with each beat, more than 100,000 times a day, these arteries twist and flex with such force that small tears appear on their inner walls. Too much homocysteine in the blood, often a genetic condition, may also cause injury. Excessive stress hormones and the nicotine from cigarette smoke are likewise potentially injurious.

Whatever the cause, the body rushes blood cells to the wound site whenever injury occurs. Cholesterol mixed in with the blood cells is deposited at the site. As it accumulates, plaque is formed. The more cholesterol, the greater the opportunity for plaque to take hold, but it is *injury to the artery wall* that provides the place for cholesterol to collect.

Wherever injury occurs, inflammation naturally follows as part of the body's repair process. But inflammation can cause a rupture in the soft protective cap that covers some plaque. When that happens, cholesterol is exposed to the bloodstream and a dangerous blood clot is formed. The clot closes off the artery channel, denies blood to the heart and is the actual trigger for most heart attacks. It's no wonder, then, that a person whose blood clots easily has an increased risk of heart attack.

Suddenly cholesterol is only one in a group of interrelated factors that together play a causal role in a heart attack. In other words, you should know your cholesterol numbers. But if that's *all* you know, you may be woefully short of information needed to gauge your true cardiac risk. In fact, scientists have identified more that 250 risk factors for the disease. That's a daunting number, to be sure, but easier to live with when you remember that not all markers are created equal. For instance, while one study done several years ago suggested

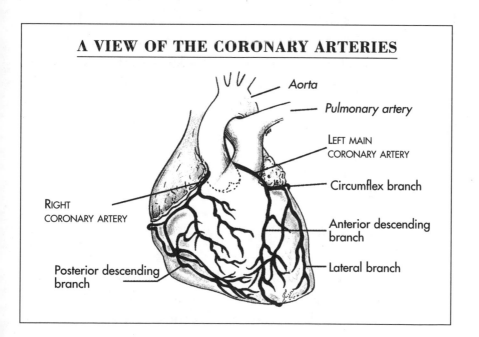

A VIEW OF THE CORONARY ARTERIES

Aorta

Pulmonary artery

LEFT MAIN
CORONARY ARTERY

Circumflex branch

RIGHT
CORONARY ARTERY

Anterior descending
branch

Posterior descending
branch

Lateral branch

GOING BALD?

According to a Harvard study of 22,000 male doctors, men who are losing the hair on the crowns of their heads have up to a 36% greater risk of experiencing heart problems. (Men with receding hairlines are not at increased risk.) Researchers speculate that high levels of testosterone may explain the association between baldness and heart disease.

that diagonal earlobe creases may be an indicator of heart disease, worrying about your earlobes when you ought to be lowering your high blood pressure would be pretty silly.

At the same time, you should know that cardiac markers tend to cluster and may "feed" on one other. Multiple factors do not simply add to your risk; instead, there is a geometric progression that significantly increases the chances of heart disease with each additional factor. According to the Framingham Heart Study, if you *only* smoke or *only* have high cholesterol or *only* have high blood pressure, you have twice the risk of heart disease as someone without any of these markers. But if you have two of the three markers, your risk goes up four times. And if you have all three, your risk is eight times greater. Even a small increase in one risk factor becomes more significant when combined with other risk factors.

Listed below are 10 of the most important cardiac markers, selected not only because of their direct links to heart health but also because each one of them can largely be controlled by making the right lifestyle changes.

Cholesterol and other lipids	Diabetes
Coronary inflammation	Syndrome X
Blood clotting	Aerobic capacity
Weight	Smoking
Blood pressure	Personality

And if you have any doubts about the preeminent role of lifestyle, consider the following facts. Of the six billion people who walk the face of the earth, five billion are not concerned about a heart attack.

It is not prevalent in their societies. Italians, for example, do not have high rates of heart disease. Nor do Africans or the people of Japan. But Italian-Americans do, as do African-Americans and Japanese-Americans. Was there a change in the genetic makeup of their families when they arrived in the United States? Not likely. What changed was their lifestyle.

Here's what we can say about Americans today:

■ The fat and caloric content of our diet is too high.

■ Half the population has high cholesterol.

■ More than a third of the population is obese; indeed, the proportion of adults who are classified as obese rose 49% between 1991 and 1998!

■ Cigarette smoking remains prevalent among younger females, minorities and blue-collar workers.

■ Stress is a chronic problem.

■ Adults and children are leading increasingly sedentary, inactive lives.

But we *can* change the trend. Harvard's Dr. JoAnn Manson did one study that followed nearly 86,000 women. She found that heart-healthy habits, rather than medical intervention, accounted for most

PREDICTING THE FUTURE

Markers for coronary heart disease are extremely predictive. In one of the most comprehensive studies of its type, researchers at Northwestern University Medical School and at the Medical College of Wisconsin spent 20 years looking at the cardiac risk factors of more than 11,000 men aged 18 to 39 and about 9,000 men aged 40 to 59. What they found was that the same factors in older men could be used to predict the future risk of heart disease in younger men. Based on these findings, researchers concluded that critical cardiac markers, when seen in young men, have a powerful effect on long-term risk for death from coronary disease.

of a 31% drop in heart disease over a 14-year period. And more importantly, she discovered that moderate changes in one marker produced multiple risk reductions. For instance, many who started an exercise program also increased HDL cholesterol, lowered blood pressure, lost weight and reduced blood sugar. The findings were so clear that Dr. Manson was able to chart the reduction in heart attack risk from positive behavior changes:

BEHAVIOR	REDUCTION IN HEART ATTACK RISK
Stop smoking	50% to 70% lower risk within 5 years of quitting
Reduce blood cholesterol	1% reduction in cholesterol produces a 2% to 3% drop in risk
Manage high blood pressure	1 mm Hg reduction in diastolic pressure produces a 2% to 3% drop in risk
Exercise regularly	Active lifestyle reduces risk by 45%
Maintain ideal weight	Results in a 35% to 55% lower risk, compared with those who are obese

SPEAKING FROM EXPERIENCE

What's the secret of success in making healthy lifestyle changes? In a word, persistence. Many people try for a while, but results come so slowly that they quit and go looking for something easier. What they don't realize is that, if they'd managed to hang on just a little bit longer, they could have achieved an improved coronary risk factor profile.

Heart health is a marathon, not a sprint. In other words, it's what you do over the long term that really counts. Don't worry about one particular point in the race when you may not have stayed the course. Just get back on track and keep going. —B.F.

Seattle cardiologist Steve Yarnall explains the situation this way: "You don't have to be a scientist to understand that the grease you sandblast from your oven and soak off your dishes isn't something you want in your arteries. You don't have to be a physiologist to understand that regular, moderate physical activity is preferable to no exercise. And you don't have to be a genius to figure out that setting fire to tobacco leaves and inhaling the smoke doesn't make a whole lot of sense." Fortunately, by using the Heart Savers in each step of this book, you *can* eat a better diet, exercise regularly and manage stress.

1. CHOLESTEROL AND OTHER LIPIDS

Nothing is more closely identified with heart disease and heart attacks than cholesterol. And rightly so. Too much cholesterol in the blood tends to clump together on the inner walls of coronary arteries, combining with fibrous tissue to form sludge-like bumps that thicken artery walls and reduce blood flow to the heart. Still, cholesterol is not the be-all and end-all of heart disease. Nor is it toxic. It occurs naturally as a soft, waxy substance in all cells and in limited amounts (the approximately 1,000 milligrams the average body makes a day) is necessary for good health. Only when it is *excessive*, a condition called hypercholesterolemia, do we have a problem.

Total Cholesterol

In 1981, the *New England Journal of Medicine* published a study in which rhesus monkeys, which have a basic metabolism not unlike ours, were fed a typical high-fat American diet. The animals showed a significant rise in blood cholesterol; after two and a half years, a number of them suffered heart attacks and died (something that would be unlikely in the wild). Autopsies showed that multiple coronary artery blockages had developed, similar to those in humans with severe coronary artery disease. Researchers concluded that as cholesterol rose, so did the likelihood of arterial plaque.

More recent studies involving humans suggest the same conclusion. The Framingham Heart Study, one of the largest ongoing cholesterol studies in the world, has evaluated over 6,000 men and women since 1948. Its data show that the higher the total cholesterol, the greater the risk of heart attack. The Multiple Risk Factor Intervention Trial (MRFIT), which included more than 350,000 men aged 35 to 57, also found a correlation between cholesterol level and death rate. The risk of a fatal heart attack began to rise gradually at a cholesterol level of 150, increased more steeply after 200 and began to soar at 230.

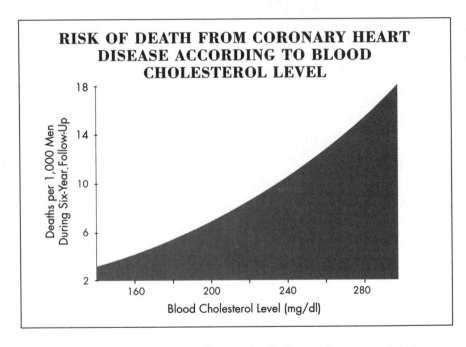

Research also suggests that high cholesterol early in life is predictive of heart attack death later in life. One study examined over 1,000 male medical students in 1947. Forty years later, those cholesterol levels were compared with their current risk of heart disease, heart attacks and death. Subjects in the highest quarter of the group in 1947 had six times the risk of a heart attack as compared with those in the lowest quarter. Dr. Michael Klag, director of the study, explains, "This was a young, healthy, lean population. It's remarkable how strong the relationship is between blood cholesterol at age 22 and cardiovascular disease 40 years later."

But just as increased cholesterol predicts increased heart attack risk, decreased levels forecast a reduction in risk. The Scandinavian Simvastatin Survival Study (4S) found that lowering cholesterol can prevent heart attacks and reduce death in men and women who already have heart disease and high cholesterol. In this study, more than 4,400 patients were divided into two groups. One group took a cholesterol-lowering drug; the other group, a look-alike placebo. The group using drug therapy reduced their total cholesterol by 25% and their LDL cholesterol by 35%; cholesterol in the second group remained unchanged. After a five-year follow-up, 622 patients in the placebo group had suffered at least one heart attack, whereas only 431 of the group with lowered cholesterol did—a difference of more than 30%. Moreover, treated patients were much less likely to need coronary bypass surgery or angioplasty. This was also the first trial to show that lowering cholesterol reduces major coronary events in women.

Other studies, including the West of Scotland Coronary Prevention Study and the Air Force/Texas Coronary Atherosclerosis Prevention Study, have concluded that lowering cholesterol produces similar benefits for people without heart disease, greatly reducing the risk that they will develop coronary heart disease.

In addition, there is evidence that lowering cholesterol can result in *coronary regression*, a shrinking in the size of plaque. When rhesus monkeys with coronary plaque were fed a low-fat diet, a reduction of blood cholesterol took place—along with a 35% to 75% reduction in plaque size. Angiographic studies on humans also suggest that a reversal (albeit small) in the disease process is possible when cholesterol drops significantly, often causing plaque to shrink at the rate of 1% to 2% per year.

9

At first glance, this may not seem significant. But the disease may progress at the rate of 2% to 4% a year when cholesterol stays high, so the net gain from lowering cholesterol may be as much as 6% a year. Furthermore, once plaque begins to shrink, the tendency for clotting seems to be much less. The heart attack rate is then diminished even before much reversal has been demonstrated.

At least 10 trials have examined the link between cholesterol reduction and disease reversal. The late Dr. David Blankenhorn at the University of Southern California and Dr. Greg Brown at the University of Washington directed two of the most important. Each trial used a combination of low-fat eating and drug therapy to reduce cholesterol. In both trials, the majority of patients with lowered cholesterol showed a slowing of disease progression. Less cholesterol in the blood simply meant less cholesterol available for plaque to build and the disease to progress. But a more important finding was that when cholesterol improved (LDL fell to below 100 and HDL rose to 45 or more) coronary regression was achieved in 16% to 30% of patients.

Trials involving intensive dietary and lifestyle changes alone, without drug therapy, have produced similar results. Dr. Dean Ornish at the Preventive Medicine Research Institute conducted one notable study in which 48 men and women, all with coronary arteries between 40% and 100% clogged, were counseled to quit smoking, exercise aerobically for 30 minutes three times a week and use stress dissipation techniques. Twenty-six members of the group followed the American Heart Association's recommended diet, in which 30% of their calories came from fat. The other 22 people ate a strict vegetarian diet with only 8% of calories from fat, exercised moderately for at least three hours a week, meditated regularly for stress management and met

CHOLESTEROL AND ALZHEIMER'S DISEASE

A Finnish study of almost 1,500 people showed that one of the factors contributing to Alzheimer's is the amount of blood flow to the brain. Subjects with high cholesterol were over two times more likely to develop the disease than those with normal cholesterol.

twice weekly in support group sessions. When coronary arteries were evaluated after a year, the first group showed a drop in cholesterol of only 13 points, with their disease staying the same or worsening. But the second group experienced an average drop of 55 points, with the vast majority showing less disease. More importantly, 17 of the 22 people in this group demonstrated angiographic evidence of regression. Again, a significant lowering of cholesterol resulted in a shrinkage of plaque.

Newer studies have concentrated on the effect of lowered cholesterol on *plaque stabilization*. In the modern view of heart disease, this may be of even greater importance than regression, since we now know that the nature of the plaque—is it stable or unstable?—has more to do with heart attacks than its size. Studies suggest that reducing blood cholesterol tends to dry out plaque, which makes it less likely to rupture. "What appears to happen first is that lowering cholesterol tends to stabilize the plaque," says Dr. John LaRosa, formerly at George Washington University. "So, even though the opening hasn't changed that much, the plaque is no longer susceptible to clotting, spasm and hemorrhaging—the things that cause the closing off of the blood vessel and trigger the heart attack. This is a major health benefit."

Whether you're hoping to prevent heart disease or to stabilize or reverse the disease, medical experts agree that for every 1% decrease in total cholesterol, your chance of having a heart attack decreases 2% to 3%. But you must realize that the reverse is also true. If your blood cholesterol rises 1%, the frequency of heart attack increases similarly. According to Dr. William C. Roberts, whatever your total cholesterol is, reducing that number by about 40 points cuts your risk of a first or subsequent heart attack *in half*.

Total Cholesterol: Know Your Number, Know Your Risk

You and your doctor can't determine your cardiac risk or formulate a response strategy unless you know your cholesterol number. The amount of cholesterol you have in your bloodstream is expressed as the number of milligrams (mg) of cholesterol in one deciliter (dl) of blood. For example, a person with 210 milligrams of cholesterol in a deciliter of blood has a cholesterol level of 210 mg/dl, popularly expressed as a cholesterol "count" of 210. But as we'll discuss later, you really need to know more than that, which is why you should request a standard lipid profile that includes triglycerides, LDL cholesterol and HDL cholesterol. In general, all adults over age 20 should have a lipid profile done at least once every five years. If parents or grandparents had heart disease before age 55, testing at a younger age may be appropriate. Also, if you have heart disease, or if you have two or more major cardiac markers (smoking, high blood pressure, obesity, diabetes, sedentary lifestyle), you should be retested annually.

While the nonfasting "finger stick" cholesterol test typically used at shopping malls and health fairs is a practical way to screen large numbers of people, readings can vary from the gold-standard fasting laboratory test by 30 to 50 points. In general, if you have a "finger stick" reading over 200, have your doctor check it against a fasting laboratory test.

It's important to use a laboratory that your physician trusts to give reliable measurements. Not all laboratories are standardized or well regulated, and test results can vary. In addition, certain factors can affect your cholesterol number:

- Smoking before a test may cause higher readings.
- Not fasting for 12 hours before a test may cause elevated readings.
- Lying down for a test may cause lower readings; sitting up tends to cause slightly higher readings.
- Morning levels are usually higher than those measured later in the day.
- Exercise, stress, dieting, body weight change, medications and phases of a woman's menstrual cycle can affect readings.

This is why a single cholesterol reading is not the whole story—and why you should have a second measurement done within eight weeks of the first. If the second reading is within 30 points of the first, use the average of the two values. Otherwise, have a third test performed and use the average of all three tests.

The National Cholesterol Education Program, in collaboration with the American Heart Association and other medical authorities, has issued guidelines for total cholesterol:

TOTAL CHOLESTEROL	RISK CLASSIFICATION
Below 200*	Desirable
200 to 239	Borderline high
240 and above	High
Your number: _____	Your risk: _____

*In particular, heart patients and those who have two or more risk factors should strive for a level no higher than 200, preferably in the 150-to-160 range.

If your total cholesterol is over 200, you are not alone. The American Heart Association estimates that 98 million Americans are at increased risk for coronary heart disease because of high cholesterol. In fact, about 25% of all Americans over 20 years of age have a cholesterol count over 240, putting them at high risk for heart attack. By comparison, the average adult in China has a cholesterol level of 125.

LDL Cholesterol

In the case of cholesterol, the whole is less important than the sum of its major parts (LDL and HDL). For example, take two women, both 50 years of age and both of whom have an identical total cholesterol value of 210. The first woman has an LDL of 105, whereas the second has an LDL of 155. Provided that all other factors are equal, the second woman is clearly at greater risk of developing heart disease, even though their total cholesterol value is the same.

Just like oil in water, waxy cholesterol is insoluble in blood. In order to be transported, it must first be combined with fat and protein molecules. The resulting chemical package, called a lipoprotein, is nature's vehicle for moving cholesterol throughout the body. Most lipoproteins contain cholesterol and triglycerides in their core, with protein and fat forming an outer coat. Various types of lipoproteins have different sizes, shapes and functions, contain different amounts of cholesterol, triglycerides and protein, and are usually classified on the basis of their density or compactness. One of the most important is low-density lipoprotein, or LDL cholesterol.

Predominantly made of fat and very little protein, LDL transports about 60% to 80% of the body's cholesterol through the bloodstream. Circulating in the blood for several days after its creation, LDL is taken up by body cells as building blocks for hormones and cell parts. But the cells may not require all the cholesterol that is delivered. The excess floats in the blood, collects on artery walls, causes inflammation and produces plaque. Much of the problem stems from the fact that LDL is an unstable chemical package that comes apart quite easily. Should it penetrate an artery wall and "unravel," unused cholesterol can be released and deposited in susceptible blood vessels. LDL is commonly called "bad" cholesterol because of its major role in the clogging process.

Since many experts believe that LDL is a more accurate marker of cardiac risk than total cholesterol alone, LDL is now viewed as an independent risk factor: the higher your LDL, the greater your risk for arterial buildup. Or put another way: for every increase of one milligram of LDL, the risk of heart attack increases by 2%. For people with cardiovascular disease, the American Heart Association and the American College of Cardiology now recommend lowering LDL cholesterol to less than 100 as *the number one goal* in lipid management. Indeed, a recent landmark study showed that in patients with stable coronary disease, aggressive LDL lowering (via statin drug therapy) was at least as effective as angioplasty and usual care in reducing the incidence of subsequent cardiac problems. According to Dr. Claude Lenfant, director of the National Heart, Lung and Blood Institute, lowering the level of LDL can reduce the short-term risk for heart disease by as much as 40%.

LDL Cholesterol: Know Your Number, Know Your Risk

The National Cholesterol Education Program created the following scale to assess cardiac risk from LDL cholesterol:

LDL CHOLESTEROL	RISK CLASSIFICATION
Below 100*	Optimal
100 to 129	Near optimal
130 to 159	Borderline high
160 to 189	High
190 and above	Very high
Your number: _____	Your risk: _____

*Heart patients and those with other forms of cardiovascular disease (such as carotid artery disease or peripheral arterial disease), diabetes and/or multiple risk factors should strive for this level.

Some authorities suggest that an LDL cholesterol goal of less than 100 for everyone, regardless of other risk factors or a history of cardiovascular disease, would greatly simplify the guidelines and dramatically improve our health.

Here's the bottom line: the more LDL cholesterol you have in your blood, the greater your risk of coronary heart disease. And if your LDL is 130 or greater, you have a cardiac marker that raises heart disease risk, no matter what your total cholesterol may be.

Lipoprotein(a)

As testing has become more sophisticated, subcomponents of LDL are being identified as cardiac markers in their own right. One, lipoprotein(a), or Lp(a), may be an underlying cause in a quarter of premature heart attacks; it is the most common family lipid disorder in people who develop heart disease younger than 60 years of age. Studies by Stanford University and the Jewish Hospital of Cincinnati show that elevated levels of Lp(a) enhance the oxidation of LDL,

15

thereby promoting the entry of this harmful form of cholesterol into the artery walls. In addition, Lp(a) seems to increase inflammation and clotting, thus dealing heart health a double whammy.

Lp(a) is genetically determined and can vary in individuals by a factor of 1,000. But as Dr. Ronald Krauss says, "It's clear that at high levels—starting at 30—Lp(a) is associated with heart disease and stroke." In studies involving 5,200 people, researchers found that those with the highest levels of Lp(a) had a 70% greater risk of having a heart attack over 10 years than those with the lowest levels. And the Heart and Estrogen/Progestin Replacement Study (HERS) found that women with the highest Lp(a) levels had 54% greater risk of heart problems than those at the lowest levels.

See your doctor to find out if an Lp(a) blood test is advisable. Certainly people with known heart disease, a strong family history and/or multiple risk factors should consider doing so as a preventive effort. You can get it done as part of your lipid profile testing.

Your number: _____   ____ Below 30 (desirable)*
                               ____ Above 30 (higher risk)
*Many experts recommend a level no higher than 20.

As of now, dietetic treatment can do little to lower Lp(a), although some studies suggest that eating fish frequently may help. If your Lp(a) is over 30, your doctor may advise drug therapy. Niacin or a fibric acid derivative such as gemfibrozil (Lopid) can effectively reduce Lp(a).

Estrogen has also been shown to lower Lp(a), but prescribing hormone replacement therapy as a means of control is not currently recommended. Also, reducing LDL cholesterol to below 100 (usually with a statin drug) may get Lp(a) down. Most doctors believe the best treatment for this marker is a heart-healthy lifestyle: control cholesterol, triglycerides, blood pressure, diabetes and weight with a low-fat diet and exercise; don't smoke; and dissipate your stress.

Apolipoprotein B

Apolipoprotein B is another LDL component now considered a cardiac marker. Apo B, the protein part of a low-density lipoprotein, transfers cholesterol from the lipoprotein to the cells for use or to the liver for excretion. If the balance is correct—that is, if the amount of Apo B matches up to the amount needed by the cells—there is no health issue. However, any excess Apo B will circulate in the bloodstream and deposit cholesterol in artery walls. Says Dr. Arthur Moss of the University Medical Center in New York, "The cholesterol itself is an innocent passenger. It's Apo B that determines whether cholesterol is used correctly, is eliminated or ends up as plaque."

Early research shows that Apo B may predict heart risk better than LDL level, but much more exploration is needed. At this point, talk with your doctor to determine if it may be a concern for you. Your level can be measured with an Apo B test, which requires a blood draw. A risk classification has been established for men and women in milligrams per deciliter as follows:

MEN	RISK CLASSIFICATION	WOMEN
Below 52	Desirable	Below 49
52 to 109	Normal	49 to 103
110 and above	High	104 and above
Your number: _____	Your risk: _____	

Apo B is in large part genetically determined, so taking control of your manageable lifestyle factors becomes even more important.

Pattern B Particles

A new breed of cholesterol test, the advanced lipid test, has uncovered another cardiac marker: the size and number of LDL particles.

It turns out that smaller LDL particles, called Pattern B, tend to adhere more easily to blood vessel walls and produce blockages. This makes them more dangerous than larger particles, called Pattern A.

It is estimated that Pattern B is found in about 30% of the American public, particularly in families with a history of heart disease.

Depending on the particle types that make up LDL, two people with the same count could have different risks. Take two men, both of whom have an LDL of 130. One has normal LDL particles, Pattern A. The other has small LDL particles, Pattern B, and a lot of them. Though their LDL is the same, the man with the smaller particles would have a greater cardiac risk than the man with the larger particles.

The size of LDL particles is, to a large extent, genetically determined, so there may not be much that can be done about them. Nonetheless, recent research suggests that the appropriate treatment is exercise, reduction of body weight and fat stores, and niacin—three of the least expensive therapies for heart disease.

In summary, individuals with small, dense LDL are at a three-fold increased risk of developing heart disease. However, affected individuals often have many other metabolic abnormalities (such as high triglycerides, obesity, insulin resistance, diabetes, low HDL cholesterol); therefore, this association cannot be used as conclusive evidence that Pattern B itself increases the risk of heart disease.

As of this writing, Pattern B is not routinely tested. Some experts believe that in the future such testing may be beneficial for those people with "borderline" lipid levels, who need to know whether or not they should get further medical help. As a general rule, triglyceride levels above 200 indicate Pattern B; if triglycerides are below 100, Pattern B is unlikely.

HDL Cholesterol

High-density lipoprotein, called HDL, is known as "good" cholesterol. Made up of protein and very little fat, HDL forms a stable package; since it does not unravel when it comes in contact with an artery wall, the cholesterol it carries does not become available for deposit.

Furthermore, HDL actually assists in undoing the damage wrought by LDL. It acts as a scavenger, picking up excessive LDL from artery walls and transporting it back to the liver for removal from the body. Because HDL helps to prevent cholesterol from building up on the walls of the arteries, a high HDL level is considered cardio-protective.

While HDL averages only about 25% of total cholesterol, it is crucially important as a cardiac marker. Low HDL, defined as below 40 for men and 45 for women, is considered a predictive risk factor. A high level of HDL, defined as 60 or higher, is associated with lower risk. It is estimated that for every one milligram increase in HDL, there is a 4% decrease in cardiac risk.

HDL Cholesterol: Know Your Number, Know Your Risk

The National Cholesterol Education Program has proposed the following scale of HDL cholesterol to approximate cardiac risk:

HDL CHOLESTEROL	RISK CLASSIFICATION
60 and above*	Low
40 to 59	Moderate
Below 40	High
Your number: _____	Your risk: _____

*According to the National Cholesterol Education Program, an HDL level of 60 or above is cardioprotective.

Average HDL levels are 45 for men and 55 for women. Female sex hormones, particularly estrogen, tend to raise HDL levels, a difference that in part explains the lower rates of heart disease in women of childbearing age. However, as women enter menopause and estrogen plummets, so does protective HDL. A low level of HDL cholesterol is taking on growing importance as a risk factor, especially if it's under 40.

KNOW YOUR RATIO

While HDL and LDL are independent markers for heart disease, the ratio of total cholesterol to HDL can be helpful in estimating cardiac risk. To calculate your HDL ratio, divide your total cholesterol by your HDL number. For example, someone with a total cholesterol of 250 and an HDL of 50 has an HDL ratio of 5. According to the American Heart Association, the following chart illustrates the relationship between ratio and risk:

HDL RATIO	RISK CLASSIFICATION
Below 3.5*	Optimal
3.5 to 5.0	Average
5.1 to 6.0	Borderline high
Above 6.0	High
Your ratio: _____	Your risk: _____

*HDL ratio for men should not be above 4.5, and for women not above 4.0.

Triglycerides

Most of your body's fat is in the form of triglycerides. Almost all is stored in fat tissue for energy, but a small portion is found in the bloodstream as a component of lipoproteins. Like cholesterol, at normal levels triglycerides play a positive role in good health. But more than 26 studies have shown that elevated triglycerides are a predictor of coronary heart disease and of a high rate of heart attack, particularly in women who are also overweight, hypertensive and diabetic. In addition, high triglycerides are often accompanied by other risk factors, such as high blood pressure and low HDL, that raise heart disease risk. The bundling of these factors is reflected in a cardiac marker dubbed "Syndrome X" (see pages 48–50).

Triglycerides, measured by a blood test, are expressed as the number of milligrams in one deciliter of blood. The normal triglyceride range is from 50 to 150, depending on age and sex, but obesity and overweight, physical inactivity, cigarette smoking, excess alcohol intake, high carbohydrate diets (greater than 60% of calories), several diseases (such as Type 2 diabetes), certain drugs (such as higher doses of beta-blockers), various genetic disorders, and liver and kidney disease all contribute to higher triglyceride numbers.

Triglycerides: Know Your Number, Know Your Risk

Doctors once thought that triglycerides were not really an issue unless they were over 400, which could lead to pancreatic disease. But research at Baylor University by Dr. Antonio Gotto found that much lower levels—between 200 and 250—were associated with an increased risk of heart disease. For that reason, the American Heart Association now recommends keeping your triglycerides below 150 and, if possible, under 100. The National Cholesterol Education Program has issued the following risk classifications:

TRIGLYCERIDES	RISK CLASSIFICATION
Below 150	Desirable
150 to 199	Borderline high
200 to 499	High
500 and above	Very high
Your number: _____	Your risk: _____

2. CORONARY INFLAMMATION

Remember the skinned knee you had as a child? Remember how it turned red and felt hot to the touch? That's because white blood cells congregated at the site of the wound. The proteins that were then released, which enabled the wound to heal, produced inflammation that lasted until healing was under way.

It's the same with injuries to the coronary arteries. These arteries flex and twist each time the heart beats, causing minute fissures in the artery lining; since the heart beats more than 100,000 times a day, there is nothing we can do about these wear-and-tear injuries, all of which may cause inflammation. Genetic makeup can also produce arterial injuries; for example, some people have high levels of an amino acid called homocysteine in their blood, which, in excess, can damage artery walls. And finally, certain lifestyle habits promote arterial wounds. Each time a smoker inhales, nicotine and carbon monoxide are released into the bloodstream, irritating the artery walls. Stress, which causes adrenaline and other powerful hormones to race through the blood vessel system, can also cause injury.

The danger here is that chronic inflammation destabilizes plaque, which makes it easier for the protective cap to rupture, releasing cholesterol into the bloodstream. Then a blood clot is formed, which can stanch blood flow to the heart or brain. As Harvard Medical School researcher Dr. Paul Ridker says, "We have learned that coronary heart disease is very much an inflammatory disease, the same way that arthritis and lupus are inflammatory diseases." The implications of this are enormous. Dr. Ridker estimates that between 25 and 35 million healthy middle-aged Americans have normal cholesterol but above average inflammation, putting them at risk of heart attacks and strokes.

Homocysteine

A good way to estimate your inflammatory response is to check your homocysteine level. When you eat meat or vegetable protein, your body initiates a series of biochemical reactions that ultimately lead to the production of homocysteine. In proper amounts, homocysteine in the blood is not a health threat. But an inadequate dietary intake of the B vitamins (especially folate) or certain genetic defects can elevate homocysteine levels.

High homocysteine, a condition called hyperhomocysteinemia, damages the linings of blood vessels, triggering the growth of cells that form the framework of plaque. It also promotes the breakdown of LDL cholesterol within the plaque, which can lead to blood clots. At one time experts speculated that high homocysteine was not the cause of arterial damage but the result of damage already done. If that were the case, then reducing homocysteine in the blood would not provide any coronary protection. Newer research suggests the opposite conclusion: lowering homocysteine may reduce cardiac risk.

Dr. Kilmer McCully, a pathologist, first uncovered the role of homocysteine in heart disease in 1969. While performing autopsies on children who had died of a genetic overabundance of homocysteine, he discovered that they had had severe atherosclerosis—a condition usually found in elderly people. But there was one critical difference: the children had no plaque on their artery walls. Dr. McCully also found a deficiency in folic acid and vitamins B_6 and B_{12}. Further studies on adults showed that many heart disease victims had total cholesterol levels under 200. Dr. McCully theorized that excess homocysteine was a constant irritant to vessel walls, scarring and thickening arteries over time and providing circulating cholesterol with sites on which to stick and build up plaque. Cholesterol was part of the heart disease equation but not the cause. High homocysteine was.

To bolster his position, Dr. McCully cited population studies on cholesterol. He argued that northern Europeans did not suffer more heart disease than southern Europeans because of a diet richer in fat. Indeed, studies showed that northern Europeans had much higher levels of homocysteine than their southern counterparts, perhaps because northerners eat fewer fruits and vegetables, sources of the all-important B vitamins that regulate homocysteine levels.

Numerous studies now support Dr. McCully's position:

■ A study of nearly 15,000 male physicians aged 40 to 84 found that high homocysteine tripled their heart attack risk.

A LINK TO OTHER RISK FACTORS

A study of Norwegian men and women revealed that elevated homocysteine levels are associated with other major coronary risk factors. People who smoke cigarettes or live a sedentary lifestyle, for example, have higher homocysteine levels than nonsmokers and exercisers.

■ The Harvard Nurses' Health Study found that postmenopausal women with high homocysteine levels had twice the risk of heart attack as compared with those with moderate levels.

■ Some studies show that 10% of coronary heart disease can be ascribed to high homocysteine and that elevated levels can double, triple or *quadruple* the risk of heart attack even when cholesterol numbers are normal.

■ A 1995 analysis of all relevant studies to date demonstrated that the risk of heart disease increased progressively as homocysteine levels rose.

But not all the data are negative. Multiple studies have found that reducing homocysteine levels with three B vitamins—folic acid, B_6 and B_{12}—reduces cardiovascular risk substantially.

The exact process by which high levels of homocysteine contribute to coronary heart disease is not fully known. In addition, elevated homocysteine promotes blood clotting, which increases the chance of heart attack and stroke. About 20% to 40% of people with coronary heart disease have elevated homocysteine. Research shows that for every 10% rise in homocysteine, there is about the same rise in the risk of developing severe coronary heart disease.

Homocysteine: Know Your Number, Know Your Risk

At present, there are no professional guidelines to determine who should be tested for elevated homocysteine. Most doctors test patients who have had a heart attack, bypass surgery or other signs of heart disease (such as chest pain), or a strong family history of atherosclerosis. But because it is a strong marker, many physicians are now screening for homocysteine as part of a standard lipid panel. Some experts suggest that it can provide more information about the state of a patient's heart health than a cholesterol test alone.

Homocysteine is determined with a blood test called Abbott Homocysteine, which describes your level as the number of micromoles per liter of blood (μmol/l). Physicians consider 5 to 15 μmol/l to be a "normal" range, although heart disease risk begins to rise at 9. As the level of this marker goes up, so does the likelihood of heart disease. Studies suggest that a 5 μmol/l increase in homocysteine indicates the same increase in risk as a 20 mg/dl rise in total cholesterol level.

HOMOCYSTEINE LEVEL	RISK CLASSIFICATION
Less than 5	Desirable
5 to 9	Normal
10 to 30	Moderate
31 to 100	High
Above 100	Severe
Your number: _____	Your risk: _____

C-Reactive Protein

Produced by the liver and present in the blood during episodes of acute artery inflammation, high-sensitivity C-reactive protein (CRP) is another important marker for heart attack and stroke. A number of studies confirm its significance:

■ The Harvard Physicians' Health Study found that high CRP levels predicted a first heart attack in healthy men six to eight years in advance. Those with the highest level of CRP in their blood had three times the risk of a heart attack compared with those with lower levels.

■ In the Nurses' Health Study, those with the highest levels of CRP had more than four times the risk of heart attack or stroke even if they were nonsmokers with normal cholesterol and no family history.

■ A study reported in the *New England Journal of Medicine* found that the risk of heart attack rises in people as their cholesterol or CRP climbs, but is highest in people who have both high cholesterol and elevated CRP. Out of 12 risk factors studied, CRP was the strongest predictor of future cardiovascular events.

**CRP: Know Your Number,
Know Your Risk**

Heart attack risk begins to rise with CRP levels such as 0.55 to 0.99 milligrams per deciliter (mg/dl). Levels above 2.5 are associated with a two-to-fourfold increase in cardiac risk. Your doctor may use your test results to check further for coronary heart disease, particularly if your cholesterol is also elevated.

According to a study in the *New England Journal of Medicine*, the following is a risk guideline for CRP:

TOTAL CRP	RISK CLASSIFICATION
Less than 0.70	Lowest
0.70 to 1.1	Low
1.2 to 1.9	Average
2.0 to 3.8	Higher
3.9 to 15.0	Highest
Your number: _____	Your risk: _____

Testing for CRP as part of your lipid profile is especially appropriate if you have multiple cardiac risk factors, an indication of early heart disease or a strong family history. Ask your doctor to order a high-sensitivity CRP (hs-CRP) test as opposed to the standard CRP test used for arthritis. An hs-CRP test usually costs about $30 and is widely available, but many physicians may not automatically include it in their blood test order. This may change in the future.

3. BLOOD CLOTTING

After elevated cholesterol sets the stage for heart disease by forming artery-clogging plaque, inflammation moves in to destabilize the plaque, causing its cap to rupture and exposing the inner part of soft cholesterol to the bloodstream. Then the third player enters—blood clotting, or coagulation.

A HEART DISEASE BUG?

Researchers are finding that coronary inflammation, much like stomach ulcers, can result from low-grade bacterial or viral infections such as gingivitis and herpes. These infections can trigger the body's immune system response, which causes inflammation to take place as part of the natural healing process, thereby accelerating atherosclerosis.

More than a decade ago, researchers reported that traces of *Chlamydia pneumoniae* were often found in cholesterol-clogging deposits within the arteries. They were unable to determine whether this bacterium existed there as an innocent bystander or was produced by inflammation within the artery, but a number of studies have supported the latter theory. For example, rabbits that were fed a high-fat, high-cholesterol diet and infected with chlamydia showed worse plaques than animals merely fed an unhealthy diet.

In another study, frequent users of certain antibiotics (tetracycline or quinolones) showed a reduced risk (30% to 55%) of heart attack when compared with people who didn't use these drugs. The researchers cautioned, however, that their study did not prove that taking the drugs caused the reduced risk.

The exposed cholesterol causes a blood clot, called a thrombosis, to form on the plaque. This combination of clot and plaque seals off the artery opening, choking off the blood supply and causing a heart attack. According to Dr. Scott Goodnight, a cardiovascular disease expert at the University of Oregon Health Sciences Center, "The actual heart attack is caused by a blood clot more than 95% of the time."

Coagulation occurs when white blood cell fragments known as platelets come together to form a clot or clots. The more these cells aggregate, the greater the number of blood clots and the larger they become. Therefore, a tendency for blood to clot easily is an important cardiac marker.

Beyond your personal experience with shaving nicks, how do you know whether or not your blood coagulates easily? Some experts recommend screening for fibrinogen, a protein in the blood that promotes clotting and inflammation. High levels of fibrinogen are often accompanied by other risk factors such as overweight, high triglyceride levels and diabetes, and several recent studies suggest that increased fibrinogen is an independent factor for heart disease. (Conversely, people with low levels of this clotting factor are known to have a reduced risk of cardiac problems, even if they have elevated cholesterol levels.)

One relevant investigation, based on a follow-up of 2,600 individuals from the Framingham Offspring Study, reported that participants with the highest levels of fibrinogen had more than twice the risk of coronary heart disease and heart attacks as participants with the lowest levels of fibrinogen. The researchers who carried out the study suggested that fibrinogen's function in helping to form blood clots after an injury may be similar to the clotting that occurs in coronary arteries, leading to heart attacks.

Excess fibrinogen is often found among the constellation of metabolic abnormalities that characterize the marker known as Syndrome X (see pages 48–50). Some researchers speculate that elevated fibrinogen may be the lethal link that makes other risk factors so dangerous to heart health.

ALCOHOL AND INFLAMMATION

A recent German study reported that both heavy drinkers and non-drinkers had higher concentrations of CRP and other inflammatory markers than did moderate alcohol consumers, who had the most appropriate levels of the markers.

In addition to inhibiting inflammation, moderate alcohol consumption may lower blood concentrations of fibrinogen, which promotes blood clots.

Clotting: Know Your Number, Know Your Risk

As with the tests for cholesterol and other lipids, blood is drawn and evaluated to test fibrinogen levels. The following scale approximates relative clotting risk in milligrams of fibrinogen per deciliter of blood (mg/dl):

FIBRINOGEN	RISK CLASSIFICATION
Below 200	Desirable
200 to 400*	Borderline high
Above 400	High
Your number: _____	Your risk: _____

*This is considered a "normal" range.

4. WEIGHT

No nation in the history of the world has experienced the obesity problem that we now have in the United States. Compared with people of normal weight, obese people have a 50% to 100% greater risk of premature death, and yet the American waistline continues to expand. Well over half of our adult population is either overweight or obese. Indeed, the typical man weighs 20 to 30 pounds too much and the typical woman is overweight by 15 to 30 pounds. In addition, a small but substantial group of about six million Americans are morbidly obese, tipping the scales at 100 or more pounds in excess of the norm.

To make matters worse, surveys show that Americans are in denial about their weight. Only 39% of adults consider themselves overweight or obese.

It's tempting to blame these staggering numbers on genetics, but research suggests that what we weigh is largely determined by how we live. Ours is a fast-food, couch-potato culture that makes it all too easy to put on extra pounds.

A Dangerous Lifestyle

First and foremost, we eat too much. "Portions are getting larger, particularly at restaurants," says Dr. Denise Bruner, president of the American Society of Bariatric Physicians. "Dinner plates used to be 10½ inches in diameter; now they're closer to 12½. At fast-food places, you can supersize for a few pennies more." In addition, many people concerned about fat in their diet are overeating fat-free and low-fat foods. And finally, the American sweet tooth now gets to taste 34 teaspoons of sugar a day from food and beverages, especially soda. This has contributed to a gain in average daily calorie consumption from 1,839 a decade ago to 2,200 today.

The second problem is that we don't get enough exercise. Everyone from the surgeon general on down recognizes regular physical activity as necessary for weight loss, but less than one-third of Americans follow suit.

The tragic bottom line is that overweight and obesity among both adults and children in the United States are costing an estimated 300,000 lives every year. Says columnist George Will, "Although Americans spend more than $30 billion a year on weight-loss products or programs, obesity is, strictly speaking, epidemic. Scientists

SPEAKING FROM EXPERIENCE

We've learned that even 5 or 10 pounds of extra weight can undermine cardiac health. An eight-year study of more than 115,000 women aged 30 to 55 revealed that those who were as little as 5% overweight were 30% more likely than their leaner counterparts to develop heart disease. That risk increased to 80% in those who were moderately overweight, while those who were obese were over 300% more likely to develop heart disease.   —*B.F.*

for the Centers for Disease Control and Prevention reported that in 1991 only four states had obesity rates of 15% or higher. Today, 37 do, and the obesity rate is increasing in every state and among all racial and ethnic groups." In fact, the CDCP has announced that obesity is spreading "with the speed and dispersion characteristic of a communicable disease."

Consider the following:

■ The surgeon general recently warned that obesity may soon surpass smoking as the nation's principal cause of preventable death.

■ Actuarial studies have found that the death rate from all causes increases as weight rises, and this risk becomes substantial for people who are obese, defined as weighing 30% or more above ideal weight.

■ "Five of the 10 leading causes of death in the United States are linked to weight," says cardiologist Dr. Charles H. Hennekens of Harvard Medical School.

■ The overweight condition of Americans increases the risk of kidney disorders, gout, gallstones, osteoporosis, arthritis, breathing problems, back pain, certain cancers and—no surprise, you knew we'd get there—heart disease.

The Cardiac Risk

Weight problems and obesity in particular are directly linked to high blood pressure, increased cholesterol and triglycerides, lower HDL cholesterol and their consequences: heart disease and stroke. According to the National Institutes of Health, an estimated one-quarter of cardiovascular disease can be attributed to obesity. Dr. Kenneth Cooper, head of the Cooper Clinic in Dallas, Texas, regards obesity as one of the top cardiac risk factors: "Obese people are three times more likely to have high blood pressure and four times more likely to

> ### PORKY PETS
>
> The next time you think about tossing Fido a piece of steak, think again. About 60 million dogs and cats in the United States are overweight. "Our pets often reflect our lifestyles," says veterinarian Kimberly Rudloff. "If we're couch potatoes, so are they."

have diabetes. In addition, they are two times more likely to die from heart disease than are people of normal weight."

Obese people, as compared with their leaner counterparts, have higher levels of plasminogen activator inhibitor-1, a substance that can cause artery-blocking blood clots. Obesity also may heighten inflammation in the arteries, thus increasing the risk for clotting. Says Dr. Paul Ridker, an expert on C-reactive protein, "Overweight and obese people tend to have higher levels of C-reactive protein than people of normal weight. Even an extra 10 or 20 pounds can raise CRP and contribute to a heart attack."

And finally, fatty acids released into the blood by fat stored in the body have been shown to trigger irregular heartbeats, which in extreme cases may lead to sudden cardiac death.

SHRINKING DRESS SIZES

A woman's size 8 today was, on her mother and grandmother, a size 10. That's because clothing designers now use dress size as a marketing tool, knowing that women are more likely to buy clothing for their size 10 (or 12) body if it says size 8.

Abdominal Obesity

The link between overweight and heart disease is particularly strong if the excess weight is carried around the middle. Says Dr. William Castelli, former director of the Framingham Heart Study, "People with wide hips and flat bellies may be overweight, but the extra weight does not seem to increase their cardiac risk as much as that of people with narrow hips and potbellies. Abdominal obesity, which is more of a male problem, is predictive of coronary disease."

Potbellies make many men appear "apple-shaped," while many more women could be described as "pear-shaped." Perhaps because abdominal fat is more metabolically active than fat stored in thighs, hips and buttocks, "apples" are three to five times more likely than "pears" to suffer heart attacks. Potbelly fat is a strong predictor and reason enough to determine if it's penalizing your cardiac health. "You can do this simply by measuring your waist," says Dr. Scott

Grundy of the University of Texas Southwestern Medical Center. "Position a soft tape measure around your waist, just above the navel. The American Heart Association defines a high-risk waistline as 35 inches or more for women and 40 inches or more for men. Studies show that people with these measurements were three times more likely to have high blood cholesterol levels, four times more likely to be in poor physical condition and seven times more likely to be diabetic than people with smaller waists."

Weight: Know Your Number, Know Your Risk

The National Institutes of Health recommends using body mass index (BMI) to measure your weight. BMI describes body weight relative to height and is equal to weight in kilograms divided by height in meters squared. Alternatively, you can estimate BMI from pounds and inches. Simply multiply your weight in pounds by 705, divide by height in inches, then divide by height in inches again.

The Body Mass Index Table on pages 34 and 35 can save you some time. To use the table, find your approximate height in the left-hand column labeled "Height." Move across to your weight. The number at the top of the column is the BMI for your height and weight.

It is recommended that all adults have their BMI determined and assessed in light of the following guidelines:

BMI*	CONDITION	RISK
19 to 24.9	Healthy weight	Desirable
25 to 29.9	Overweight	Borderline high
30 to 39.9	Obese	High
40 to 54	Very obese	Very high
Your BMI: _____	Your risk: _____	

*BMI usually correlates very well with body fat, although very muscular people may have a high BMI without excess body fat. In that case, there is no added health risk.

33

BODY MASS INDEX TABLE

BMI	19	20	21	22	23	24	25	26	27	28	29	30	31	32	33	34	35
	HEALTHY WEIGHT						OVERWEIGHT					OBESE					
Height (feet/ inches)	Body Weight (pounds)																
4'10"	91	96	100	105	110	115	119	124	129	134	138	143	148	153	158	162	167
4'11"	94	99	104	109	114	119	124	128	133	138	143	148	153	158	163	168	173
5'0"	97	102	107	112	118	123	128	133	138	143	148	153	158	163	168	174	179
5'1"	100	106	111	116	122	127	132	137	143	148	153	158	164	169	174	180	185
5'2"	104	109	115	120	126	131	136	142	147	153	158	164	169	175	180	186	191
5'3"	107	113	118	124	130	135	141	146	152	158	163	169	175	180	186	191	197
5'4"	110	116	122	128	134	140	145	151	157	163	169	174	180	186	192	197	204
5'5"	114	120	126	132	138	144	150	156	162	168	174	180	186	192	198	204	210
5'6"	118	124	130	136	142	148	155	161	167	173	179	186	192	198	204	210	216
5'7"	121	127	134	140	146	153	159	166	172	178	185	191	198	204	211	217	223
5'8"	125	131	138	144	151	158	164	171	177	184	190	197	203	210	216	223	230
5'9"	128	135	142	149	155	162	169	176	182	189	196	203	209	216	223	230	236
5'10"	132	139	146	153	160	167	174	181	188	195	202	209	216	222	229	236	243
5'11"	136	143	150	157	165	172	179	186	193	200	208	215	222	229	236	243	250
6'0"	140	147	154	162	169	177	184	191	199	206	213	221	228	235	242	250	258
6'1"	144	151	159	166	174	182	189	197	204	212	219	227	235	242	250	257	265
6'2"	148	155	163	171	179	186	194	202	210	218	225	233	341	249	256	264	272
6'3"	152	160	168	176	184	192	200	208	216	224	232	240	248	256	264	272	279
6'4"	156	164	172	180	189	197	205	213	221	230	238	246	254	263	271	279	287

36	37	38	39	VERY OBESE														
				40	41	42	43	44	45	46	47	48	49	50	51	52	53	54
172	177	181	186	191	196	201	205	210	215	220	224	229	234	239	244	248	253	258
178	183	188	193	198	203	208	212	217	222	227	232	237	242	247	252	257	262	267
184	189	194	199	204	209	215	220	225	230	235	240	245	250	255	261	266	271	276
190	195	201	206	211	217	222	227	232	238	243	248	254	259	264	269	275	280	285
196	202	207	213	218	224	229	235	240	246	251	256	262	267	273	278	284	289	295
203	208	214	220	225	231	237	242	248	254	259	265	270	278	282	287	293	299	304
209	215	221	227	232	238	244	250	256	262	267	273	279	285	291	296	302	308	314
216	222	228	234	240	246	252	258	264	270	276	282	288	294	300	306	312	318	324
223	229	235	241	247	253	260	266	272	278	284	291	297	303	309	315	322	328	334
230	236	242	249	255	261	266	274	280	287	293	299	306	312	319	325	331	338	344
236	243	249	256	262	269	276	282	289	295	302	308	315	322	328	335	341	348	354
243	250	257	263	270	277	284	291	297	304	311	318	324	331	338	345	351	358	365
250	257	264	271	278	285	292	299	306	313	320	327	334	341	348	355	362	369	376
257	265	272	279	286	293	301	308	315	322	329	338	343	351	358	365	373	379	386
265	272	279	287	294	302	309	316	324	331	338	346	353	361	368	375	383	390	397
272	280	288	295	302	310	318	325	333	340	348	355	363	371	378	386	393	401	408
280	287	295	303	311	319	326	334	342	350	358	365	373	381	389	396	404	412	420
287	295	303	311	319	327	335	343	351	359	367	375	383	391	399	407	415	423	431
295	304	312	320	328	336	344	353	361	369	377	385	394	402	410	418	426	435	443

WHERE YOU LIVE MATTERS

According to *Men's Fitness* magazine, some cities foster fitness and weight control while others cultivate overweight. Sunny San Diego, where apparently everyone runs on the beach, topped the magazine's list of "fittest" cities. In contrast, Houston ranked among the fattest cities in the United States.

SOME OF THE FITTEST	SOME OF THE FATTEST
San Diego	Houston
Seattle	Columbus, Ohio
Minneapolis	Mesa, Arizona
Denver	Kansas City, Missouri
Boston	Phoenix
Virginia Beach, Virginia	Cleveland
Portland, Oregon	Chicago
Washington, D.C.	Philadelphia

5. BLOOD PRESSURE

Blood pressure, the force needed to move blood through the vascular system against the resistance of the artery walls, is often compared to the pressure inside an ordinary garden hose. When the nozzle of the hose is opened, the water pressure in the hose decreases. But if the nozzle is tightened or more water is added, the pressure increases.

High blood pressure is usually attributed to a narrowing of arteries and their smaller vessels (the arterioles), to a loss of elasticity, or to both. Resistance creates pressure, causing the heart to work harder just to keep the blood moving. This added stress, both on the heart and on the vascular system, can lead to the bulging and rupture of an artery (called an aneurysm), hardening of the arteries, stroke, heart attack, kidney failure, congestive heart failure and death. Constant high blood pressure affects the artery linings, causing sufficient trauma to create arterial injury and inflammation. This circumstance in turn causes even more narrowing of artery openings, so the heart is less likely to receive an adequate supply of blood. Then it has to expend more energy, which means it needs more oxygen, resulting in a no-win situation.

Afflicting about 63 million Americans (and more common in African-Americans than in Caucasians), high blood pressure represents a major public health threat. Every year, it kills 45,000 Americans outright and contributes to the deaths of an additional 210,000. One study done at the Boston University School of Medicine estimates that 9 out of 10 middle-aged Americans will, at some point, develop high blood pressure.

High blood pressure is a predictive, primary risk factor for heart disease and stroke. People with high blood pressure are up to five times more likely to have a heart attack and more than twice as likely to have a stroke than people with normal blood pressure. Yet, according to Dr. Sidney Smith, past president of the American Heart Association, 79% of hypertensive patients do not receive adequate treatment. Indeed, half of all people with high blood pressure don't even know they have the condition and end up suffering needlessly in their ignorance.

Like coronary heart disease itself, high blood pressure progresses silently, increasing year after year with no overt symptoms other than, perhaps, some nonspecific complaints: dizzy spells, chest pains, swelling in ankles and feet, headaches, changes in vision, leg cramps, loss of concentration. Then quite suddenly, usually in middle age, hypertension appears. By this time, however, it's usually too late to repair the damage done. Chronic illness and death may ultimately occur.

In addition, people with high blood pressure are twice as likely to develop Type 2 (non-insulin-dependent) diabetes as are those with normal blood pressure. High blood pressure is also linked to age-related macular degeneration, a progressive loss of vision due to the deterioration of nerve tissue in the retina.

Blood Pressure: Know Your Numbers, Know Your Risk

Blood pressure is expressed as two numbers representing millimeters of mercury (mm Hg). The top number represents *systolic pressure*, which is taken when the heart beats—at that moment when blood is pumped out of the heart in one big burst of peak pressure and the aorta expands to handle the flow. The bottom number is the *diastolic pressure*, registered between heartbeats when the pressure falls to its lowest point as the heart relaxes back to its normal size and refills with blood. Normal systolic pressure is 120 mm Hg and normal

THE POWER OF INTIMACY

A study at the State University of New York at Oswego has found that spending a little quality time with your significant other, regardless of what you do together, seems to have a calming influence on a person's blood pressure. Researchers theorize that the familiarity of an intimate relationship sends out a "safety signal" that lowers blood pressure.

"This does not mean that single people are doomed to high blood pressure," says lead study author Dr. Brooks Gump. "Rather, the findings suggest that comfortable relationships—close friends included—have a soothing effect on blood pressure." While it is unclear what such a short-term change in blood pressure means to health, we do know that temporary flare-ups in blood pressure can take a cardiovascular toll. It may well be that the calming influence of a partner acts as a counterbalance and eventually benefits the heart.

diastolic pressure is 80 mm Hg, typically expressed in figures as 120/80 and verbally as "120 over 80."

Blood pressure, however, varies naturally with weight, activity, body position, age and even time of day. Because of such fluctuations, you would not be considered to have high blood pressure unless you had three elevated readings in a row. Furthermore, if you're anxious about having your blood pressure taken, you may develop what's called "white-coat hypertension"—a temporary condition responsible for a whole set of misdiagnoses. That's why some doctors use ambulatory blood pressure monitoring, in which the patient wears a blood pressure cuff that inflates periodically over a 24-hour period; attached to the cuff, a monitor the size of a tape recorder stores the readings as they're taken. This technique is also useful for evaluating the effectiveness of blood pressure medications, as well as the relationship between blood pressure and abnormal symptoms (such as dizziness) during the day.

> ## HYPERTENSION AND MEMORY LOSS
>
> If left untreated, high blood pressure in midlife can cause memory loss later in life. The Framingham Heart Study found that for every increase of 10 points of systolic pressure in middle age, there was a 7% or greater risk of impaired cognitive skills 20 years later.

So, let's say you're tested and your doctor tells you that you have high blood pressure, or hypertension. What does this mean? Only that the pressure in your arteries is consistently above the normal range—generally agreed to be 140/90. (If you have diabetes, another important cardiac marker, even lower blood pressure is recommended, ideally less than 130/80.) The higher your numbers, the greater the risk.

For many years it was thought that the bottom number (diastolic pressure) was more important. Doctors suggested that this number reflected the minimum pressure to which the arteries are constantly exposed and found it to be less variable than the top number (systolic pressure), so systolic hypertension was often undertreated. But now, study after study shows that the percentage of people who experience heart attacks or strokes increases with both elevated systolic and diastolic pressure. Which of these two numbers should be used to diagnose the presence and severity of hypertension? The common-sense answer is, of course, both.

The following standards have been established by the National Institutes of Health for assessing high blood pressure:

BLOOD PRESSURE READING

SYSTOLIC	DIASTOLIC	RISK
Less than 120	Less than 80	Optimal
Less than 130	Less than 85	Normal
130 to 139	85 to 89	High normal
140 to 159	90 to 99	Stage 1 hypertension
160 to 179	100 to 109	Stage 2 hypertension
180 and above	110 and above	Stage 3 hypertension

RISK RANGES

Your systolic pressure:

_____ Below 130 (lower-risk range)

_____ 130 and above (higher-risk range)

Your diastolic pressure:

_____ Below 85 (lower-risk range)

_____ 85 and above (higher-risk range)

The ranges above are used so that you can determine whether or not this marker is a cardiac risk for you. Obviously, risk is more easily estimated at the extremes. A person with a systolic pressure of less than 120 has a lower risk, while one who has a reading higher than 180 is already showing advanced hypertension. But what about borderline risk? Is someone with a systolic pressure of 139 "safe" while a person with a systolic pressure of 141 is "at high risk"? The line is not that clear. Ask your doctor for more specific information on your number and your risk.

RECOMMENDED ACTIONS

For healthy people over 18 years of age, the following actions are recommended, based on an initial blood pressure check:

BLOOD PRESSURE READING

Systolic	Diastolic	WHAT TO DO
Less than 130	Less than 85	Recheck in 2 years
130 to 139	85 to 89	Recheck in 1 year
140 to 159	90 to 99	Confirm within 2 months
160 to 179	100 to 109	See your doctor within 1 month
180 or higher	110 or higher	See your doctor immediately

If your systolic and diastolic readings cross categories, follow the recommendations for the shorter follow-up time. If you have questions or concerns, talk with your doctor.

Also, understand that just because your blood pressure isn't high, this doesn't mean it's low enough. High blood pressure doesn't suddenly occur at 140/90. Instead, the risk for heart disease rises along a continuum as blood pressure increases. Researchers examining records of 7,000 people in the Framingham Heart Study found that over a 10-year period those with high-normal blood pressure were about twice as likely to suffer a heart attack as compared with people with optimal blood pressure.

It's important to have your blood pressure checked regularly. If your readings are usually within normal range, keep on doing what you're doing to avoid an upward climb. But if they're consistently elevated, talk with your doctor about methods to control your blood pressure. This is crucial. According to the Framingham Heart Study, a man in his thirties with a diastolic pressure between 85 and 94 has a five times greater risk of a heart attack than a man with a diastolic pressure below 70. But the opposite is also true: for every one-point drop in diastolic blood pressure, there is a 2% to 3% drop in heart attack risk. Therefore, aggressive management of blood pressure is a prudent measure. As blood pressure expert Dr. Sheldon G. Sheps has observed, "You shouldn't be satisfied unless your blood pressure is controlled."

Three major trials have, in recent years, examined the effects of aggressive blood pressure treatment in persons aged 60 and older with isolated systolic hypertension. Subjects were randomly assigned to drug treatment with antihypertensive medications or to a placebo group that received a look-alike (but inactive) pill. Those in the treatment group had markedly fewer cardiovascular events over the follow-up periods.

6. DIABETES

About 16 million Americans have diabetes, a condition that disrupts the way the body uses glucose, a sugar molecule that comes from the food we eat. For the body to absorb glucose, a hormone called insulin, which is produced by the pancreas, is necessary. But in people with diabetes the pancreas does not produce insulin (or produces too little of it) or the body does not properly use the insulin that is produced. As a consequence, glucose builds up in the blood and eventually begins to appear in the urine. Over time, high glucose levels can cause devastating results such as stroke, high blood pressure, blindness, kidney disease, nerve damage and amputation. Diabetes is the fourth leading cause of death (often prematurely) in the United States. And it is a definite marker for heart disease, especially among women, in part because diabetes predisposes people to high blood pressure and a poor lipid profile.

Even though diabetics have heart disease death rates about two to four times higher than nondiabetics, most people who suffer from this disease are unaware of their increased cardiovascular risk. In one recent survey by the American Heart Association, diabetics identified loss of vision and amputation as the most serious complications of their disease. Only one-third of those surveyed named heart disease as a serious complication.

There are three main types of diabetes. *Type 1 diabetes*, previously called insulin-dependent or juvenile-onset diabetes, occurs in childhood or early adulthood—often in children who have a diabetic parent or sibling. While the genetic component is strong, Type 1 diabetes can also result from other diseases of the pancreas and may be set off by an environmental trigger such as a virus, toxin or food. People with Type 1 have a severe shortage of insulin; their pancreas produces little or none at all. Since the absence of insulin means glucose cannot be used for energy, the body burns fat for its energy, causing ketones (substances formed by the breakdown of fat) to build up in the bloodstream. Before the development of injectable insulin, children with diabetes usually died young. Now they can live relatively normal lives.

Type 2 diabetes, previously called non-insulin-dependent or adult-onset diabetes, accounts for 90% to 95% of all cases of diabetes. It usually strikes people in their forties or older, although it

---

COMMON SYMPTOMS OF DIABETES

Type 1 and Type 2 diabetes have many symptoms in common. One difference is that the symptoms of Type 1 tend to come on suddenly, while those of Type 2 appear quite gradually.

Frequent urination

Increased hunger and thirst

Weight loss

Headaches; blurred vision

Weakness and fatigue

Irritability

Infections, especially yeast infections

Slow healing of cuts or bruises

Tingling or numbness in the hands or feet

Recurring skin, gum or bladder infections

is increasingly showing up in overweight, sedentary young people—some still in their teens. Genetics can play a role in the development of Type 2 diabetes. (It has been found that certain populations, including African-Americans, Hispanic/Latino Americans, Asian-Americans, Pacific Islanders and Native Americans, have a higher incidence.) However, the main factor in the development of Type 2 diabetes is obesity.

Type 2 diabetics produce some insulin, but their bodies have developed a resistance to it; as time passes, these individuals require more insulin than the pancreas can produce, and the buildup of glucose in the bloodstream damages blood vessels and organs. Some quick-weight-loss diet books, in an attempt to justify their pop science, have claimed that insulin resistance leads to overweight. Scientific evidence, however, shows the reverse to be true. *Overweight leads to insulin resistance.* This points to a major link between overweight and the onset of Type 2 diabetes.

SPEAKING FROM EXPERIENCE

There's some terrifying information out there about the weight and health of our kids. The fact is that there have never been so many overweight and obese American children and adolescents. The typical 12-year-old today weighs 11.7 pounds more than his or her counterpart in 1973. In the last decade the obesity rate in white children has increased by 50%; in Hispanic-American and African-American kids, it has doubled.

One result of this excess weight is that record numbers of children have Type 2 diabetes. Until a few years ago, it was called adult-onset diabetes. Now, because so many children have it, it's simply called Type 2 diabetes. —*J.P.*

To be clear: over 85% of Type 2 diabetics are overweight. Burgeoning obesity is the central reason that more Americans are contracting Type 2 at a younger age. But this situation can be reversed. You can lower your risk of getting full-blown diabetes by at least 80% if you lose as little as 5% of your body weight and exercise as little as 30 minutes a day.

A third type of diabetes is *gestational diabetes*, which affects 3% to 5% of pregnant women in the United States. In this condition, hormones from the placenta block the normal action of insulin in the body, creating insulin resistance. Because certain complications arising from gestational diabetes can be quite serious, every pregnant woman is tested for it.

Diabetes: Know Your Number, Know Your Risk

It's important to know your estimated risk for diabetes, particularly if you have a family history. Experts recommend that all adults over the age of 45 be tested for diabetes every three years.

The routine diagnostic test for diabetes is the fasting blood glucose test, which can be administered as part of your lipid panel. (Fasting means not eating for at least eight hours prior to blood sampling.) Researchers at the National Institute of Diabetes and Digestive and Kidney Diseases suggest that morning, rather than afternoon, is the optimal time for administering a blood glucose test because of the so-called "dawn

EXERCISE LOWERS HEART ATTACK RISK

About 75% of diabetics die of heart attack or stroke. About half of the higher-than-normal risk of cardiovascular disease in diabetics comes from just two factors: high blood pressure and low HDL. But researchers from the Framingham Offspring Study have now found that people with elevated levels of insulin are more prone to blood clots, thereby increasing their risk of heart attack and stroke. By making the body more receptive to the effects of insulin, exercise may improve a person's ability to dissolve clots and thus reduce cardiovascular risk.

phenomenon"—blood glucose levels of diabetics are highest in the morning hours.

Results of the fasting blood glucose test are represented as milligrams of glucose in one deciliter of blood. The American Diabetes Association suggests that the following scale be used for an estimation of risk:

GLUCOSE	RISK CLASSIFICATION
Below 110	Desirable
110 to 125*	Borderline high
Above 125**	Confirmed diabetes
Your number: _____	Your risk: _____

*This relatively new risk category, called "impaired fasting glucose," indicates glucose values greater than desirable or normal but less than the level that is diagnostic of diabetes. Doctors are trying to learn how to predict which people with this condition will end up with diabetes. If you fall into this risk category, work with your doctor on a program to reduce your own risk.

**A fasting blood glucose of 126 or higher indicates diabetes. Previously, a value of 140 was the standard. In some instances, doctors will elect to perform an oral glucose tolerance test, in which case a glucose value of 200 or more indicates a diagnosis of diabetes.

According to the Cleveland Clinic's Dr. Byron Hoogwerf, blood glucose levels can vary from hour to hour. Consequently, if the fasting blood glucose level is even slightly elevated (110 to 125), he recommends a follow-up blood test called hemoglobin A1c, or simply HbA1c.

In a nutshell, HbA1c testing measures the amount of glucose attached to red blood cells. The higher your blood glucose, the more sugar your red blood cells will accumulate over time. Because red blood cells typically live 90 to 120 days, this test reveals your "average" blood sugar during that time. For people without diabetes, target

HbA1c numbers range from 4% to 6%. Diabetics should strive for a value below 7%.

Today, HbA1c testing can be done in a doctor's office using a blood sample from a finger stick. Diabetics should probably have an HbA1c test every six months; insulin-dependent diabetics should aim for three-month intervals. Your doctor can best determine the frequency that is most appropriate for you. Comparing the test results with your current blood glucose level offers a more accurate picture of diabetes control. The following chart provides an example of how the two measurements may relate to one another, as well as the level of control.

GAUGING YOUR LEVEL
OF DIABETES CONTROL

Average Blood Glucose	Diabetes Type 1 or 2	HbA1c
mg/dl	Level of Control	%
360 —	POOR CONTROL	— 14
240 —		— 10
	MARGINAL CONTROL	
210 —		— 9
	GOOD CONTROL	
150 —		— 7
	GOAL	
90 —		— 5

Think of your HbA1c test as a quarterly stock market report. Some days the market rises, other days it falls. By getting a quarterly report, you get a better picture of what the market has been like over the past three months.

7. SYNDROME X

Syndrome X, also known as metabolic syndrome, is a combination of cardiac risk factors believed to be a product of insulin resistance. As discussed in the previous text on diabetes, our bodies convert the food we eat into glucose, which insulin transports to cells where fuel is needed. The cells, however, are protected by receptors that act as "gates," controlling which substances are allowed in. Normally, insulin is the "key" that opens these gates and allows glucose to enter the cells.

Unfortunately, these receptors can become resistant to insulin's action, probably as a result of weight gain and physical inactivity. If this occurs, the pancreas pumps out more insulin in an attempt to force glucose into the cells. This scenario, if repeated over time, is thought to trigger a series of metabolic abnormalities culminating in Syndrome X. The condition directly damages the coronary arteries, contributing to the buildup of plaque and promoting blood clots.

Syndrome X affects an estimated 60 to 75 million Americans. It shows up as excess fibrinogen as well as elevated levels of plasminogen activator inhibitor-1 (PAI-1), a substance that slows clot breakdown, and a dangerous combination of cardiac risk factors including high triglycerides, low HDL, abdominal obesity and elevations in blood pressure, blood sugar and uric acid. It is widely believed that this cluster of metabolic abnormalities speeds the development of coronary heart disease, particularly in women and diabetics.

People with Syndrome X typically have a moderate level of total cholesterol, often under 200, so the syndrome may be overlooked in a medical exam. For example, data on a 51-year-old male in the Framingham Heart Study produced the following lipid profile:

Total cholesterol	195
LDL cholesterol	108
HDL cholesterol	32
Triglycerides	264

Because his total cholesterol was under 200 and his LDL level was "desirable," it might be assumed that this man had a low cardiac risk. In fact, the man had coronary heart disease that was likely attributable to Syndrome X. Says Dr. Castelli, "In Framingham, we've found that when triglycerides are high and HDL is low, the predictive risk of heart attack doubles . . . even when total cholesterol is in line. We've also found that when you fatten up in the abdomen, you start to move your triglycerides and HDL toward Syndrome X. And when you add in high blood pressure and diabetes, the effect is disastrous."

Syndrome X: Know Your Profile, Know Your Risk

In 2001, the National Cholesterol Education Panel published the following risk profile for Syndrome X:

Is your HDL number below 40 (men) or below 50 (women)?	Yes _____	No _____
Is your triglyceride number over 150?	Yes _____	No _____
Is your waist size 35 inches or above (women) or 40 inches or above (men)?	Yes _____	No _____
Is your blood pressure consistently 130/85 or greater?	Yes _____	No _____
Are you a diabetic (a fasting glucose of 110 or greater)?	Yes _____	No _____

If you answered "yes" to two of the five questions above, you probably have a Syndrome X profile. If you answered "yes" to three or more, you definitely have a Syndrome X profile.

High triglycerides and low HDL, obesity, diabetes, high blood pressure—all are fairly common health problems and each increases cardiac risk. But in combination as part of Syndrome X, they can be deadly. A recent study followed more than 6,000 heart patients for 8 to 10 years after bypass surgery. It found that among people who had three or four of the characteristics of Syndrome X, the risk for death in the 10 years after surgery increased by 1.5 to 3 times compared with people with none of the conditions. The risk rose even more for women—a 5 to 12 times increase in the 10-year death rate.

But it doesn't have to be that way. The risk factors that in combination can create Syndrome X are modifiable with healthy lifestyle changes and, if necessary, drug therapy.

8. AEROBIC CAPACITY

People who demonstrate strength, stamina and flexibility—what we think of as physical fitness—are most often in better overall health than those who can't heft a child or touch their toes. But that doesn't mean they're in good cardiovascular health. Much more important is their aerobic capacity, which is both a critical cardiac marker and a predictor of longevity.

Aerobic, which means "with oxygen," describes activities that cause the heart and lungs to process oxygen at a steady rate over a period of time. Brisk walking, jogging and swimming develop stamina and endurance, the ability to keep on going without placing undue strain on the cardiovascular system. Regular aerobic exercise develops aerobic fitness, the ability to work the muscles hard—but not so hard that the heart and lungs can't keep up with the oxygen demand.

In order to understand the benefits of aerobic fitness, we need to back up and examine what enables us to work and play. Through a series of chemical reactions, the food we eat is converted into energy reserves. Much more energy is formed if plenty of oxygen is available to body tissues—and that depends on the volume of blood the heart pumps per minute and the amount of oxygen the tissues extract from the circulating blood. These two variables determine the level of aerobic fitness. But since there is little difference from one person to another in the amount of oxygen that is extracted by the tissues, we know that aerobic fitness is largely reflective of the pumping effectiveness of the heart.

Quantifying Aerobic Fitness

People who run or jog, go out for a brisk walk or participate in a spinning class know very quickly if they have aerobic fitness. If you can run steadily for 30 minutes, for instance, you can probably call yourself aerobically fit. But if you have to stop to catch your breath 10 minutes into your walk, it's a safe bet that you haven't achieved aerobic fitness.

This type of casual determination is not sufficient, however, for evaluating your aerobic fitness as a cardiac marker, because it fails to measure your oxygen consumption. The gold standard in this case is a progressive treadmill test done with sophisticated equipment that involves having you breathe through a mouthpiece or face mask. It factors your breathing and heart rates with your final speed and the grade of the incline, or the number of minutes achieved in the test. The results are expressed in *metabolic equivalents (of task)*, or METs, a numerical rating of the body's ability to produce energy needed to perform certain activities.

One MET equals the amount of oxygen required for sitting at rest or lying down. The more effort it takes for a given activity, the greater the number of METs expended. Walking at a pace of two miles per hour, for instance, expends about 2 to 3 METs, the same as playing the piano or pitching horseshoes. Boosting your walking speed to four miles per hour calls for about 5 METs, about the same as needed for gardening or washing windows. And jogging at the speed of five miles per hour requires about 8 METs, about the same as climbing stairs or downhill skiing.

The highest MET level you can achieve during an exercise stress test is referred to as your maximal MET level. Average men and women have an 8 to 12 MET capacity. This means that at maximal exercise, they can consume 8 to 12 times the amount of oxygen that they take in at rest. Older or unfit persons or heart patients generally average 5 to 8 METs. In contrast, marathoners and other highly trained endurance athletes have been measured at 15 to 20 METs or more.

Increasing your maximal MET level is crucial for cardiac health and longevity, as demonstrated in a series of landmark studies by Dr. Steven Blair and colleagues at the Cooper Institute. In one study, more than 13,000 healthy men and women were given a medical examination and a treadmill stress test. At the time, none of the subjects exhibited any evidence of heart disease or cancer. During a follow-up period averaging more than eight years, nearly 300 of the participants had died. The study concluded that, in general, the higher the subjects' initial level of fitness, the lower the subsequent death rate from heart disease or cancer. This was true even after statistical adjustments were made for age, coronary risk factors and family history of heart disease.

Interestingly, there appeared to be no further decrease in mortality associated with fitness levels higher than 9 to 10 METs. Moreover, the greatest reduction in death risk for men occurred as they progressed from the lowest level of aerobic fitness (6 or less METs) to the next lowest level (7 METs). These findings suggest that even a

SPEAKING FROM EXPERIENCE

It's not that hard to find excellent physical activities of moderate intensity, which generally correspond to 3 to 6 METs. There are recreational activities—brisk walking (three to four miles per hour), biking, dancing fast, golf (pulling a cart or carrying clubs). There are also activities that are useful and productive—washing or waxing your car, washing windows or floors, raking leaves, ordinary home care, general cleaning, mowing the lawn with a power mower, home repair or painting.

Or, if you want, you can have fun *and* feel righteous at the same time by working in the garden or doing conditioning exercises, general calisthenics, lap swimming or water aerobics.　　　　*—B.F.*

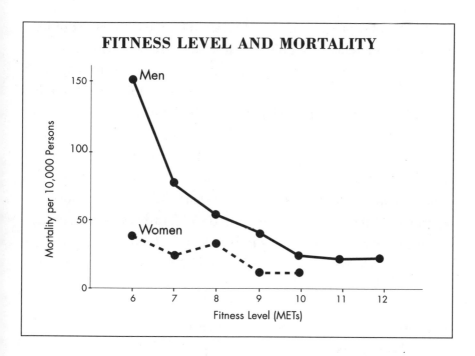

FITNESS LEVEL AND MORTALITY

slight improvement in aerobic capacity among the most unfit sub-stantially reduces heart disease mortality.

In a subsequent study, Dr. Blair followed nearly 10,000 men who were given two treadmill tests about five years apart. Approximately five years after the second test, deaths from all causes were examined. The highest death rate occurred in men who were rated "unfit" at both examinations; the lowest death rate was in men who were rated "highly fit" both times. However, men who improved from the "unfit" to the "fit" category between the first and second examinations had an intermediate death rate, supporting the hypothesis that improved aerobic fitness leads to decreased mortality.

More recently, these researchers examined the risk of dying among people who had one or more of the major cardiac markers: low aerobic fitness, cigarette smoking, high blood pressure, over-weight or obesity, and elevated blood cholesterol. Low aerobic fitness proved to be the strongest predictor of subsequent mortality. Men and women who had low fitness levels were twice as likely to die during the eight-year follow-up period. In addition, the protective effect of high aerobic fitness remained, even for those who had other risk factors.

Dr. Victor F. Froelicher, a world-renowned cardiologist at Stanford University Medical Center, explains it this way: "Aerobic capacity seems to be an independent predictor of mortality. A low exercise capacity of less than 4 METs indicates a higher mortality group, regardless of the underlying extent of coronary heart disease or cardiac impairment. On the other hand, an aerobic fitness level greater than 10 METs designates a group with excellent survival, regardless of their cardiac history. If 10 METs truly exerts a 'protective effect' that obviates any survival benefit from coronary bypass surgery, this has enormous implications for cost containment and medical care."

Aerobic Capacity: Know Your Numbers, Know Your Risk

Knowing your aerobic fitness level in METs is important in determining whether or not this cardiac marker is a risk for you. But being exercise-tested with a face mask can be an inconvenience, and the test itself requires complicated equipment, technical expertise and frequent calibration. So how can you estimate your fitness level in more practical ways?

One method is a simpler treadmill stress test that allows doctors to predict or estimate peak METs from the speed and grade or time achieved. The graph on page 55 illustrates one of the most common treadmill protocols, invented by Dr. Robert Bruce. The first stage of the Bruce protocol starts at 1.7 miles per hour and 10% grade. Then, every three minutes, the speed and grade are increased until the subject exhibits abnormal signs or symptoms, suggesting that the test be stopped, or until the point of exhaustion for the subject. Needless to say, such tests should never be attempted without medical clearance, continuous electrocardiographic monitoring and a physician being immediately available.

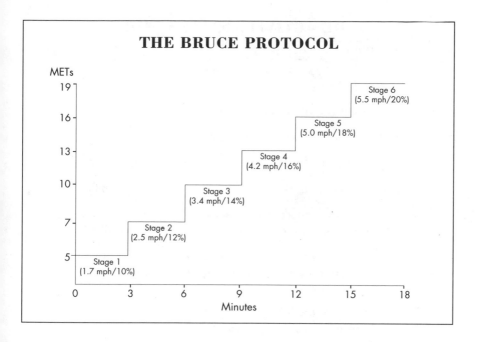

A 50-year-old man who is able to achieve 9 minutes, or stage 3, corresponding to 3.4 mph and 14% grade, has an estimated fitness level of 10 METs. This individual would be classified as "low risk." In contrast, the man who poops out after only 1½ minutes at stage 1 would be classified as "high risk," suggesting that his mortality rate is greater than average.

Although standard treadmill testing remains popular as a medical evaluation, it is quite costly (about $300 to $500 per test), time-consuming and not without risk.

Another method of estimating MET capacity is the use of a patient questionnaire like the Duke Activity Status Index, shown on the following page. For our purposes, the Duke questionnaire is a great way to determine whether or not aerobic fitness is a marker that puts you at increased cardiovascular risk; if so, you may want to consult with your doctor about the appropriateness of a treadmill stress test. The key to the usefulness of this questionnaire lies in answering each of the questions as honestly as possible.

DUKE ACTIVITY STATUS INDEX

CAN YOU:	POINTS
1. Take care of yourself, i.e., eat, dress, bathe and use the toilet?	2.75
2. Walk indoors, as around your house?	1.75
3. Walk a block or two on level ground?	2.75
4. Climb a flight of stairs or walk up a hill?	5.50
5. Run a short distance?	8.00
6. Do light work around the house like dusting or washing dishes?	2.70
7. Do moderate work around the house like vacuuming, sweeping floors or carrying groceries?	3.50
8. Do heavy work around the house like scrubbing floors or lifting or moving heavy furniture?	8.00
9. Do yard work like raking leaves, weeding or pushing a power mower?	4.50
10. Have sexual relations?	5.25
11. Participate in moderate recreational activities like golf, bowling, dancing, doubles tennis or throwing a baseball or football?	6.00
12. Participate in strenuous sports like swimming, singles tennis, football, basketball or skiing?	7.50

Total points: _____

Add up the points for each question to which you answered "yes." Your aerobic fitness, expressed as METs, can be approximated by using the following formula:

METs = (0.43 × total points + 9.6) divided by 3.5

As an example, if your total is 28.7 points, your equation would be: 0.43 × 28.7 = 12.34 + 9.6 = 21.94 divided by 3.5 = 6.26 METs.

Now check your own MET level against the scale below:

AEROBIC FITNESS	MORTALITY RISK
4 or less	High
5 to 9	Average
10 or more	Low
Your METs: _____	Your risk: _____

Put simply, aerobically fit people generally live longer than their unfit counterparts. And it's not that hard to achieve. An exercise program can increase a sedentary person's maximal MET level by 10% to 30% in just three months. And most people who engage in only moderately intense exercise for at least 30 minutes a day can attain a "cardioprotective" fitness level of 9 to 10 METs or more.

9. SMOKING

Responsible for more than 500,000 deaths annually, smoking is the single most preventable cause of death in the United States. According to the American Lung Association, if a person starts smoking before age 20, each cigarette costs him or her about 20 seconds of life. For a two-packs-a-day smoker, this means throwing away more than eight years.

Most people assume that the greatest health risk from smoking is cancer. And while it's true that smoking leads to more than 150,000 cancer deaths each year, the impact of smoking on the risk of heart disease is much greater. Smoking contributes to about 40% of all cardiac deaths.

Smokers are twice as likely as nonsmokers to have a heart attack and are five times more likely to die from sudden cardiac death. In one study, the mortality from coronary heart disease in those smoking 25 or more cigarettes per day was nearly triple that of nonsmokers. It's the same for stroke. Results from the Harvard

Physicians' Health Study of more than 22,000 doctors show that the risk of stroke among smokers is twice that of nonsmokers.

When combined with other risk factors such as high cholesterol or hypertension, the effect of smoking is compounded and lethal. Indeed, autopsy studies illustrate that coronary heart disease is far more severe and extensive in smokers than in nonsmokers. This increase is due to the inhalation of toxic compounds. A lighted cigarette gives off several hundred compounds, some in gaseous form and some in particles. The gases, which constitute 60% of cigarette smoke, include carbon monoxide, cyanide, ammonia, nitric acid, acetone and acrolein. The particulate compounds, which are inhaled as tar, produce ammonia, benzopyrene and at least 10 other known carcinogens, as well as the toxic chemical nicotine.

WHAT WERE THEY THINKING?

According to a 2002 CNN poll, 32% of American men and 22% of American women said they believe you can smoke and still stay healthy.

Scientists are not certain how these compounds work to produce coronary heart disease, but studies show carbon monoxide and nicotine to be the chief culprits. To begin with, keep in mind that a single cigarette contains 640 times the amount of carbon monoxide that OSHA would allow in any industrial plant in the country, according to studies at UCLA by Drs. George Sieffert and Wesley Moore. Then consider carbon monoxide's effects on the body:

■ As it moves through the bloodstream, artery walls become injured (pitted and cratered) and irritated. This causes inflammation, which increases cardiac risk.

■ It can irritate arteries to the point where they spasm and constrict, causing blood flow to be interrupted. This condition can also trigger malignant heart rhythms, causing sudden cardiac death. Cigarette smokers have two to four times the risk of SCD as nonsmokers.

■ It increases the viscosity of blood, causing the platelets to become "sticky" and more likely to clot. The propensity to clot seriously increases the risk of heart attack.

■ Since its presence in the blood tends to reduce HDL cholesterol by 10% to 20% in regular smokers, it not only elevates risk but decreases protection as well.

The nicotine in cigarette smoke increases cardiac workload by increasing the heart rate by up to 15 to 25 beats a minute and raising blood pressure by 10 to 20 points. To maintain the increased workload, the heart needs more oxygen. In the blood of smokers, however, what's delivered is more nicotine and carbon monoxide. The consequence is an enormous strain on the cardiac muscle that can lead to a heart attack.

But there's hope for those who can give it up. Research shows that within two to three years of quitting, former smokers reduce their risk of heart attack and stroke to levels similar to those of people who never smoked. And within five years of quitting, former smokers have a 50% to 70% lower risk of heart attack than current smokers.

Smoking: Know Your Number, Know Your Risk

The risk of cardiac and other health problems increases with the number of cigarettes smoked and the length of time a person has been a smoker. But the reverse is also true: risk can diminish with smoking reduction or cessation. The following scale approximates the cardiac risk from smoking:

CATEGORY	RISK
Non-tobacco user*	Optimal
Former tobacco user (at least four months tobacco-free)*	Lower
Cigar and/or pipe smoker or 1 to 10 cigarettes daily	Moderate
11 to 39 cigarettes daily	Higher
40 or more cigarettes daily	Extremely high
Your risk: _____	

*Nonsmoking is the only "recommended" category. All other categories place the individual at progressive levels of increased risk: the more cigarettes smoked, the greater the risk.

Choose Your Poison

Cigarettes pose the greatest smoking hazard, but other forms of tobacco are also injurious. Cigar and pipe smokers have a higher risk of heart disease than nonsmokers. This is probably due to the fact that cigar and pipe smokers actually *do* inhale, even though most of them think they don't.

Smokeless tobacco is now used by millions of Americans, the largest percentage being men under 24 years of age who tend to think they're avoiding the health risks of cigarette smoking. The fact is that snuff and chewing tobacco contain nicotine, usually in more concentrated levels than in cigarette smoke. The body absorbs nicotine through the nasal passages and the lining of the mouth, rather than the lungs, but the result is the same: a kick in the heart rate and blood pressure, producing strain on the cardiac muscle. Smokeless tobacco is *not* a safe alternative.

Secondhand smoke, or passive smoking, is another significant cardiac factor. A study at the University of California Medical School in San Francisco found that wives of cigarette smokers are three times more likely to suffer heart attacks than women whose husbands never smoked. And one Japanese study suggests that just half an hour of exposure to secondhand smoke can damage coronary artery walls, impair the arteries' ability to dilate and reduce normal blood flow to the heart.

10. PERSONALITY

In the past few years, a new cardiac marker has attracted the attention of both scientists and health professionals. Traditional cardiac markers such as smoking, high cholesterol and high blood pressure were found to account for less than 50% of the heart attacks that occur in the United States, and these days research is being focused on a link between psychosocial variables—personality and behavior—and a rise in stress hormones that increase artery inflammation and blood pressure. Chronic stress, Type A personality (especially some of its components), anger/hostility, depression and social isolation not only have a direct negative influence on cardiac health, but also increase the power of the other, more traditional markers.

Chronic Stress

If there is a common element to modern life, it is that we are a hurried, harried and "stressed-out" society. Most people simply do not have enough time for their overcommitted, overscheduled and workaholic lives. Chronic stress hits everyone, from the mother trying to balance her personal and work life, to the elderly couple dealing with extensive medical bills, to the 55-year-old worker who has been "downsized," to the investor watching the NASDAQ dive, to the high schooler trying to get into an Ivy League college.

Unbridled stress has a significant influence on cardiac health. Its adverse effects include:

- Surges in heart rate and blood pressure
- Increases in cholesterol and homocysteine
- Promotion of artery wall inflammation
- Constriction of coronary arteries, which can result in heart attacks
- Heart rhythm irregularities, which can trigger sudden cardiac death
- Increases in blood clotting

In addition, people under stress tend to smoke, eat high-fat food and lead sedentary lives. If their weight goes up, which is likely, so do their triglycerides, body mass index and waist circumference, as well as their chances of getting diabetes.

An eight-year study of day-of-the-week variations in heart attack incidence showed the incredible impact of stress: significant peaks were found between 7 and 10 o'clock on Monday mornings, when the occurrence of heart attacks was 21% higher than during the rest of the week. The low was on Saturdays.

Acute emotional distress has also been implicated in the occurrence of fatal heart attacks among people with coronary heart disease. For example, on the first day of the Iraqi missile attacks on Israel during the Persian Gulf War in 1991, there was an abrupt 58% increase in cardiac deaths among the Israeli population. Similar findings were noted in a comparison of the county coroner's records for the days immediately before and after the massive Los Angeles earthquake of 1994 with the records for corresponding periods in 1991, 1992 and 1993.

Type A Personality

Type A personality, a behavior pattern that makes people prone to coronary heart disease and heart attack, was first identified in the 1960s by San Francisco doctors Meyer Friedman and Ray Rosenman, who saw it as an external manifestation of internal stress. Characteristically, Type A individuals are hard-driving competitors who feel that they have to do everything themselves. They are involved in an incessant struggle to accomplish more and more in less and less time against the perceived opposition of other people or things. They are combative, relentless "doers," impatiently steamrolling over any obstacles that may appear to stand in their way. Someone once described the perfect Type A coat of arms: a clenched fist wearing a stopwatch.

Type A people, who make up about 50% of the population, are often society's heroes and leaders, people who "get things done"—but frequently at the cost of their cardiovascular health. Studies such as the Western Collaborative Group Study have found that the risk of heart attack is five to seven times greater for a Type A than for a more relaxed Type B. While further research is necessary (some experts believe that particular components of Type A behavior—notably anger and hostility—are more closely linked to coronary artery disease than others), Type A personality is considered an independent risk factor.

Women and Type A

Type A personality is not and never has been an exclusively male trait. It was initially identified with males because most of the early research was on men. Today we know that Type A women under stress act no differently than Type A men and suffer similar health consequences. Psychologist Margaret Chesney has found that Type A women tend to make lifestyle choices that foster poor health habits: in general, they smoke more, exercise less, are more overweight, consume more caffeine, feel angry more often and get less sleep than Type B women.

Employed women are more A-prone, but housewives are not immune. Studies at the University of Kansas show that housewives structure their home environments to be as stressful as some work environments, attempting to "do it all themselves." Many found

TYPE D BEHAVIOR

Historically, we've been concerned about the classic Type A personality—combative, time-driven people who literally push themselves to heart attacks. But now doctors are looking at a new category, Type D, as in "distressed." Type D personalities demonstrate negative feelings about virtually everything. In other words, the glass is always half empty, never half full.

We've known that negative emotions, particularly depression, significantly increase the risk of developing heart disease while lowering long-term survival of cardiac patients. But new studies suggest that pessimistic people, "negative thinkers" who worry over trivial, everyday events, are four times more likely to have a heart attack than more positive thinkers. In addition, people who become easily worried over small problems and who continually bottle up their distress are far more likely to die during a heart attack than people who handle stress more easily and who express their emotions openly.

homemaking more taxing and reported less satisfaction in their marriages. These traits—taxing work and lack of marital satisfaction—are the same as those reported in other studies on Type A men and on career women.

Type A: Know Your Personality, Know Your Risk

A number of simple, effective tests have been developed to assess propensity for Type A behavior. A good example is the following self-scoring test, adapted from Dr. Andrew Goliszek's book *60 Second Stress Management*. This 30-question test asks you to describe yourself and your feelings on a rising scale (1 = never; 5 = always). The higher the total score, the greater the Type A tendency. While not clinically exact, this test will give a global representation of whether or not Type A behavior is a risk for you.

TYPE A BEHAVIOR TEST

Read each statement below and grade yourself on how you would respond to each situation using the following:

1 = never   2 = seldom   3 = sometimes   4 = usually   5 = always

1. I become angry whenever I have to stand in line for more than 15 minutes. _____

2. I handle more than one problem at a time. _____

3. It's hard finding the time to relax and let myself go during the day. _____

4. I become irritated or annoyed when someone speaks too slowly. _____

5. I try hard to win at sports or games. _____

6. When I lose at sports or games, I get angry with myself and/or others. _____

7. I have trouble doing special things for myself. _____

8. I work much better under pressure or when I have to meet a deadline. _____

9. I find myself looking at my watch when I'm sitting around and not active. _____

10. I bring work home with me. ____

11. I feel energized and exhilarated after being in a pressure situation. ____

12. I feel like I need to take charge in order to get things moving. ____

13. I find myself eating quickly regardless of whether I have time or not. ____

14. I do things quickly regardless of whether I have time or not. ____

15. I interrupt what people are saying when I think they are wrong. ____

16. I'm inflexible and rigid when it comes to changes at work or at home. ____

17. I become jittery and need to move whenever I'm trying to relax. ____

18. I find myself eating faster than the people I'm eating with. ____

19. At work, I do more than one task at a time in order to feel productive. ____

20. I take less vacation time than I'm entitled to. ____

21. I find myself being very picky and looking at small details. ____

22. I become annoyed at people who don't work as hard as I do. ____

23. I find that there aren't enough things to do during the day. ____

24. I spend a good deal of my time thinking about my work. ____

25. I get bored very easily. ____

26. I'm active on weekends either working or doing projects. ____

27. I get into arguments with people who don't think my way. ____

28. I have trouble "rolling with the punches" whenever problems arise. ____

29. I interrupt someone's conversation in order to speed things up. ____

30. I take everything I do seriously. ____

Total: ____

SCORE	PERSONALITY TYPE
100 to 150	Type A
76 to 99	Type A/B
30 to 75	Type B

Scores of 90 and above are associated with a greater risk of cardiovascular problems.

SPEAKING FROM EXPERIENCE

Looking back to the time before my bypass surgery in 1977, I can see that I demonstrated many of the classic characteristics of Type A personality:

■ *Feeling a great sense of urgency.* Time always seemed to slip away—I just never seemed to have enough of it. When the end of day came, I seldom had completed the 30 or 40 items that were on my daily "to do" list. (I actually used to cheat. I'd make a list in the morning that always included one or two things I'd already done. Then I could cross them out right away!) Type A's are always in a hurry, making a fetish of being punctual, and they're greatly annoyed if somebody keeps them waiting. I used to set my watch ahead, making me constantly behind schedule, in order to induce more self-pressure to be on time. Recently I read an article by Dr. Argir Kirkov Hadzhichristov, a Bulgarian doctor who studies people who live to be 100 or more. None of them wears a watch!

■ *Doing two or more things at once.* I would talk on the phone while signing letters, watch television while reading a book, and let my brain follow a completely different train of thought when I was chatting with someone.

■ *Acting as if I were constantly on deadline.* Type A's do everything fast. They even eat rapidly and will never linger at the dinner table. They dislike routine jobs at home because they think their time is too valuable. I used to show my impatience by interrupting people to answer questions before they were asked (a behavior I've worked hard to overcome). Type A's do not delegate well at all. If the job is not being done precisely as they would do it, they step in and take over.

■ *Not being able to sit still.* I was constantly tapping and drumming my hands and feet. My speech was way too rapid, my words and gestures clipped, my smiles tense and tight. Type A's walk quickly and drive too fast. They just have to keep moving, preferably at top speed.

■ *Measuring success in terms of numbers*—dollars, sales calls, size. The Type A's first thought upon seeing a Michelangelo painting will be: *How much is it worth?*

■ *Turning hobbies into competitive events.* When my children were young, I built model cars for fun and relaxation. But then I entered a competition and won. Soon I was building more and more cars and competing every weekend! Type A's play to win, even with children. Some sons of Type A's reach adulthood without ever having beaten their fathers in a single game of one-on-one basketball. Winning is success; losing is disaster. As one psychologist observed, "Never enter a fun-run with Type A's. They will kill for a T-shirt or a blue ribbon."

■ *Feeling guilty about relaxing and doing nothing.* Type A's take a briefcase on vacation or climb into a hammock with a sheaf of projects. And when at the beach or on a mountain peak, their overwhelming concern about starting back by a certain time will overshadow the beauty surrounding them.

■ *Feeling insecure.* Type A's have a constant fear that sooner or later they won't be able to cope in a given situation and will lose status in the eyes of people whose opinions matter to them. Fear of failure keeps them struggling to achieve more without ever savoring their accomplishments.   *—J.P.*

Most health professionals do not believe that Type A behavior can be totally changed in a society that teaches it's better to wear out shoes than sheets, the early bird gets the worm and a man's reach should exceed his grasp. As long as our society views Type A behavior as a desirable personality trait, it will be encouraged. The basic problem, as Ralph Waldo Emerson wrote, is that "solitude is impractical and society is fatal."

Nonetheless, a decrease in the intensity of Type A behavior *is* attainable and well worth the effort in terms of cardiovascular health. In a study conducted at Stanford University, 600 cardiac patients received intensive behavioral training to change Type A behavior—how to slow down, be more patient and have a more positive outlook—along with advice on diet and exercise. Only 12.9% of this group suffered a second heart attack. A second group of similar size received diet and exercise information only, with no instruction on modifying Type A behavior. More than 21% of this group experienced a second heart attack. A third group of 90 patients received no instruction at all; 32% had a second heart attack. Says Dr. Carl Thoresen, a professor at Stanford, "This study clearly tells us that changing these destructive Type A habits can affect the chances of a second heart attack."

Anger and Hostility

Are you the kind of person who becomes visibly upset when you're cut off in traffic by another car? Do you interrupt others in the middle of a sentence or feel a flash of irritation when you're interrupted? Do you become enraged when someone yells into a pay phone right next to your ear or exceeds the maximum number of items permitted in the supermarket express line?

If so, accept the fact that these behaviors may be hazardous to your health.

Duke University scientists have shown that hostile people— those with high levels of cynicism, anger and aggression—are at a much higher risk of developing heart disease and other chronic illnesses. Other researchers believe that dominant personality may also be problematic. "Having a dominant personality or a high level of irritability are two personality traits that make one prone to heart disease," says Dr. Aaron Wolfe Siegman of the University of Maryland. "We found that people with a dominant personality had a 47% higher risk of heart disease, and those easily irritated had a 27% increase in heart disease, compared with their less domineering, more easygoing counterparts. There is something about anger that thickens the walls of the heart and coronary arteries." These findings held true even after accounting for other risk factors including cholesterol, diabetes, obesity and smoking.

Feeling angry from time to time is normal. Things happen in life that make us mad. Some people express anger readily,

WOMEN AND ANGER

Generally, men tend to get angry, blow up, get it over with and move on. Women often avoid anger or pretend it's not there, and this "anger diversion" actually creates more stress.

According to Dr. Deborah Cox of Southwestern Missouri State University, women divert anger by containing it, biting their tongue to keep from saying what they feel. "Women also internalize anger by absorbing guilt and blame meant for others with whom they're angry," says Dr. Cox. "If we feel unable to talk directly about anger to the person with whom we're angry, the next most likely target is ourselves." Many women become so afraid of their own anger that they lose their ability to *know* when they're angry.

And finally, some women externalize their anger by abusing and insulting others. While this may seem like a way to "get anger out," spilling it irresponsibly onto others—particularly children—is never a productive response.

shouting loudly and gesturing wildly at the slow driver in the fast freeway lane. Others fume silently over imagined slights. When anger is incurred by a specific event (as opposed to things in general) and is appropriate (a modest level for a moderate amount of time), then it usually is not a health risk. But if anger surfaces too frequently, too intensely and lasts too long each time it makes its presence felt, and if chronic hostility begins to take on the look of a personality trait, a commensurate rise in health risk is triggered, particularly for cardiovascular disease. Getting so angry that your "blood boils," it seems, may stress your heart and cause your arteries to clog, too.

Anger triggers a variety of physiological responses. When you're angry, your muscles tense, your breathing becomes shallow and rapid, your heart races and your blood pressure rises. In addition, stress chemicals such as epinephrine are released into the bloodstream. All these responses are normal. But if anger is chronic, it can penalize your heart, particularly if you already have coronary artery disease.

Heart attack risk is almost three times greater in people with high levels of anger than in those who control it. A study directed by Dr. Peter Angerer of the University of Munich in Germany followed 150 people with diseased arteries and found that over a two-year period the subjects who reported high levels of expressed anger, particularly those with low levels of social support, were significantly more likely to have their coronary heart disease worsen. In addition, Dr. Murray Mittleman and associates at Beth Israel Deaconess Medical Center in Boston reported that the risk of a heart attack increased in the two hours following an episode of anger, suggesting that anger was a trigger that doubled and even tripled the risk of heart attack.

How does chronic anger penalize the heart? No one is certain, but it is thought that high levels of stress chemicals injure the coronary artery walls and over time provide deposit sites for artery-clogging cholesterol. These chemicals can also stimulate arterial inflammation, blood clotting and high blood pressure, and evoke potentially lethal heart rhythms.

Anger and Hostility: Know Your Personality, Know Your Risk

The following test, from the Arnot Ogden Medical Center, will help you to assess your general tendency to "fly off the handle." You will score a value of "1" if the statement is never true for you, "2" if it's rarely or sometimes true, "3" if it's often true and "4" if it's always true. Add up your scores to find your total.

NEVER	RARELY	OFTEN	ALWAYS
1	2	3	4

It doesn't take much to get me mad.

1	2	3	4

People tell me I should calm down.

1	2	3	4

I blow up at terrible drivers.

1	2	3	4

If I'm upset, I'll hit the dog or the cat.

1	2	3	4

People call me hot-headed.

1	2	3	4

I'm furious about the way I get treated at restaurants or stores.

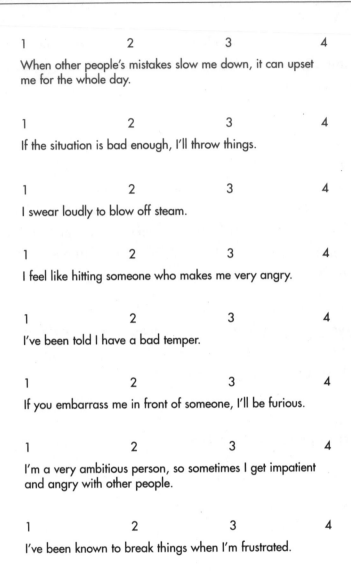

| 1 | 2 | 3 | 4 |

When other people's mistakes slow me down, it can upset me for the whole day.

| 1 | 2 | 3 | 4 |

If the situation is bad enough, I'll throw things.

| 1 | 2 | 3 | 4 |

I swear loudly to blow off steam.

| 1 | 2 | 3 | 4 |

I feel like hitting someone who makes me very angry.

| 1 | 2 | 3 | 4 |

I've been told I have a bad temper.

| 1 | 2 | 3 | 4 |

If you embarrass me in front of someone, I'll be furious.

| 1 | 2 | 3 | 4 |

I'm a very ambitious person, so sometimes I get impatient and angry with other people.

| 1 | 2 | 3 | 4 |

I've been known to break things when I'm frustrated.

If you scored 18 or below on this test, you have a high temper threshold and are able to stay calm in situations that would frustrate many others. This is a big help in managing your stress levels. If you scored 19 to 27, you get angry about as often as most other people. If you scored 28 to 35, there's a good possibility that you're under too much stress or it may be that getting angry has become a habit; take this score seriously and begin to make changes now, before it adversely affects your health.

If you scored over 35 on the test and continue with the same behaviors and attitudes, you risk serious stress-related disease. It may be helpful to speak to a counselor about ways to deal with your anger.

Depression

Doctors have associated heart attacks and clinical depression for some time, usually in that sequence. After all, who wouldn't be depressed after a heart attack? But new research is showing that depression may be more than a consequence of heart disease; it may actually be a *cause* of it.

- Depression is reported to precede a heart attack in up to 50% of cases.

- Depression has also been associated with an increased number of cardiovascular events after an initial heart attack or following coronary bypass surgery. In two recent studies, patients who were depressed were three to five times more likely to die during the first year after suffering a heart attack than were nondepressed patients.

- A study of about 4,500 elderly people free of coronary disease found that the risk of heart disease and death increased by 40% and 60%, respectively, for those who became depressed when compared with those who did not become depressed.

- Scientists at the Johns Hopkins Medical Centers found that, everything else being equal, people who have some depression symptoms are twice as likely to suffer heart attacks as those with no symptoms, and people diagnosed with major depression were 4.5 times as likely.

- After a person suffers angina or a heart attack, depression is a better predictor of prognosis than many other known risk factors for

DEPRESSION AND GENDER

According to a study published not long ago in the *International Journal of Psychiatry in Medicine*, women tend to report symptoms of depression in this order: self-disappointment, irritability, hopelessness, dissatisfaction, sleep difficulties. Men tend to report symptoms in this order: dissatisfaction, difficulties completing work, fatigue, irritability, hopelessness, self-disappointment.

heart disease. People with major depression are up to eight times more likely to die within one and a half years than those with mild to moderate depression symptoms.

■ If depression turns to hopelessness, studies show an increased risk of coronary mortality. A study of 1,000 men found that those who felt hopeless had a 20% greater increase in heart disease than those who were more hopeful.

One reason for the link between depression and cardiac risk is that depression contributes to poor lifestyle choices. Depressed people are more apt to eat poorly, be sedentary, drink, smoke and use drugs. Depressed heart patients are also less likely to see their physician or take prescribed medications. "It may also be that stress hormones play a role," says clinical psychologist Dr. Judith Schwartzman. "Depression can be thought of as an extreme and prolonged response to stress. Many of the physiological changes that happen when you are in fight-or-flight mode, such as an increase in cortisol,

HIGH ANXIETY

Intense psychological stress resulting from high anxiety levels can cause alterations of the heart's rhythm and trigger sudden cardiac death. Data show that men who have high anxiety levels are up to six times more likely to experience sudden cardiac death than are men of calmer disposition. That's three times greater than the increased risk of sudden cardiac death from smoking.

Anxiety is an inappropriate manifestation of one of our most ancient instincts—to flee danger when it confronts us. Just how it increases cardiac risk is yet to be determined, but researchers hypothesize that anxiety triggers not only fear but also a host of physiological responses, including increased heart and breathing rates. What makes anxiety a medical condition is its presence in the absence of any real danger, often when there is no cause whatever for fear.

also happen when you are depressed." Heart disease and depression may have common origins. "You get mood changes with heart disease," says Dr. Schwartzman. "And people also often experience something called vital exhaustion, which essentially means they're worn out, shortly before heart disease surfaces. But is it a symptom of early heart disease or of depression? It could be either."

On the positive side, people with depression symptoms who have had one heart attack can greatly reduce their chance of a second heart attack by managing stress. "We found that people who walked regularly as a stress dissipation technique after an initial heart attack benefited from the exercise and the social contact and support," says Dr. François Lesperance of the Montreal Heart Institute. "Lack of walking is a symptom of more severe depression. The coronary survivor's true best friend is a dog. Then they'd have to be out walking about an hour a day."

Recently, investigators in the Standard Medical Intervention and Long-Term Exercise (SMILE) Study randomly assigned 156 patients with major depression to three groups: those who received exercise training, those who received drug treatment and those who received both. Most of the patients demonstrated a reduction in depressive symptoms, with no significant group differences at the end of four months of treatment. Patients who continued to exercise on their own tended to maintain their improvement after the termination of formal treatment.

Depression: Know Your Personality, Know Your Risk

How do you know if depression is a problem for you? The following screening test, adapted from the Harvard Department of Psychiatry National Depression Screening Day Scale, commonly called the HANDS™ questionnaire, is designed to help identify individuals who are likely to be suffering from a depressive disorder that may require treatment.

DEPRESSION SCREENING TEST

1. I feel sad most of the time.   Yes _____   No _____

2. I don't enjoy the things I used to.   Yes _____   No _____

3. I sleep too little or too much.   Yes _____   No _____

4. I don't feel like eating or
I eat too much.   Yes _____   No _____

5. I can't make decisions.   Yes _____   No _____

6. I have difficulty concentrating.   Yes _____   No _____

7. I feel hopeless.   Yes _____   No _____

8. I feel worthless.   Yes _____   No _____

9. I get tired for no reason.   Yes _____   No _____

10. I think about killing myself.   Yes _____*   No _____

Scoring:

If you answered yes to four or more of these questions, *and you have felt this way every day for two weeks or more,* you may be suffering from clinical depression and should consult a health care professional for a complete evaluation.

*If you answered yes to question 10, seek help immediately, regardless of your answer to any of the other questions.

To find the location of a facility in your community that offers free depression screenings, visit <www.mentalhealthscreening.org> or call 1-800-520-NDSD (6373).

Social Isolation

Numerous studies show higher cardiovascular death rates among people who are socially isolated. One of the first studies to identify the importance of social networks in buffering the deleterious effects of heart disease involved a small town in eastern Pennsylvania called Roseto. Health researchers were startled to find a strikingly lower death rate there than in neighboring towns. From 1955 to 1961, Roseto had 157 cardiovascular deaths per 100,000 population, while three neighboring towns averaged over 600 cardiovascular deaths. After careful analysis, researchers concluded that social support and close family ties were the primary reasons for Roseto's lower rate. They also predicted that, over time, social ties would diminish and cardiovascular death rates would rise, a prediction that proved true over the next 20 years.

Since the Roseto report, a number of scientific investigations have confirmed this effect. For example, a six-month mortality rate of 16% was noted among patients who lived alone after their heart attack vesus 9% for those living with others.

Another study, conducted by Dr. Redford Williams and colleagues at Duke University, showed that married patients with heart disease fared far better than their unmarried counterparts. But the people with the highest death rate were unmarried patients who had no close family or friends. These patients had a five-year survival rate of just 50%, compared with 82% for those who had a spouse, a confidant or both.

It remains unclear how social isolation harms health. Perhaps lonely people are less likely to get rapid medical assistance. Another possibility is that those without social ties may not seek medical attention, take prescribed medications or be encouraged to follow their doctors' advice. Or it may be that social isolation produces an injurious mental and physical effect. Much research is still to be done. Then again, there may be a lot more to Barbra Streisand's contention that "people who need people are the luckiest people in the world."

Your Cardiac Marker Profile

The first step in the Piscatella Protocol is to take all the information you've gained about yourself in relation to the 10 controllable heart-health markers and create your own risk profile. Individually and in concert, these markers wield considerable influence over your cardiac destiny.

Recommended marker values (identified by asterisks) reflect the optimal levels, representing the lowest cardiac risk. It's important to understand that these values are not hard-and-fast. We cannot say that people with a total cholesterol of 240 will definitely have a heart attack any more than we can label people with a cholesterol of 199 as "home free." But cardiac risk *is* greater for the individual with the higher cholesterol number. And that's why your cardiac marker profile is so significant—it can help you to evaluate your own risks.

1. Cholesterol and Other Lipids/Lipoproteins

TOTAL CHOLESTEROL	RISK
Below 200 mg/dl*	Desirable
200 to 239 mg/dl	Borderline high
240 mg/dl and above	High

Your number: _____ Your risk: _____

LDL CHOLESTEROL	RISK
Below 100 mg/dl*	Optimal
100 to 129 mg/dl*	Near optimal
130 to 159 mg/dl	Borderline high
160 to 189 mg/dl	High
190 mg/dl and above	Very high

Your number: _____ Your risk: _____

HDL CHOLESTEROL	RISK
60 mg/dl and above*	Low
40 to 59 mg/dl	Moderate
Below 40 mg/dl	High
Your number: _____	Your risk: _____

TRIGLYCERIDES	RISK
Below 150 mg/dl*	Desirable
150 to 199 mg/dl	Borderline high
200 to 499 mg/dl	High
500 mg/dl and above	Very high
Your number: _____	Your risk: _____

2. Coronary Inflammation

HOMOCYSTEINE	RISK
Less than 5 µmol/l*	Desirable
5 to 9 µmol/l	Normal
10 to 30 µmol/l	Moderate
31 to 100 µmol/l	High
Above 100 µmol/l	Severe
Your number: _____	Your risk: _____

C-REACTIVE PROTEIN	RISK
Less than 0.70 mg/dl*	Lowest
0.70 to 1.1 mg/dl	Low
1.2 to 1.9 mg/dl	Average
2.0 to 3.8 mg/dl	Higher
3.9 to 15.0 mg/dl	Highest
Your number: _____	Your risk: _____

3. Blood Clotting

FIBRINOGEN	RISK
Below 200 mg/dl*	Desirable
200 to 400 mg/dl	Borderline high
Above 400 mg/dl	High

Your number: _____   Your risk: _____

4. Weight

BODY MASS INDEX	RISK
19 to 24.9 kg/m^2*	Desirable
25 to 29.9 kg/m^2	Borderline high
30 to 39.9 kg/m^2	High
40 to 54 kg/m^2	Very high

Your number: _____   Your risk: _____

WAIST CIRCUMFERENCE	RISK

Men

Less than 40 inches*	Lower
40 inches and above	Higher

Women

Less than 35 inches*	Lower
35 inches and above	Higher

Your number: _____   Your risk: _____

5. Blood Pressure

SYSTOLIC	DIASTOLIC	RISK
Less than 120 mm Hg*	Less than 80 mm Hg*	Optimal
Less than 130 mm Hg*	Less than 85 mm Hg*	Normal
130 to 139 mm Hg	85 to 89 mm Hg	High normal
140 to 159 mm Hg	90 to 99 mm Hg	Stage 1 hypertension
160 to 179 mm Hg	100 to 109 mm Hg	Stage 2 hypertension
180 mm Hg and above	110 mm Hg and above	Stage 3 hypertension

Your number: _____   Your risk: _____

6. Diabetes

FASTING GLUCOSE	RISK
Below 110 mg/dl*	Desirable
110 to 125 mg/dl	Borderline high
Above 125 mg/dl	Confirmed diabetes

Your number: _____   Your risk: _____

7. Syndrome X

FACTORS

Is your HDL number below 40 (men)
or below 50 (women)?   Yes _____ No _____

Is your triglyceride number over 150?
                         Yes _____ No _____

Is your waist size 35 inches and above
(women) or 40 inches and above (men)?
                         Yes _____ No _____

Is your blood pressure consistently
130/85 or greater?   Yes _____ No _____

Are you a diabetic (a fasting glucose
of 110 or greater)?   Yes _____ No _____

"YES" ANSWERS	RISK
None*	Desirable
1 to 2	Borderline high
3 to 5	Confirmed Syndrome X

Your number: _____ Your risk: _____

8. Aerobic Capacity

MET LEVEL	RISK
(Treadmill testing or Duke Activity Status Index)	
4 METs or less	High
5 to 9 METs	Average
10 METs or higher*	Low

Your number: _____ Your risk: _____

9. Smoking

CATEGORY	RISK
Non-tobacco/user*	Optimal
Former tobacco user* (at least 4 months tobacco-free)	Lower
Cigar and/or pipe smoker or 1 to 10 cigarettes daily	Moderate
11 to 39 cigarettes daily	Higher
40 or more cigarettes daily	Extremely high

Your number: _____ Your risk : _____

10. Personality

TYPE A PROFILE TEST SCORE	PERSONALITY TYPE
100 to 150	Type A
76 to 99	Type A/B
30 to 75	Type B

Your number: _____ Your personality: _____

There is presently insufficient data to categorically link heart disease with a specific personality type. Not all type A's have heart attacks; not all Type B's are free of heart disease.

However, the consensus is that people with Type A personality (especially certain components, e.g., anger / hostility) are at increased risk and should be considered as such for the purposes of this assessment.

ANGER PROFILE TEST SCORE	LEVEL OF ANGER
18 or less*	Desirable
19 to 27	Average
28 to 35	High
36 and above	Severe

Your number: _____   Your anger level: _____

As with Type A personality, there is insufficient data to link numeric results from the anger profile test to incidence of heart disease. However, some experts believe that high and severe levels of anger demonstrate increased cardiovascular risk, and that is how you should evaluate your score for the purposes of this assessment.

DEPRESSION TEST SCORE (HANDS QUESTIONNAIRE)	RISK
Less than 4	Average
4 or higher	Elevated

Your number: _____   Your risk: _____

NOTE: Another assessment, using several of these markers, for calculating the risk of developing heart disease over the next 10 years can be obtained using estimates of the Framingham Risk Score. It is available on the NHLBI Web site <www.nhlbi.nih.gov> and has been validated in white and black men and women without known heart disease.

YOUR ASSESSMENT SUMMARY

Is this a risk for you?

CRITICAL MARKERS	YES	NO
Total cholesterol		
LDL cholesterol		
HDL cholesterol		
Triglycerides		
Homocysteine		
C-reactive protein		
Fibrinogen		
Body Mass Index		
Waist circumference		
Blood pressure		
Diabetes		
Syndrome X		
Aerobic capacity		
Smoking		
Type A personality		
Anger		
Depression		

Time for Action

IRST OFF, DON'T PANIC. If your profile exceeds the recommended values in any category—that is, if you've identified a risk—keep in mind that you can make things better simply by taking action. Remember, each step you take is a step in the right direction: according to the Harvard Nurses' Health Study, published in the *New England Journal of Medicine*, as many as four out of five heart attacks could be prevented if people followed a heart-healthy lifestyle.

But how to do that? To start with, the most important thing you can do is make the commitment. On the following pages you'll find the first 13 Heart Savers, designed to help you mitigate your risks. Read them carefully. Take them to heart. Decide to control your destiny.

WATCH YOUR CHOLESTEROL NUMBERS

If your total cholesterol is 200 or above, it's too high and you need to take action to bring it down. A healthy diet is the first line of defense and can be as effective as state-of-the-art drug therapy. Center your diet on foods that can lower cholesterol, such as soy foods and whole grains and vegetables rich in soluble fiber. Limit foods rich in saturated fat (red meat, for example, and whole-milk dairy products) and trans fat (such as hydrogenated margarine). Until recently, the American Heart Association recommended a diet of no more than 30% of calories from fat, but today the emphasis is on reducing saturated and trans fats. The AHA now says you can get up to 35% of your total calories from fat (unless overweight is an issue), but less than 10% of these calories should come from a combination of saturated fat and trans fats.

Some experts still advise a diet lower in total fat for cardiac health. Dr. Dean Ornish, among others, suggests a 10%-fat diet—certainly effective in bringing down cholesterol but very difficult to follow. Dr. Gerhard Schuler of Heidelberg University in Germany recommends more moderate fat levels. "A 20%-fat diet lowers cholesterol," he says, "and is much easier to achieve in the real world."

If diet and exercise do not improve your cholesterol after six months, it may be time to consider drug therapy. Some of the most widely used cholesterol-lowering medications include statin drugs, bile acid sequestrants and nicotinic acid. (See pages 317–22 for more information.) One study of more than 6,000 subjects was cut short a year before its intended end date because those receiving a statin drug had a 40% lower incidence of heart attacks. According to Dr. William C. Roberts, "Statin drugs are to atherosclerosis what penicillin was to infectious diseases." Talk with your doctor about the pros and cons of cholesterol-lowering drugs.

REDUCE YOUR LDL LEVEL 2

Get your LDL level as low as you can, ideally below 100. Again, the first line of defense is dietary change. Step 4 of our protocol offers numerous tips for modifying your diet, but to begin with, here are some simple yet effective ways to get your LDL level under control:

■ Moderate caloric intake and increase physical activity to lose weight.

■ Cut down on foods rich in saturated fat, trans fat and dietary cholesterol (all animal foods).

■ Increase foods rich in complex carbohydrates (such as fruits and vegetables), soluble fiber (oat bran, oatmeal and beans), bioflavonoids (strawberries and eggplant), antioxidants (vitamins C and E and beta-carotene), and sterol or sterol esters (Take Control, Benecol and other cholesterol-lowering margarines).

■ Substitute soy protein for animal protein. Studies suggest that this could lower LDL and total cholesterol by 8% and 9%, respectively.

In addition, you may want to talk to your doctor about drug therapy, particularly statins. Many doctors are now recommending that heart patients and others at high risk start drug therapy along with dietary change immediately. Studies confirm that statins reduce the risks of heart attack, stroke, bypass surgery or balloon angioplasty by 20% to 30% with minimal side effects. Other investigators have reported that veins and arteries used in bypass surgery reclog 40% more slowly in patients with low LDL levels.

3 INCREASE YOUR HDL LEVEL

Exercise, moderate alcohol consumption, losing weight and drug therapy all can increase your HDL (much more on those later), but here's a preview of what you should know:

■ *Exercise, exercise, exercise!* A regular program of exercise is effective in boosting HDL concentration. The nice thing about it is that you don't have to be a fanatic. Researchers at Stanford University have reported that approximately 1,000 calories of additional energy expenditure— equivalent to walking or running 8 to 10 miles weekly— may represent the "threshold" exercise dosage required for increasing HDL cholesterol. So, first see your doctor about an exercise program, then get started.

■ *Moderate alcohol consumption* has been shown to boost HDL. The key is "moderate," since the risks of heavy drinking (increased triglycerides, hypertension, cancer, stroke, liver disease, accidents) outweigh the potential cardiac benefits. The Brigham and Women's Harvard Study found that the form of alcohol you drink doesn't matter; wine, beer and hard liquor have equally beneficial effects on raising HDL cholesterol.

■ *Lose weight* if you're overweight. Choose monounsaturated oils (such as olive oil) over polyunsaturated oils (such as corn oil) and saturated fats. Vitamin E may also modestly raise the HDL level.

■ *Quit smoking!*

■ *Drug therapy* can be effective. Niacin, many statin drugs and gemfibrozil (Lopid) have been shown to elevate HDL. The best counsel if your HDL is low is to talk to your doctor about an appropriate course of action.

BRING DOWN YOUR TRIGLYCERIDES

There are many things you can do to lower your triglyceride level: moderate your caloric intake; cut down on foods rich in sugar, saturated fat and trans fat; increase your consumption of fish and healthful oils; eat foods rich in fiber; moderate alcohol; exercise regularly; don't smoke; and utilize drug therapy if necessary. The message is familiar, but here are some additional facts to consider:

■ A loss of just three to five pounds can reduce triglycerides by as much as 30%.

■ In this case, some fats are good—notably the omega-3 fatty acids found in salmon, sardines and tuna.

■ Drug therapy has proven effective. If your triglycerides are above 400, and especially if they exceed 1,000, you're likely to have a high rate of cardiovascular complications and are at risk of developing acute pancreatitis, a serious inflammatory condition. Confer with your doctor about medication. Niacin, fibric acid derivatives such as gemfibrozil (Lopid) and fenofibrate (Tricor), and statin drugs can help.

MANAGE YOUR HOMOCYSTEINE LEVEL

If your homocysteine number is elevated, you need to take action. Even though your level may be genetically influenced, there are a number of positive steps you can take:

■ *Get your vitamins.* Elevated homocysteine is often found in people whose diet contains inadequate amounts of folic acid (folate), vitamin B_6 or vitamin B_{12}, elements needed to break down homocysteine in the body. A 1995 analysis of 38 studies led scientists to a startling conclusion: "13,500 to 50,000 heart disease–related deaths in the United States could be prevented annually if people would simply get more folate." Good food sources include citrus fruits, leafy green vegetables, broccoli, asparagus, eggs, legumes, fortified cereals, bananas, chicken and pasta. And talk to your doctor about taking a multivitamin supplement with 400 micrograms of folic acid, 2 milligrams of B_6 and 6 micrograms of B_{12}. If diet and supplements don't cause your homocysteine level to drop in six weeks, consider raising the level of supplements. Don't do this on your own. Always work with your doctor.

In a 14-year study of 80,000 women, Harvard researchers found that those who consumed the highest levels of folic acid and vitamin B_6 had a 45% lower risk of heart disease than those who consumed the lowest amounts. All of the ramifications of this are not yet clear, but it makes sense to check that you're getting enough B vitamins.

■ *Consider aspirin therapy.* Aspirin has been found to reduce the inflammatory effect that is associated with excessive homocysteine.

■ *Consider drug therapy.* Statin drugs, such as Pravachol, not only lower cholesterol but also produce an anti-inflammatory response beneficial to cardiac health. Again, talk with your doctor.

6 MANAGE YOUR CRP LEVEL

If your levels of C-reactive protein are high, you have to cover the basics first: eat a low-fat diet, control your cholesterol and other lipids, stop smoking, lose weight if needed, control your blood pressure and any diabetes, manage stress and, very important, exercise regularly. A just-released study from Finland showed that moderate-intensity exercise can reduce levels of CRP. Men in the exercise group showed a 16% reduction in CRP, compared with a 2% reduction in the sedentary control group.

Beyond that, aspirin therapy has been found to be very effective as an anti-inflammatory agent, and early studies suggest that some statin drugs may lower CRP levels. For example, the Cholesterol and Recurrent Events Trial showed that pravastatin (Pravachol) lowered CRP and reduced cardiac events independent of its cholesterol-lowering effects. These trial findings lend support to the notion that statin drugs may confer cardioprotective benefits that go well beyond their cholesterol-lowering ability. See your doctor about treatment options.

If the inflammatory process is in fact a causative factor in heart disease, the treatment of America's number one killer could change dramatically. In the future it's possible that patients might be treated with antibiotics to prevent infections that cause inflammation and that CRP levels might be routinely measured to assess coronary risk. It's an exciting area of current cardiovascular research.

CONTROL YOUR FIBRINOGEN LEVEL

At this time there are no established medical treatments for lowering fibrinogen, but if your classification is borderline or high, it makes sense to take normal risk-reducing steps (such as changes in diet and exercise). You should also discuss aspirin therapy with your doctor. Aspirin's anticoagulant ability lessens the chance of clots forming and blocking narrowed arteries. Some studies suggest that niacin can also be very effective.

KEEP YOUR WEIGHT DOWN

While excess weight can cause cardiac risk to soar, maintaining an ideal body weight can reduce heart disease risk by an amazing 35% to 55%. If that's not inspiration enough, note that even a 10% loss of body weight can provide major health benefits in overweight and obese individuals.

A huge chunk of this book is devoted to helping you devise a plan of eating for a lifetime. But before you get started, it's important to understand that it is not "weight" that you want to lose, but extra "body fat." Theoretically at least, losing body fat is pretty simple: you must burn more calories than you take in—3,500 calories per pound of body fat, to be exact. In other words, if you can cut 500 calories a day, you'll lose a pound a week. You can do that by reducing your caloric intake, increasing calories burned in exercise, or both.

Here's a preview of what you should know before you start a diet:

■ *Don't crash-diet.* Fads like the "high-protein" diets might help you lose a few pounds in the short run, but they may not be safe for your heart. Many are exceptionally high in fat, including the dangerous artery-clogging saturated fat that can greatly accelerate your risk of heart disease. In addition, crash diets do not work in the long run; such diets may ultimately cause you to regain lost weight and even put on more pounds.

■ *Don't rely on "fat-burning" products* that promise to melt pounds without exercise or dietary change, even if endorsed by celebrities. These people get paid very well for their testimonials. If it's too good to believe, it probably means it doesn't work.

■ *Develop an active lifestyle.* For weight reduction, the American College of Sports Medicine recommends a daily expenditure of more than 300 calories. Researchers at the University of Pittsburgh School of Medicine think even more is necessary. They examined data on over 3,000 Americans who have lost weight and kept it off and found that such people burned an average of 2,800 calories a week, or 400 calories a day. That equates to one hour of brisk walking daily. Adding strength training to exercise programs may further increase metabolism.

SPEAKING FROM EXPERIENCE

It seems that there's a new weight-loss diet or product introduced every day—rubber suits, metabolic powders, diet books, even machines that exercise for you! With so many such products, you'd think America would be a nation of skinny folks. Instead, we're fatter than ever. The truth is that fad diets and fast-weight-loss programs seldom lead to long-term success in weight control. And they often can be a health hazard. I think most people know in their heart of hearts that controlling weight for a lifetime requires more than dieting. It takes a change in behavior, a commitment to being physically active, a new way of eating and dealing with stress effectively. These are lifetime goals, not something to do for a week or two.   —*J.P.*

■ *Watch ballooning portion size.* Says Dr. Brian Wansink of the University of Illinois, "We are seeing portion distortion, especially in restaurants. . . . Studies show that 67% of Americans eat everything on their plates, no matter what the size. Supersizing has gotten to the point where many can't remember what's a normal serving size."

■ *Plan sit-down meals.* Don't rush.

■ *Drink five to eight glasses of water daily.* Avoid high-calorie drinks such as alcohol and soft drinks.

■ *Keep a food journal.* People eat less when they account for it in writing.

■ *Take your time.* One to two pounds of body-fat loss a week doesn't sound like much, but it adds up to success.

■ *Don't eat while watching television.* Studies show that people who are distracted while eating tend to consume more calories.

MONITOR YOUR BLOOD PRESSURE

Fewer than 5% of patients with hypertension have a definable cause: perhaps a narrowing of a blood vessel supplying a kidney, hormonal disturbances or a congenital narrowing of the aorta, the major blood vessel exiting the heart. Indeed, the causes of most high blood pressure are not fully understood. Genetics plays a part, since hypertension can be inherited, but lifestyle is much more important. Sometimes high blood pressure develops or is made worse by certain over-the-counter medications like decongestants, diet pills and non-steroidal anti-inflammatory drugs such as ibuprofen. Overweight and obesity are critical indicators. So is excessive salt intake (particularly in women), because too much salt can cause the body to retain too much fluid, increasing blood volume and causing pressure to rise because the heart is working harder. The caffeine in coffee can also cause an increase in blood pressure.

On the other hand, healthy eating promotes control. Increasing antioxidant consumption—more fruits, vegetables and nuts—and decreasing sodium-rich foods can reduce blood pressure.

Chronic emotional stress is another factor that can cause blood pressure to rise. When you're under stress, your arterioles narrow, causing a temporary increase in blood pressure. When stress is occasional, such an increase usually does not present a heath problem. But when stressful events take place too frequently, stress hormones continue to constrict arterioles and send blood pressure upward. Studies by the late Dr. Robert S. Eliot, author of *Is It Worth Dying For Anyway?* show that about 20% of Americans can be classified as "hot reactors" who respond to chronic stress with skyrocketing blood pressure. Over time the result can be the permanent establishment of a new and higher blood pressure level.

Excessive alcohol consumption is also a factor. A 12-year study of 325 Japanese men, all of whom had normal blood pressure at the start, found that those who drank the most had nearly twice the risk of high blood pressure as nondrinkers. Light drinkers had the lowest risk, demonstrating once again the power of moderation.

If lifestyle modifications do not sufficiently reduce blood pressure, you may want to consult with your doctor about drug therapy. Some medications help relax and dilate vessels to facilitate blood flow. Others can help eliminate excessive fluid and salt. Commonly recommended drugs include diuretics, beta-blockers, calcium channel-blockers, ACE inhibitors and vasodilators. The choice of medication depends on the individual and other medical conditions that may be present. Another important consideration is which drug(s) lower blood pressure effectively with the fewest side effects. If drug therapy is appropriate, be sure to take your medication regularly.

10 DEAL WITH DIABETES

It is critical to your cardiac health to prevent diabetes or, if you have it, to manage it well. And here the news is good: "Recent studies show that now, for the first time, there is scientific proof that one could prevent the development of Type 2 diabetes with a lifestyle prevention program early on," says Dr. Robert Sherwin of Yale University. "Research by the

National Institutes of Health shows that people at high risk can cut their odds of developing Type 2 diabetes by 58% simply by doing two things—walking 30 minutes a day and losing weight."

Recommendations include:

■ *Manage your weight.* Being at a healthy weight reduces the risk for Type 2 diabetes. In addition, diabetics who lose as little as 5 to 10 pounds decrease their heart disease risk to that of a non-diabetic, overweight person.

■ *Eat a healthy, balanced diet* that includes adequate protein, carbohydrates (vegetables, fruits and grains in particular), reduced fat (especially saturated and trans fats) and adequate fiber (20 to 35 grams a day).

■ *Be physically active.* An activity as simple as regular gardening or walking can reduce your risk—but it should be regular. Twelve years of data from the Harvard Nurses' Health Study showed that those women who worked out regularly were half as likely to develop diabetes as those who skipped exercise. Says Dr. David A. Simmons of the University of Pennsylvania Medical School, "That's because muscles at work are able to take up sugar directly from the bloodstream without any signals from insulin. When muscle cells are inactive, they need insulin to turn on the pump. So, if you exercise, your insulin goes a lot further."

■ *Don't smoke.* Diabetics are prone to peripheral vascular disease, a narrowing of the arteries of the lower extremities. Nicotine causes arteries to constrict, so smoking is particularly harmful for diabetics.

■ *Stay upbeat and positive.* Psychological factors can influence blood glucose levels. As Dr. Patrick Lustman of the Washington University School of Medicine explains, "Depression affects diabetics in part because patients are less likely to take care of themselves if they're depressed. But we are also finding that depression is a chronic stressor and, as such, can independently cause blood sugar to rise. A positive mental attitude improves diabetes management."

■ *Turn to family and friends for support.* It's much easier to start walking if a spouse or a friend goes along; it's easier to eat right if everyone is eating the same meals.

■ *Take preventive medication, if necessary.* New research shows that glucophage (Metformin) can prevent as well as treat diabetes. It reduces insulin resistance, increases glucose uptake by the cells and improves the body's glucose control mechanisms. High-risk people who took the drug for three years reduced their risk of diabetes by almost a third. See your doctor for more information.

 ## 11 BE SMART ABOUT SYNDROME X

When Syndrome X strikes, there are key steps that you can take to reduce insulin resistance and improve the metabolic abnormalities that are associated with this condition:

■ *Eat the right foods.* According to Dr. Gerald M. Reaven of the Stanford University School of Medicine, the "ideal" diet to combat Syndrome X supplies 45% of calories from carbohydrates, 15% from protein and 40% from fat. The latter should primarily include foods rich in mono- and polyunsaturated fats, such as fish, nuts and seeds, and canola, corn, olive, safflower, soybean and sunflower oils, as opposed to saturated fats. A high-fiber diet is also extremely helpful in fighting Syndrome X, adds Dr. Dennis Sprecher of the Cleveland Clinic.

■ *Lose weight.* Shedding pounds lessens insulin resistance. In the ongoing Framingham Heart Study, weight losses of just four or five pounds produced beneficial results in people with Syndrome X. Other recent studies have shown that insulin resistance falls an average of 20% for each 10 pounds of weight loss in overweight individuals.

■ *Move!* Regular exercisers use insulin more efficiently than their sedentary counterparts. For the vast majority of middle-aged and older adults, a goal of 30 minutes a day of moderate exercise can be achieved by P.O.W. (plain old walking) at a pace of 2.5 to 4.5 miles per hour.

■ *Don't smoke.* Not smoking decreases insulin resistance.

■ *Consider medications.* If lifestyle changes aren't enough, triglyceride-lowering medications, which may reduce the likelihood of abnormal blood clotting and boost HDL levels, should also be considered. These include nicotinic acid, gemfibrozil (Lopid) and fenofibrate (Tricor), which have the added benefit of lowering LDL cholesterol. The latter drugs can, in rare cases, cause damage to the liver, which should be periodically checked. Because many people with Syndrome X also have high blood pressure, selected antihypertensive medications, including those that may simultaneously increase insulin sensitivity, might also be helpful. Talk with your doctor about which medications might be best for you.

GIVE UP SMOKING 12

In terms of cardiac risk, smoking is a black-and-white issue. If you smoke, you are much more likely to develop coronary heart disease and have a heart attack than if you do not smoke. But smoking is an addiction, and addictive habits are hard to break. It certainly takes more than cognitive understanding about the hazards of smoking to cause a change in habits. There are, however, some practical actions you can take:

■ *Get help.* Your doctor, the American Heart Association, the American Cancer Society and the American Lung Association can point you to groups and programs and treatments that work.

■ *Start a regular exercise program.* In addition to dissipating stress and burning up nervous energy (triggers for smoking), physical activity causes the release of endorphins, which promote feelings of well-being and relaxation.

■ *Go crunchy.* Many smokers find that crunchy, low-fat whole foods such as apples, carrots and celery help to dissipate the craving to smoke by keeping the hands and mouth occupied.

■ *Drink water.* Staying hydrated cuts down on the craving for nicotine.

■ *Avoid those cigarette moments.* If your craving is worst after dinner, take a walk instead.

ACCENTUATE THE POSITIVE

D welling on how difficult it is to give up smoking and how many people are unsuccessful can undermine your efforts to change. Instead, focus on the hundreds upon hundreds of successful smoking cessation programs throughout this country. Such programs generally produce quit rates of 15% to 25% in the general population that smokes. Ever higher quit rates have been reported for people with smoking-related diseases, with up to 70% of patients quitting one year after a heart attack when provided with an intensive nurse-managed program.

Consider the whole new generation of medical aids, including the nicotine patch. Think positive. Some 50 million Americans have quit smoking, and more are choosing to do so every day. What successful quitters have in common is that they all took the same first step: deciding to live without cigarettes. This decision is fundamental if you are to view the process as an opportunity for self-improvement rather than as a painful ordeal marked by nothing but deprivation.

COPE WITH STRESS

It's a given that chronic stress is part of the fabric of contemporary American society. The modern era of high-speed living, with its increased demands from family and job commitments, contributes to a hectic lifestyle. Most people are simply out of time and deeply feel the stress of overcommitted, overscheduled and workaholic lives. We're multitasking, working on weekends, grocery shopping or doing laundry at nine P.M., commuting longer distances (while using a cell phone so that no time is wasted!) and answering late-night e-mails. As a result, contemporary American life is characterized by pressures, time demands and lack of balance.

In addition, we're bombarded by "bad" news: terrorism, the spread of AIDS, an unpredictable economy. There seems to be so much out of our control that contributes to a ceaseless stress that saps our strength and threatens our health.

At the same time, support organizations of the past are not always available to us today. Organized religion and the educational system have their own challenges. The extended family, once a bulwark against the world, has broken up and moved all over the country, leaving many of us feeling alone and helpless. It should be no surprise that in a National Family Opinion poll, 80% of Americans interviewed stated that they "need less stress in their lives."

Unfortunately, the daily events that cause stress cannot be avoided. It is not possible to remove the stressors from modern life. There will always be traffic jams, jangling telephones, e-mails to answer, overdrawn checking accounts, sick children and an up-and-down stock market. The key to success is learning how to *respond* to chronic stress rather than react to it. You do have the ability to take action to manage your stress more effectively. It all starts with a decision to take charge. Mental and physical activities such as regular exercise, keeping a journal, deep breathing and creating a realistic perspective will give you the tools to handle your stress and take control of your life.

Step 2
Manage Daily Stress

Making Sense of Stress

WHEN YOU'VE WRITTEN AND LECTURED extensively for more than two decades on the positive effects of diet and exercise on cardiac health, it's hard to admit that you've been neglecting something equally important. But that's the position we find ourselves in. Recent research and experience have convinced both of us that stress management is crucial to cardiac well-being. Even more importantly, they've convinced us that you can't expect people—including cardiac patients—to stick to an exercise and diet plan if they're under chronic stress. They can't. And they won't.

Stress can have a terrible impact on the heart. It causes increases in cholesterol, blood pressure and homocysteine. It promotes arterial inflammation. It constricts arteries and promotes abnormal heart rhythms, which in extreme cases can result in sudden cardiac death. It increases blood clotting.

But its *indirect* impact is just as devastating.

Stress drives people to make poor lifestyle decisions. Strung-out people smoke. They're "too tired" to work out. They eat high-fat foods and sit around the house, both of which promote weight gain with increased triglycerides, body mass index and waist circumference, as well as diabetes. Stress causes people to become supercompetitive and driven, to feel a heightened sense of time urgency, to be angry, hostile and depressed.

Simply put, stress places people at much higher risk for heart disease. It also helps to explain why people who know what to do for a healthy heart (and that means most of us) don't do it. We know we're supposed to eat a lean, balanced diet. Exercise regularly. Not smoke. But we eat fatty food, sit on our duffs and stoke our bad habits *because of chronic stress*. This is why Step 2 of the Piscatella Protocol—right after risk assessment—concerns stress management. When you've got that figured out, and only then, you'll be in a position to better manage exercise and diet successfully.

WHAT IS STRESS?

S tress is any circumstance that imposes special physical or psychological demands on us or throws off our equilibrium. Or, as defined by Dr. Wayne Lesko of the Center for Stress Management in Arlington, Virginia, stress is "anything that causes us to change."

"Not all stress is bad. Some stress is good," says Dr. Esther Sternberg of the National Institutes of Health. Positive stress, or *eustress*, is often reflected in a confident attitude and superior performance. Athletes, for example, use it to "get up" for a big game, but all of us feel its effect; when we're under pressure, we experience heightened energy and motivation levels that enable us to function at our optimum. A certain amount of stress also makes life interesting. With too little stimulation, we tend to become bored and frustrated.

On the other hand, too much stress pushes us into overdrive. It's not unlike the strings on a violin: when they're too loose, the sound they make is poor; too tight, and the strings break. "Stress can be the spice of life," says Dr. Mark Ketterer, a clinical psychologist at Henry Ford Hospital in Detroit, "or the kiss of death." It's the latter possibility we're worried about.

Dr. Hans Selye's research in the 1930s was the first to link negative stress, or *distress*, to a common biological response that could result in illness. For example, a downsized worker experiences acute

SLEEPLESS NIGHTS, FOGGY DAYS

A mericans are sleep-deprived workaholics. According to the National Sleep Foundation, only about a third of us are sleeping the recommended seven to eight hours a night, and 40% say they have trouble staying awake on the job. Instead of working to live, we are living to work, a practice that is having a profound impact on escalating stress levels.

stress at the sight of a pink slip. Yet so does a 15-year-old at cheer-leading tryouts. The situations differ greatly, but the physical responses to acute stress—tightness in the neck, a pounding heart, a knot in the stomach, dry mouth, shallow breathing—are surprisingly similar. Dr. Selye found that humans are equipped to deal with acute stress if it's only occasional and not prolonged. But chronic stress can lead to illness—from headaches to heart attacks.

Unfortunately, modern society tends to produce constant distress. From morning to night (and sometimes throughout the night), many people experience a continuum of stressful events. Some are serious—death, divorce, terrorism. But others are more trivial—being delayed in a bank line or even doing something "fun" like shopping for the "perfect" Christmas gift. Research suggests that the

Holiday Stress

Are people more stressed—and more at risk—during the winter holidays than during other times of the year? Yes. There's even a name for the condition, which is characterized by rapid heartbeat, lightheadedness and palpitations: "holiday heart syndrome."

Eating and drinking too much, shopping and preparing for holiday festivities, and partying with relatives and friends are all tough on health. "Everything becomes exaggerated this time of year. It's like cramming for a test, where people are trying to be sociable, to do a lot of entertaining, to do in a couple of weeks what they might want to do all year long," says cardiologist Dr. Stephen Winters. "This results in a kind of performance pressure that can lead to increased stress."

Doctors suggest better planning to minimize stress. "Ask yourself basic questions when you plan your day," suggests Dr. Winters. "Do you really want to go to the mall on a busy Sunday afternoon? Do you need to make two trips through the buffet line at an afternoon party?" If the answer is no, don't do it.

cumulative effect of life's trivial hassles—the parking tickets and traffic jams—is often harder on health than a life-threatening family medical crisis. "The human body," says Dr. Pamela Peeke of the University of Maryland, "was never meant to deal with prolonged chronic stress. We weren't meant to drag around bad memories, anxieties and frustrations. When we do, long-term stress takes its toll. We end up with health problems."

The presence of distress in American society can actually be quantified:

- The Centers for Disease Control and Prevention estimates that 60% to 70% of all disease and illness is stress-related.

- Eighty-nine percent of adults state that they experience high stress levels.

- According to the American Academy of Family Physicians, St. John's wort and other herbal remedies for altering mood are one of the fastest-growing segments of alternative medicine.

- Alcoholism is linked to stress. There are almost 15 million alcoholics in the United States.

- People under chronic stress are more likely to abuse drugs in an effort to reduce that stress, according to a report in the *Journal of Psychopharmacology*.

- One in four people suffers from sleep deprivation as a direct result of stress.

- The American Academy of Child and Adolescent Psychiatry identifies an overload of stress leading to depression as a key element in tripling the suicide rate of people 15 to 24 over the past 25 years.

- More than 25% of adults have high blood pressure due to or aggravated by stress.

- An estimated 75% to 90% of visits to physicians are stress-related.

- Job stress costs American businesses about $300 billion annually in absenteeism, compensation claims, mental health claims, health insurance and direct medical expenses, and reduced productivity and retention.

■ According to the American Medical Association, over half of the national medical bill can be attributed to an unhealthy, stressful lifestyle.

■ A 1998 study of 46,000 employees found that 25% felt nervous or stressed very often during the preceding three months.

■ About 60% of women say that job stress is their number one problem.

■ Middle-aged men who feel stressed at work are much more likely to develop atherosclerosis than men with low levels of stress.

Is increased stress an inevitable hazard of modern life? Perhaps, when you think about 60-hour work weeks, long commutes, chirping cell phones, late-night e-mails, lost weekends and an uncertain economy. But in many ways life was more stressful 200 years ago, when children routinely died before reaching adulthood. The challenge we face is to master not the threats themselves, but our all-too-human response to them.

An additional problem for many women working outside the home is that they are also primarily responsible for running the home. They "punch out" of their outside job, only to "punch in" at a second one as homemaker. Even in this day of more sensitive males, studies show that women still perform the vast majority of household tasks. This is further complicated by female child-rearing responsibilities, an aspect of society that has remained unchanged. Men and women alike still see the mother as having the primary role in child-rearing. It is estimated that nearly 60% of women employed outside the home have children under six years of age. Even with good child care (not always easy to find), working women often feel guilty about leaving their children with someone else. This problem is even greater for single mothers. Many women, attempting to build two "perfect" worlds with limited time and energy, run themselves ragged and into Type A lifestyles.

Physical Responses to Stress

Stress itself is not a health hazard; it's our response to it that's potentially dangerous. The physiological changes due to stress were first described by Harvard University's Dr. Walter B. Cannon, who labeled them the "fight or flight" syndrome. To understand this response, picture yourself in the following situation. It's 20,000 B.C., and you're asleep in a cave in the middle of the night. Suddenly you're awakened by the low growl of a saber-toothed tiger. Well before you're fully awake, your brain sends a biochemical message to your body in the form of stress hormones—cortisol, adrenaline and norepinephrine—to put it on notice that quick action will soon be taking place.

Stored fats and sugars immediately pour into your bloodstream to provide fuel for energy. Your breathing quickens to meet anticipated oxygen needs. Your heart rate and blood pressure increase in preparation for carrying extra oxygen. Activity in your digestive system slows down to make extra blood available to your muscles and extremities. Blood-clotting mechanisms become activated in anticipation of injury. In short, all senses are primed, all muscles are tensed, all systems are go. You're ready to either take a stand and fight the tiger or take flight to save your skin.

This is a very appropriate response to external physical danger if your goal is to survive the next 20 minutes. It is not, however, a healthy response to the emotional stress that all of us face in modern society. While contemporary life has changed greatly from

KILLER DEBT

A recent Ohio State University study suggests a connection between health and the strain of debt. Dr. Paul J. Lavraks, director of the study, says, "We found that people who are stressed about debt, particularly from credit cards, tend to be in worse physical condition than those without money worries. We've known that such folks tend to be more likely to smoke and be overweight. What was a surprise was that we found heart attack to be the single most prominent health problem stemming from credit-card debt."

prehistoric times, our physiological makeup has not. The stress caused by a traffic light produces virtually the same bodily response as a confrontation with a saber-toothed tiger—a response that is no longer appropriate to the stimulus.

The hormone cortisol gets the body all worked up, heart racing and muscles tensed, but in modern society there are few ways for the stress to be released. "Fight or flight" is no help with a jangling telephone or a vaguely threatening note from the IRS. In the modern world, we do not respond to a nagging boss with a spear; we grin and bear it. In the modern world, stress is not a situation that is soon over. It is continual and chronic. And it is detrimental to your heart. Every heartbeat at elevated blood pressure takes its toll on the coronary arteries. The excess fats and sugars released for energy are not metabolized right away, so they stay in the bloodstream, contributing to arterial deposits and diabetes. And, as already noted, ongoing stress can cause arterial inflammation, which can lead to a heart attack.

Stress can also foster overweight and obesity. People under stress often have lower levels of serotonin (a brain chemical that boosts mood) and higher levels of cortisol, a combination that promotes overeating of high-fat, high-calorie foods. There is another problem as well. "We found that women in particular who have high levels of cortisol after a stressful event tend to eat more sweets," says Dr. Elissa Epel of the University of California at San Francisco. "Emotional eaters have trouble keeping the weight off." Since one facet of the stress

STRESS AND FORGETFULNESS

Researchers have found that elevated levels of the stress hormone cortisol can impair verbal declarative memory, or the ability to remember words, details and phone numbers. Every day for four days, volunteers in one study were given a dose of cortisol mimicking a mildly stressful event, a higher dose mimicking a major stress, or a placebo. About 93% of those given the higher dose of the stress hormone had more difficulty in recalling information in a paragraph read to them than did those given low doses or a placebo.

response is to use the body's fat reserves as energy, people under chronic stress are prone to storing fat in the abdomen, where it can quickly be utilized by the liver. Called "deep-belly" fat, the accumulation of fat around the middle—a potbelly—increases the risk of Syndrome X and heart disease.

The same primeval response that served ancient man so well is detrimental to the health of modern man—nothing less than a prescription for an overdose of stress chemicals. What once meant survival has become suicidal.

Emotional Responses to Stress

When a person is put under severe stress—imagine a mother seeing her toddler dart into traffic—the first emotional response is *acute alarm*. This is an emergency system that prepares the body to fight or take flight.

Too often today we feel acute alarm over less severe stressors—this time imagine a traffic light on the fritz. Indeed, acute alarm is the result of any real or perceived situation that threatens us with loss of control and incites anger and aggression. The body is prepared to fight, but how can you punch a traffic light? Instead, the intended blows are internalized. Each time this happens, powerful stress hormones are secreted and the body literally ends up stewing in its own juices.

The second emotional response to stress is *long-term vigilance*, a mental state in which we project the future and adapt to that projection. This is what separates humans from other creatures, yet many people look into the future with fear, watching and waiting for something disastrous to happen. Vigilance, a response to lack of control, can occur on a temporary basis, as in the case of accountants imagining that they won't be able to meet a tax deadline. Or it can occur as a way of life, as with air traffic controllers. Chronic vigilance can lead to a passive outlook, an "it's out of my hands" mentality that is responsible for self-doubt, a sense of failure, depression and feelings of entrapment.

The emotional response to stress dictates how we see the world and how we think it sees us. Programmed as predators, we wind up preying on ourselves. At best, the result is chronic tension. At worst, we suffer damage to the cardiovascular system that can lead to serious physical and psychological disorders and, not infrequently, to premature death.

THE STRESS OF LIFE

According to numerous polls, time is the scarcest and most coveted commodity in our modern culture. As Swedish economist Staffan Linder explains in his book *The Harried Leisure Class*, the time we need to produce and consume has by necessity reduced the amount of "free" time, which has become too valuable for us to do "nothing."

But who even has free time? Extended work hours, multitasking, longer commutes, both parents working, single-parent households, increased organized activities for children—these are just some of the factors that have produced a serious shortage of time and, for many, an increase in stress. Americans report a constant struggle to balance career, marriage and family, and an ongoing battle against fatigue. A harried and "out of control" feeling has become an ongoing challenge for many people.

Add to that the undeniable fact that life is constantly changing. People move, change jobs, get married or divorced, buy and sell houses, have children and watch them grow up. There is birth; there is death. Whether trivial or significant, happy or sad, planned or unplanned, all change stresses the body by causing it to adapt. It is the process of adaptation that the body finds stressful. Change, adaptation, stress—these elements always go together.

The body adapts to most changes fairly well. However, when change occurs too often or too rapidly, the overload has implications for your health. The relationship between the frequency of major changes in life and the predictive risk of illness has been shown in a number of study findings:

- The death rate for widows and widowers is highest during the first six months following the death of a spouse.

- The death rate from cardiovascular disease is two to three times higher for divorced women than for married women.

- Even Mondays are stressful. Most people know this intuitively, but research by Dr. Simon Rabkin of the University of Manitoba lends medical credence. Over almost 30 years, Dr. Rabkin followed 3,983 men with no previous history of cancer or heart disease. Cancer deaths were distributed evenly throughout the week, but this was not true of sudden cardiac death: Monday saw twice as high an incidence as any other day of the week.

- Just thinking about work can elevate people's stress hormones. A study conducted by University College, London, measured levels of the stress hormone cortisol in participants' saliva. Samples were taken every two hours from waking until sleep. The highest levels were found early on Monday mornings when participants were preparing to return to work.

The definitive work on stress and the predictability of illness was authored by Dr. Thomas H. Holmes at the University of Washington. He found that hospitalized patients, regardless of their illness, had one major thing in common—the occurrence of a number of life changes just prior to their hospitalization. Carrying his findings forward, Dr. Holmes developed the Social Readjustment Rating Scale, which ranks specific life events in relation to predictable illness. Some events are significant, such as divorce; some are smaller, such as being cited for a minor traffic violation. This scale also shows that stress is cumulative; just a few significant events, or a number of smaller events, can overload the adaptive system. In addition, it illustrates that events need not be negative to be stressful. Vacations, Christmas and marriage are positive but still stressful events.

Use the Holmes scale on these pages to estimate how life events may be influencing your health. Obviously, the scale cannot predict illness with certainty, but it is a good tool for raising your awareness about the potential external sources of stress in your life.

LIFE EVENTS

If one of the following events occurred in your life within the last year, give yourself the mean value in points in the *past* column. If you can reasonably expect it to happen in the year to come, give yourself the value in the *future* column.

MEAN VALUE	PAST	FUTURE	LIFE EVENT
100	____	____	1. Death of spouse
73	____	____	2. Divorce
65	____	____	3. Marital separation (or separation from any major intimate relationship)
63	____	____	4. Detention in jail or other institution
63	____	____	5. Death of a close family member
53	____	____	6. Major personal injury or illness
50	____	____	7. Marriage
47	____	____	8. Being fired from work
45	____	____	9. Marital reconciliation
45	____	____	10. Retirement from work
44	____	____	11. Major change in the health or behavior of family member
40	____	____	12. Pregnancy
39	____	____	13. Sexual difficulties
39	____	____	14. Gaining a new family member (birth, adoption, remarriage, oldster moving in)
39	____	____	15. Major readjustment (merger, reorganization; bankruptcy)
38	____	____	16. Major change in financial state (a lot worse or lot better off than usual)
37	____	____	17. Death of a close friend
36	____	____	18. Changing to a different line of work
35	____	____	19. Increase in the number of arguments with spouse
31	____	____	20. Mortgage or loan for major purpose
30	____	____	21. Foreclosure on mortgage or loan

MEAN VALUE	PAST	FUTURE	LIFE EVENT
29	___	___	22. Major change in responsibilities at work (promotion, demotion, lateral transfer)
29	___	___	23. Son or daughter leaving home (marriage, college)
29	___	___	24. In-law troubles
28	___	___	25. Outstanding personal achievement
26	___	___	26. Starting or ceasing formal schooling
26	___	___	27. Spouse starting or ceasing work outside home
25	___	___	28. Major change in living conditions (building a new home, remodeling, deterioration of home or neighborhood)
24	___	___	29. Revision of personal habits (dress, manners, associations)
23	___	___	30. Troubles with boss
20	___	___	31. Major change in working hours or conditions
20	___	___	32. Change in residence
20	___	___	33. Change to a new school
19	___	___	34. Major change in usual type or amount of recreation
19	___	___	35. Major change in church activities
18	___	___	36. Major change in social activities (clubs, movies, visiting, etc.)
17	___	___	37. Purchase of major item (auto, computer, etc.)
16	___	___	38. Major change in sleeping habits (amount or time of day)
15	___	___	39. Major change in number of family get-togethers
15	___	___	40. Major change in eating habits (amount, hours or surroundings)
13	___	___	41. Vacation
12	___	___	42. Christmas or major holiday
11	___	___	43. Citation for minor violations of the law

Chance of a physical illness in the next 12 months if your score for the past year is:

300 or more:	80%
150 to 299:	50%
Less than 150:	30%

A CHANGING VIEW

Stress is usually thought of as a modern problem, but its impact on health has been recognized for hundreds of years. Medical observations from the 18th century describe people "paled with fear," or "reddened with rage," or "weeping with joy or sorrow." Such observations also noted that people under extreme stress could go mad or pine away. In 1813 James Johnson, a London physician, was the first to note the relationship between the "wear and tear" of life and premature old age. But documentation of the impact of stress on cardiac health goes back even further. Dr. William Harvey, the first physician ever to present a theory of blood circulation, wrote in 1628, "Every affection of the mind that is attended with either pain or pleasure, hope or fear, is the cause of an agitation whose influence extends to the heart."

Despite this history, not until very recently did physicians rank the treatment of stress as a high priority. Perhaps that is because it has been hard to measure. The same event can produce totally different reactions in two people. For one, the event is upsetting and stressful; for the other, it is viewed simply as a new challenge. In addition, traditional medicine has resisted the notion that a mental condition alone could have a measurable effect on arteries and organs. As Dr. Esther Sternberg explains, "Until recently, scientists and physicians dismissed the idea that stress could make you sick. They had the same motto as the state of Missouri: 'Show Me.' Now researchers are able to do just that."

Evidence reveals that chronic stress wreaks havoc on the body. While stress is seldom listed as the official cause of death, its negative role is now undisputed. Researchers estimate that mental stress has either caused or aggravated the symptoms of 50% to 90% of all hospital patients in the United States.

Indeed, stress may be the single greatest contributor to illness in the industrialized world.

STRESS AND GENDER

Since acute stress produces the same physiological responses in both men and women, scientists have long assumed that the behavioral response of both sexes was similar. New studies, however, show that this is not the case when stress results in depression.

■ "When life's burdens lead to depression, men and women respond quite differently," says Dr. Susan Nolen-Hoeksema, a professor of psychology at the University of Michigan. "Men drink. And women think." That's not to say that men never ruminate and women never drink, but in a study of 1,300 adults aged 25 to 75, Dr. Nolen-Hoeksema found that when upset, women tend to sit and stew while men are more likely to use alcohol to take the edge off.

■ New research at UCLA Medical School indicates that women typically employ a "tend and befriend" response. When stress mounts, women are more prone to protect and nurture their children ("tend") and turn to other females for support ("befriend"), perhaps because evolution has valued behavior that leads to a higher rate of offspring survival and the passing on of desirable traits.

■ When men or women are subject to stress, a powerful hormone called oxytocin is produced by the pituitary gland. Secreted at high levels during childbirth (to aid in labor), oxytocin exerts a calming influence. Estrogen, a female sex hormone, seems to amplify this effect, while androgens, male sex hormones, tend to diminish it.

This difference in response to stress could in part explain why American women, on average, live 7.5 years longer than men. "The fact is that women have their own ways of responding to stress," says lead researcher Dr. Shelly Taylor. "We didn't realize this in the past because the vast majority of subjects in the 'fight or flight' studies were males. Women made up only 17% of participants in those studies." While much more research must be done, many health professionals are leaning toward the acceptance of this theory.

HOW STRESS WORKS AGAINST YOUR HEART

We've already hinted at some of the negative effects that stress can have on your cardiovascular health. Now it's time to get specific: chronic stress is a very tough foe to combat, and we want you to be motivated.

Stress elevates blood pressure. The "fight or flight" response causes a temporary increase in blood pressure. When stress is occasional, such an increase does not usually present a health problem, but frequent elevation of blood pressure can lead to the permanent establishment of a new and higher level. According to the late Dr. Robert S. Eliot, a noted stress expert, about 20% of Americans are "hot reactors" whose response to even mild stress is a skyrocketing blood pressure. Each time stress is encountered—often many times a day—their blood pressure rises. Over time, their blood pressure settles permanently at the higher level, elevating heart attack risk significantly.

This seems to be particularly true when there is a genetic predisposition to high blood pressure. Researchers at the University of North Carolina studied men aged 18 to 22 who had at least one parent with high blood pressure and a high response to stress themselves. Ten years later, this group had three times the risk of hypertension, compared with people who had a low response to stress. But those who underwent 10 weeks of stress management therapy were able to significantly lower their blood pressure. Says Dr. Wolfgang Linden of the University of British Columbia, "Results in many stress management studies were similar to what you would find in many hypertensive drug studies, and without side effects."

Blood pressure response to stress may also be gender-specific: women's blood pressure seems to rise less than men's in reaction to stress. But women feel stress more often, according to Dr. Ronald Kessler of Harvard University. His study of 166 married couples found that women take a holistic view of everyday life. "A man may worry if someone in his family is sick," he says. "His wife takes on the burdens of the whole neighborhood. Men take care of one thing at a time. Women put the pieces together."

Stress causes arterial inflammation. Powerful hormones travel through the bloodstream every time the body reacts to acute stress. These hormones have the ability to injure coronary artery walls, creating places where cholesterol can collect, plaque can develop and inflammation can occur. The more chronic the stress, the greater the chance for injury and inflammation.

Stress injuries may be a key determinant of whether or not blockages form on artery walls. In a study conducted by Dr. Jay Kaplan of the Bowman Gray Medical School in North Carolina, one group of monkeys was fed a low-fat diet but subjected to constant social stress. Another group was fed the same diet but lived stress-free. The stressed monkeys developed arterial injuries and extensive plaque, whereas the unstressed animals did not, even though both groups ate the same diet and had similar cholesterol levels.

Stress can elevate cholesterol. People with ongoing stress often have higher cholesterol counts. This is illustrated by a study involving a group of certified public accountants whose cholesterol was measured in April, when the group was facing tax deadlines, and again during their August vacations. The result: April cholesterol levels were much higher than those in August, even though there had been no change in the accountants' diets. Studies of auto racers produced similar results: cholesterol levels were significantly higher on the day of a race than on the day after.

DOMESTIC STRESS

A five-year study on women and stress found that family stress increases a woman's chance of a heart attack more than stress on the job. While high work stress doubled the risk of a first heart attack, women with the worst family stress were four times more likely to have a first heart attack.

In addition, a recent Swedish survey of 292 women who had suffered heart attacks revealed that those with the most marital stress averaged a three times greater risk of a second heart attack during the following five years.

Warning Signs

Chronic stress, anxiety and pressure are common by-products of the modern American lifestyle. But when does stress become so pervasive that it can injure your health? It makes sense to be aware of the physical, emotional and behavioral signs of *overstress*:

- Ringing in the ears
- Increased muscular tension; neck and back aches
- Numbness or tingling
- Chest pains; shortness of breath
- Stomach and intestinal problems
- Irregular menstrual periods
- Skin eruptions and cold sores
- Loss of self-esteem; a feeling of worthlessness
- Difficulty making decisions
- A feeling that there "just aren't enough hours in the day" to get things done; trouble meeting deadlines
- A sense of paranoia; increased sensitivity to criticism
- Feelings of fatigue and boredom, unhappiness and sadness
- A hard time concentrating or being productive or creative
- A short temper; a tendency to criticize and be argumentative
- Problems with moodiness or depression
- Poor memory
- Rigid behavior
- Poor lifestyle habits: overeating, abusing alcohol and/or drugs, being "too tired" to exercise, smoking
- Oversleeping or not getting enough sleep

Often a person under great stress can exhibit many of these warning signs simultaneously. The cruel irony is that the reaction to stress may itself produce more stress in an ever-escalating spiral. Be sure to talk with your doctor or health professional if you experience more than the occasional sign of being overstressed.

Some researchers believe this effect is caused by a reduction of the liver's capacity to prepare for cholesterol excretion. One of the physical responses to stress is the shunting of blood to the arms (to fight) and legs (to take flight) and away from internal organs. Reducing blood supply to the liver causes a slowing down of function, impairing the organ's ability to rid the body of cholesterol. This may explain why some people under chronic stress have difficulty reducing cholesterol. It's not that they produce more cholesterol than others; it's that they have a problem eliminating it.

Stress elevates homocysteine. High levels of homocysteine are thought to injure artery walls, promoting inflammation and blood clots that can cause heart attacks. Even brief periods of stress affect homocysteine levels. In a study at Ohio State University, 34 middle-aged women were given stressful challenges over a 10-minute period. Homocysteine levels in the blood increased significantly. "This was after just 10 minutes of stress," says Dr. Catherine Stoney, an author of the study. "We have to wonder about the effects of chronic stress."

Stress promotes blood clotting. This response makes good sense as part of the "fight or flight" pattern. After all, if you face a physical threat that could result in a wound, the ability to produce and sustain coagulation provides protection. But that same ability, based on an increase in the stickiness of blood platelets, also creates a higher risk for heart attacks.

Stress can trigger sudden cardiac death. Coronary arteries are often pictured as passive, rigid tubes, like PVC pipe. They are not. Lined with muscle tissue, arteries dilate and constrict rhythmically. Powerful stress hormones can cause muscle tissue to contract abruptly, producing a spasm that cuts off blood to the heart. Stress can also trigger heart rhythm irregularities. In either case, sudden cardiac death can result.

Of more than 5,000 male heart attack fatalities examined at Brigham and Women's Hospital in Boston, 30% were found not to have substantial coronary plaque at the time of death. Their deaths were attributed primarily to lethal heart rhythm irregularities or coronary spasm brought on by an episode of acute stress. Other research reveals many examples of stress-induced sudden cardiac death:

- Ten days after the assassination of President John F. Kennedy, the 27-year-old army captain responsible for the ceremonial troops at the funeral died of a cardiovascular complication.

- After 31 years of trying to bowl a 300 game, a 40-year-old man in Detroit collapsed and died of a massive heart attack about 15 minutes after finally achieving his goal.

- A 56-year-old man collapsed and died of a heart attack while celebrating his first hole-in-one.

- A man watching his favorite baseball team lose on TV got so overwrought that he suffered a fatal cardiac event.

Stress contributes to obesity. The powerful stress hormone cortisol is an appetite stimulant that historically increased food intake to supply extra energy in dealing with enemies like the saber-toothed tiger. But the stresses we face today aren't the kind you fight or run from. Instead, we usually just sit there and get upset and anxious. Meanwhile, our brain assumes we've gotten really physical with such high levels of cortisol circulating, so it gives us a big appetite for the special fuels of the stress response—fats and carbohydrates. And this means lots of extra calories. Stress hormones also cause the body to hold on to fat cells as an energy reserve, thereby hindering weight-control efforts.

Stress can also foster overweight by promoting poor lifestyle choices such as overeating and exercise avoidance. "There is increasing evidence that stress may affect weight through changes in behavior that influence health," says Dr. Jane Wardle, writing in *Psychosomatic Medicine*. "For many people, that means unrestrained, emotional eating." Anger, depression, loneliness, anxiety—any of these negative emotions can be caused or aggravated by chronic stress and can motivate a person to eat. In this case, food isn't eaten because of hunger; instead, it has become a reward or a consolation, good for whatever ails. Stressed people are unconcerned about the quality of what they eat. They choose "high-comfort" foods because of nervous energy, not even tasting them and often losing track of calories.

Experts say that people who reach for food in response to stress do so as a means of self-medication. "It's nature's way of getting you to feel better," says Dr. Judith Wurtman at McLean Hospital outside Boston. "When the right foods are eaten, they act like an edible tranquilizer." In particular, foods that are rich in carbohydrates increase levels of serotonin in the brain, and serotonin minimizes symptoms of stress. "Contrived diets that are low in carbohydrates— such as the high-protein, low-carbohydrate diets—cause a depletion of brain serotonin," adds Dr. Wurtman, "contributing to increased tension, insomnia and anxiety. Add current levels of persistent uncertainty characteristic of our society, and you have a recipe for high stress." Unfortunately, comfort foods do not provide instant relief. The effects of serotonin on the brain can take about 30 minutes to be felt. If you keep eating until you feel better, that half-hour later can also mean two or three doughnuts eaten.

In addition, overweight people can feel additional stress because they hate being overweight. Many suffer from low self-esteem, actually despising their bodies. They see their lives and their appearance as being out of control. Tension and unhappiness—the stress of the situation—drive them to overeat often to the point of bingeing. Feelings of guilt, accompanied by even lower self-esteem, soon result and the cycle begins anew.

Lack of exercise compounds the problem. Stress causes mental fatigue, a chronic feeling of tiredness that keeps many overweight people from participating in physical activities that would help to dissipate stress and renew energy levels. As a result, these people choose to be sedentary. They restrict activities that would burn fat, control weight and give them a sense of being in charge of their lives. When stress produces a cycle of overeating and underexercising, extra weight becomes a predictable result.

Time for Action

IF YOU ASK A ROOMFUL OF PEOPLE, "How many of you would like to reduce the stress in your lives?" a lot of hands will go up. If you then ask, "How many people would like to win Lotto?" more hands will go up. The truth is that the chances for one are as good as for the other. Stress is part and parcel of modern life, particularly in the United States, where a fast-paced, out-of-time lifestyle and a Type A–fostering culture combine to induce high levels of frustration, anxiety and anger. There will always be traffic jams and overdrawn checking accounts. And there will always be stress. But we do not have to succumb to it.

The secret is not to avoid stress, but to manage it; not to react to stress, but to respond to it. Effective stress management means knowing the level of stress under which you can function safely and then controlling the way in which you react to stress above that level. Woody Allen once said that death is nature's way of telling us to slow down, but we definitely shouldn't wait that long before making the decision to slow down, assess stress in terms of causes and reactions, and figure out how to manage it.

The first step is to make a decision to take control, to decide to manage your stress rather than have it manage you. As author Arlen Price has said, "Where the heart is willing, it will find a thousand ways to succeed. Where it is unwilling, it will find a thousand excuses."

Next, identify what causes you to feel stressed. Is it coming from your job, your home, or both? Are too many things happening in your life? Are you always out of time? Are you setting unrealistic goals for yourself? Do you have Type A personality traits?

And finally, do something positive about combating stress. The Heart Savers in this section are all designed to help you do that. Remember, though, it takes some flexibility to devise a stress-busting strategy. No single approach works for everybody. Jogging and meditation are great for some people, but dull, boring and stressful for others. You have to find what works for you. But even using a handful of tips on a regular basis will allow you to better cope with stress when the going gets tough.

TAKE TIME OUT TO RELAX 14

According to Dr. Herbert Benson of Harvard University, the key to handling stress lies in learning how to produce a relaxation response to offset the stress response. Anything you can do to relax your mind and body on a regular basis will enhance your chances of managing stress in your life. Set aside time for yourself in the midst of your busy schedule. You deserve it! Then look for an activity that will help you switch off and relax. Go for a walk, read a book, listen to music, soak in a warm bath, practice yoga. Never use lack of time as an excuse to keep you from practicing relaxation techniques. *Make* the time, even when your schedule is hectic. Do it for yourself, because no one else will do it for you.

RESERVE JUDGMENT 15

The Chinese character for crisis means "danger," but it can also be translated as "opportunity." This contrast in definition is basic to an understanding of stress and stress management: *it's not the event that is stressful, but the perception of the event.* Each of us sees the same event differently, as in the movie *Rashomon,* and this difference dictates whether or not the event produces stress. In other words, one person's stress can be another person's pleasure.

There's a famous anecdote that illustrates this point. An elderly, wealthy woman who lived in an elegant New York hotel was awakened at one o'clock in the morning by piano music from the adjoining suite. Boiling mad to be hearing "noise" at that hour, she called up the night manager and was told that the offender was none other than the world-renowned concert pianist Artur Rubinstein; apparently disappointed in his performance that evening at Carnegie Hall, he was replaying the entire three-hour concert. Hearing this, the woman promptly forgot her complaint, pulled up a chair next to the wall and happily listened to Mr. Rubinstein play.

Had a change of events reduced her stress? No. She had taken a highly charged, stressful event and turned it into one of deep pleasure. As author Carlos Castaneda has suggested, "Things don't change. You change your way of looking, that is all."

FOCUS ON CONCERNS, NOT WORRIES

A *concern* is a problem that can be addressed or a situation that can be changed. For example, being habitually late for work or car pool is a legitimate concern. It's a problem, but it can be addressed with an action such as setting the alarm clock for 15 minutes earlier or laying out clothes the night before. In this way, the concern is dealt with realistically, the problem is solved and the situation is de-stressed.

A *worry*, on the other hand, is immune to direct action. A good example is a woman who has been working to lose weight. She's been eating fewer calories, exercising regularly and making steady progress, until one day, in a moment of weakness, she eats a dozen Oreo cookies. Her mind turns this relatively minor slipup into a major event and time-travels to unlock unpleasant images of the past or bring up future "foul-ups." By dwelling on the incident, she feels guilty and her self-esteem suffers.

A better idea would be to zero in on the present and make it her *concern* to get back on track for weight control. Why worry about the event? It's over. It can't be undone. Worrying will not affect the outcome, but planning to eat fewer calories and exercise a few more minutes over the next couple of days will put things in perspective.

EXPECT THE UNEXPECTED

Build a cushion into your day for the unexpected. Instead of cramming your schedule, fill it to 80%, leaving 20% for traffic jams, family illness and other surprises.

KEEP A JOURNAL 18

Researchers have long recognized the health benefits that come from writing about significant personal experiences in an emotional way. Journaling is especially valuable in coping with the aftershocks of extremely stressful events such as divorce or the death of a spouse or close relative. Dr. James Pennebaker, a psychologist at the University of Texas, studied rape victims and others who experienced upsetting and traumatic events. He found that people who wrote about those experiences reduced their stress and consequently had fewer health problems than those who did not.

The same holds true for relieving daily stress—as long as you focus on feelings, not facts. You may want to start with where you were or what you were doing. But move quickly to a description of your reaction to the event and how it is affecting you. That will let you consider how those feelings square with your personal rules, values and beliefs.

The best way to get started is simply to write every day, at the same time and in a place set aside as a sanctuary. Use a notebook or computer. Some experts argue that the physical act of writing with a pen on paper is therapeutic, but we believe there are no rules. There is no right way or wrong way. Just let it rip. Even if words don't come easily to you, keep at it. The more you write, the quicker it will become second nature to you.

PRACTICE POSITIVE SELF-TALK 19

Each of us is continually involved in self-talk, a running internal conversation that interprets events and actions. Most people are generally aware of some self-talk, yet a great deal of it occurs beyond conscious awareness. If you tune in to it, however, you become more aware of what you're telling yourself. After you've done that, you can begin practicing *positive* self-talk, a technique that will help you quiet your mind and gain a healthier perspective on life.

Unfortunately, much of our self-talk consists of negative, harmful put-downs. If corrected by a boss or parent, we might say to ourselves, "Can't I do anything right? I'm always fouling things up!" These messages—not the event—trigger the stress. Indeed, whenever we tell ourselves "This is terrible," "How could they do this to me?" or "The workload is killing me," we set ourselves up for a nasty set of emotions. The procedure takes place in a step-by-step sequence of events:

A		B		C
SITUATION	→	**BELIEF**	→	**EMOTION**
(the event)		(self-talk)		(the result)

Suppose you're scheduled for an important job interview. You jump in your car and turn the key, but nothing happens. The interview is scheduled for nine A.M., and there's no way you can make it. This is the situation (A). The belief you have about the meaning of the event, your interpretation, takes the form of self-talk (B). In this instance, the talk is negative: "Mr. Brown will be disappointed in me. He'll think I'm rude and I don't care about the job. Why does this always happen to me? I'll never have such a great opportunity again." The result is, of course, skyrocketing stress (C).

But what if the self-talk is positive? "Mr. Brown will be unhappy with me because I'm late, but the battery is dead. Getting upset won't help. I'll call him to say I have to come by taxi. I won't be there on time, but I'm sure he'll understand. He's probably been caught in the same situation himself. And besides, he *wants* to talk to me. He knows I'll be a great addition to his company." This self-talk produces a very different perspective of the event and keeps it from generating overstress.

The A-B-C model illustrates how thinking influences feeling and explains why two different people can respond to the same situation with far different emotional reactions. The model also suggests that emotions can be changed by altering self-talk. This is known as *cognitive restructuring*. It calls for being aware of our negative self-talk, challenging those self-defeating comments and replacing them with positive statements that decrease or prevent a negative emotional response.

The first step toward positive self-talk is listening. Spend some time focusing on your inner monologue. Don't judge, don't apologize; just listen and learn. Then, the next time you notice a negative thought, try countering it with something positive. The trick is to stay in the moment, the zone of noncritical thinking, and not let yourself be dragged down by worries about what you did in the past or might do in the future.

CLARIFY YOUR GOALS AND VALUES 20

People who are under the greatest stress, say many psychologists, are those who drift through life without direction. They have no standard against which to measure their lives, which means that the act of living itself carries no reason and little joy. As Viktor Frankl, author of *Man's Search for Meaning*, wrote: "There is ample evidence that in many cases, depression, aggression and addiction are caused by feelings of emptiness and meaninglessness. Today, many people have enough to live on, but nothing to live for. They have the means, but no meaning."

Stress-resistant people, on the other hand, have goals that concern quality of life as well as material success. They concentrate on what is worth *being*, not just what is worth having. Sure, having goals of any sort can put us under some pressure, but when our goals are ones that make life meaningful, they work for us by allowing us to work toward them.

Dr. Robert S. Eliot used an exercise to clarify and crystallize priorities. He called it the "Six Months to Live" test. Suppose you had just six months to live and had to decide how to spend your time. You make three lists to identify 1) the things you have to do, 2) the things you want to do, and 3) the things you neither have nor want to do. Dr. Eliot recommended throwing the third list away, since the items on it are what's preventing you from doing what you really want to do. The first list should be taken care of, but once it's out of the way, the rest of the time should be spent on the second list—those things that give life meaning for you. It's important to select goals that are genuinely important and that reflect personal values, interests and talents.

WRITE YOUR OWN EPITAPH

One exercise we use in seminars may help you put your values and goals into perspective. Write your own epitaph, based on how you're presently living. Then ask yourself if that's how you'd like to be remembered. If you're a hardworking, perpetually stressed-out person who isn't home very much because of your job's travel requirements, you may end up writing "Here lies the best marketing consultant on the West Coast." If you would rather have written "Here lies a great parent and a wonderful spouse," you may realize that your true values, priorities and goals are inconsistent with how you actually live. By putting balance in your life and reducing your stress, you will find more tranquillity—and often more productivity at work!

 TRANQUILIZE WITH EXERCISE

Frequent exercisers have more positive moods and less anxiety than those who exercise little or not at all. In one study, researchers found that after 30 minutes on a treadmill, people scored 25% lower on anxiety tests and exhibited favorable changes in brain activity. "The relationship is clear across the board," says psychologist Thomas Stephen. "The more you exercise, the better your mood is and the less likely you are to be anxious or depressed."

No one is certain why this is so. One reason may be that the physical act of exercise allows the body to "throw off" tension. Anyone who runs, walks or swims regularly knows that post-exercise feeling: the body feels tired, even drained, but good and less stressed out.

Another possibility is that exercise reduces stress hormones, which is particularly important for those who suffer from chronic stress. Since these people are always geared up in a "fight or flight" mode, they generally have high levels of stress chemicals circulating in the bloodstream. When no physical response is necessary, the stress hormones bombard the coronary arteries, causing injury, inflammation and, in rare instances, sudden cardiac death. Exercise appears to burn up excess stress hormones. Obviously, the next time stress appears, the stress chemicals will reappear. With regular exercise, however, the body learns to metabolize these hormones more effectively, potentially reducing the likelihood of coronary injury.

A third possibility is that exercise stimulates the brain's production of endorphins, chemicals that produce a positive feeling and a happy, self-satisfied attitude and thus enhance one's sense of calm and well-being. Simply put, people who exercise regularly feel better about life. The result is an enhanced ability to cope with stress.

Other scientific studies support the notion that exercise can have a positive effect on emotions and moods:

■ A University of Southern California study found the effect of a 15-minute walk to be comparable to that of a strong tranquilizer in reducing tension.

■ A Duke University study showed that Type A behavior, characterized by aggressiveness and impatience, can be modified by aerobic exercise. In this study, 50 men and women aged 25 to 61 were tested to determine whether they were A or B types, then put on an exercise program (45 minutes, three times a week). After 10 weeks, the Type A's were found to be substantially calmer and more relaxed than they were at the start of the study.

■ A study in England found that regular exercise boosts people's moods and may even fight clinical depression by elevating the body's levels of phenylethylamine, a natural chemical linked to energy, mood and attention. Men in the study who exercised had levels 14% to 57% higher than those who never exercised at all. Researchers speculate that phenylethylamine may play a role in the purported "runner's high."

■ A review of research by the American Psychological Association on the effect of exercise on depression found that just five weeks of mild to moderate aerobic exercise and/or a weight training routine could boost mood. The research suggested that regular exercise can also benefit those who suffer from panic disorder.

The bottom line is that exercise makes you feel self-reliant, powerful, in control and generally better about yourself—all of which can reduce stress. Having the discipline to commit to regular exercise means *you* are in control. As clinical psychologist Dr. Kenneth R. Pelletier has observed, "When people begin to pay attention to their health, they seem to have a much better ability to look at things that used to bug them and simply be more detached. If you're taking time out of your life to exercise, you're taking a psychological stance that in itself is going to have you reacting differently to your job, your office, your sense of achievement, your career."

 BREATHE DEEPLY

When you're feeling stressed, your blood pressure increases and your muscles tense. There's little you can do about that, but you can control your breathing. And because breathing is one of the internal communications systems that tell your organs how to function, controlling your breathing can promote a relaxation response.

Deep breathing can be used as a calming technique in response to a stressful situation, or it can be practiced regularly as a stress preventive, done once or twice a day to break tension's hold. But in order to use the technique successfully, you must know how to breathe. Most people, particularly during stressful situations, tend to breathe incorrectly by expanding the rib cage. Chest breathing results in short, shallow breaths. It is constricting and actually *heightens* stress.

LEARN HAPPINESS

Although the Declaration of Independence provides for the pursuit of happiness, there are no guarantees that the pursuit will be successful. Researchers such as Dr. Sonja Lyubomitsky at the University of California contend that happiness can be learned. "It's a product of both nature and nurture," says Dr. Lyubomitsky. "About 50% of happiness comes from the genetic variables—some people are born programmed to be happy. Another 10% of happiness comes from individual circumstances. And a whopping 40% is a result of behavior modification."

On the other hand, deep breathing, also called abdominal or diaphragmatic breathing, creates a state of calm. The technique is easy to practice and can be done standing, sitting or lying down. Find a comfortable position and take deep breaths through your nose with your mouth closed. As you inhale, push out your stomach. This lowers the diaphragm. Hold the breath for a few seconds, then expel it slowly and easily through your mouth with your lips pursed, as if you were whistling or kissing. Make your exhalation twice as long as your inhalation. Both intake and expulsion should be rhythmical. If you've never practiced deep breathing, a good way to learn it is to lie on your back, relax and place two or three books on your stomach. When you breathe in and push out your stomach, the books will rise. When you exhale, their weight should press in. Once you get the hang of it, you can practice deep breathing in any position, even sitting in a comfortable chair with your feet up.

By regulating your breathing, making it slow and regular, you're actually modulating your feelings. Do it for just a few minutes and tension will lessen. The key to success, however, is daily practice. If you want to be good at using deep breathing in an emergency, you have to be good at using it in ordinary circumstances.

GET ENOUGH SLEEP

A nationwide survey by the National Sleep Foundation found that 44% of Americans reported trouble falling asleep, 48% said they wake up in the night too often and 50% said they wake up feeling unrefreshed. Chronic sleeplessness is linked to psychological distress, such as depression and anxiety. Research at Pennsylvania State University suggests that blood levels of cortisol and other stress hormones are significantly higher in insomniacs than in healthy sleepers. But it's a catch-22: getting seven to eight hours of sleep on a regular basis is critical to managing chronic stress, yet this kind of stress often keeps us awake.

So what can you do to get a good night's sleep?

■ *Avoid stimulants*. Don't drink any caffeine after two P.M. Avoid nicotine. And don't drink alcohol any later than three to five hours before bedtime.

■ *Lose excess weight*. Overweight people are more prone to snoring and other nighttime breathing problems that can interfere with sleep.

■ *Try not to nap during the day*. While napping for 15 to 20 minutes can increase alertness and productivity, a nap that lasts an hour or more can cause you to lapse into a deep sleep and wake up feeling worse than when you first fell asleep.

■ *Exercise regularly*. Studies have shown that 30 to 40 minutes of daily exercise can help some people fall asleep more easily. But remember, the best time for exercise is in the morning or afternoon, not in the evening.

■ *If you can't fall asleep, get out of bed*, no matter what time it is. Don't go back to bed until you feel sleepy.

■ *Avoid eating heavy meals*. If you have to eat a meal an hour or so before bedtime, make it a light one.

■ *Relax your mind* with meditation, deep breathing or prayer. Try not to watch TV or listen to the radio. Don't read or do work in your bed.

■ *Establish a routine.* Have a regular time for getting out of bed each morning, regardless of how many hours you've slept. Try to go to bed and get up at the same time every day, even on Saturday and Sunday.

■ *Establish a peaceful setting.* Minimize the amount of light and noise in your bedroom, and keep the temperature moderate.

■ *Take a hot bath.* Researchers found that insomniacs who took a 30-minute warm bath about an hour before bedtime slept better than they had before.

■ *Talk to your doctor.* Some over-the-counter or prescription medicines can interfere with sleep. Find out if anything you're taking could be having an effect on your ability to sleep.

DEVELOP RESILIENCY

Because differences in the perception of stress explain why some people can weather devastating experiences with serenity and others cannot, researchers are looking carefully at resiliency—the ability to get through, get over and thrive after trauma, trials and tribulations. Instead of asking why bad things happen to good people, these scientists are now focusing on how good people can best overcome bad events or situations.

Stress-resistant, resilient people often share distinctive habits of the mind. They tend to focus on immediate issues rather than global ones. Work by Drs. Suzanne Kobasa and Salvatore Maddi at the University of California at Irvine shows that many such people are stress-resistant because of "hardy" personalities. In a study of the breakup of the Bell System, Drs. Kobasa and Maddi found that the executives who flourished under the change demonstrated three attitudinal characteristics:

■ A sense of control—the belief that they can influence and shape events, and turn situations, even bad ones, to their advantage

■ A commitment to life—the belief that their actions are worth doing at full tilt since they are useful to themselves, their families and to society, and the knowledge that no one aspect of life should become an obsession

- Love of a challenge—a willingness to accept and anticipate change as natural and exciting, not threatening

No one can be successful in everything. Failure is a product of the human condition. But failing does not have to be a weakness; it can provide for tremendous growth. It isn't the failure that's important; it's how you handle it. Imagine what would have happened if certain people had allowed themselves to think of themselves as failures:

- Albert Einstein's poor performance in all his high school classes except math prompted a teacher to predict failure for him and encourage him to leave school.

- Thomas Edison's father called him a dunce and his teachers described him as "addled," warning that he "would never amount to anything."

- Sir Winston Churchill, who twice failed the entrance exams to Sandhurst, was considered "dull" by his father.

Can you learn resiliency and hardiness? Drs. Kobasa and Maddi say yes. First focus on signals from the body that something is wrong, then mentally review the situation that might be stressful. Next, mentally reconstruct the stressful situation to think about how it could have gone better or worse. This often illustrates that things did not go as badly as they might have. And finally, compensate for stress through self-improvement. When life seems out of control, taking on a new challenge can result in regaining self-esteem and a sense of accomplishment. The source of the stress—loss of a job, divorce, health problems—may be impossible to avoid. But by taking on a new task, a person is assured that he or she can still function.

If you're curious about how resilient you might be in the face of adversity, take the test on the facing page, adapted from *The Survivor Personality* by Al Siebert, Ph.D.

HOW RESILIENT ARE YOU?

Circle the appropriate numbers below to rate how much each of the following applies to you (1 = very little; 5 = very much).

1 2 3 4 5   Curious; ask questions; want to know how things work; experiment.

1 2 3 4 5   Constantly learn from own experience and experience of others.

1 2 3 4 5   Need and expect to have things work well for self and others. Take good care of self.

1 2 3 4 5   Play with new developments; find the humor, laugh at self, chuckle.

1 2 3 4 5   Adapt quickly; highly flexible.

1 2 3 4 5   Feel comfortable with paradoxical qualities.

1 2 3 4 5   Anticipate problems and avoid difficulties.

1 2 3 4 5   Increase self-esteem and self-confidence every year. Develop a conscious self-concept of professionalism.

1 2 3 4 5   Listen well; read others, including difficult people, with empathy.

1 2 3 4 5   Think up creative solutions to problems and challenges. Trust intuition and hunches.

1 2 3 4 5   Manage the emotional side of recovery. Grieve, honor and let go of the past.

1 2 3 4 5   Expect tough situations to work out well; keep on going. Help others, bring stability to times of uncertainty and turmoil.

1 2 3 4 5   Find the gift in accidents and bad experiences.

1 2 3 4 5   Convert misfortune into good fortune.

Add numbers for your score:

60 to 70: Highly resilient	30 to 39: Struggling
50 to 59: Better than most	Under 30: Seek help
40 to 49: Adequate	

MEDITATE

One centuries-old technique of meditation, which many now call repetition, involves the repeating of a single word for a concentrated but brief period of time. Designed to clear the mind and anchor it in the present, it produces an immediate calming effect on the nervous system. Studies at UCLA and Harvard University show the physiological effects of meditation. When you're asleep, your oxygen consumption is decreased by 8%. With meditation, however, it's down by 12%, an indication that your body is equally if not even more deeply relaxed. These studies also illustrate that meditation can decrease blood pressure significantly.

Start by selecting a quiet spot. Loosen your clothing and remove your shoes. Assume a comfortable sitting or reclining position, close your eyes and prepare to focus on something—an object, a word or your breathing. Empty your mind of everything else. Take a deep breath and slowly repeat a single word. In *The Relaxation Response*, Dr. Herbert Benson recommends using words or sounds that end in *m* or *n*, such as "calm" or "ocean," but any appropriate word will do. Slowly repeat the word mentally, over and over again. Other thoughts will occasionally interfere, but just let them pass through your mind.

SPEAKING FROM EXPERIENCE

I know several heart patients who are big believers in the positive effects of meditation, but frankly it's hard for me to do. As a Type A personality, I have difficulty clearing my mind. Lists of things I should be doing just seem to pop in, and the next thing I know, I'm thinking about a project instead of meditating. So for me, deep breathing, progressive muscle relaxation and exercise are more effective ways to create a relaxation response. But for many, many others, meditation is a tested and effective means to cope with daily stress.—*J.P.*

After a while, repetition will have an almost hypnotic effect and create a state of deep rest and relaxation. In a few minutes, you'll feel renewed energy and optimism. Meditation requires only 10 to 30 minutes, but is most effective when done every day at the same time.

Author Deepak Chopra says, "Meditation is not a way of making your mind quiet. It's a way of entering into the quiet that's already there—buried under the 50,000 thoughts the average person thinks every day."

LISTEN TO YOUR SPIRITUAL SIDE   26

Good family relationships, playing bridge with friends, belonging to the Elks or Rotary—all are associated with less stress. New studies are finding that having a religious faith and a sense of spirituality can also reduce stress. According to Dr. Fred Luskin of the Stanford University School of Medicine, "People who go to church, synagogue, mosque or Buddhist monastery once a week average 83 years of longevity. For those who do not go at all, longevity averages 75 years. You do the math!"

Historically the belief in a faith-health connection centered on God's healing power. Most of us have heard stories of people who, by sheer faith alone, have miraculously recovered from terminal illnesses or survived longer than thought possible by physicians. Their prayers, and the prayers of others in their behalf, caused divine intervention. And while that certainly may be true, it cannot be proven scientifically. It is a matter of faith.

More recently, however, medical studies are showing that belief in God and participation in organized religion have a measurable, beneficial health effect. More than 30 scientific studies have linked spiritual or religious commitment and more effective management of stress with better health or a longer life:

▪ A 29-year study of people aged 25 to 55 in Alameda, California, found that those who attended religious services once a week had 36% lower mortality than nonattendees.

■ Those with a religious commitment had fewer symptoms and better health outcomes in seven out of eight cancer studies, four out of five blood pressure studies, four out of six heart disease studies and four out of five general health studies.

■ One study showed that people with normal blood pressure who worship regularly are less likely to experience high blood pressure in the future.

■ Over 200 studies by Dr. Jeffrey Levin of Eastern Virginia Medical School found that a positive connection between religion and health cuts across age, sex, cultural and geographic boundaries.

According to Dr. Herbert Benson, praying elicits a relaxation response in the body similar to meditation or deep-breathing exercises. It decreases blood pressure, heart rate and breathing rate, and diffuses stress chemicals. "It is a legitimate stress-management technique," he states.

Religious faith also promotes a sense of hope and control, which provides a better ability to cope with stress and adverse events such as health problems. Research has shown that when people over 60 are hospitalized, over 50% report they use religious faith as their primary coping mechanism. Says Dr. Harold Koenig of Duke University Medical Center, "Commitment to a system of beliefs enables people to better handle the stress of traumatic illness, suffering and loss. The opposite is also true. Loss of religious faith, feelings of doubt and anger are normal when dealing with serious illness. But when people get stuck there, it creates stress that interferes with the body's ability to recover."

Attending religious services provides the social support associated with stress reduction. Says Dr. Luskin, "Social bonding is a well-documented key to health and longevity. Church, synagogue or mosque often provides an 'us' in an 'us vs. them' world. It is a family, a circle of friends. It provides community and support so helpful to allowing us to move safely through our lives. This protective effect results in less stress and better health."

Many religious people also practice "sin avoidance," staying clear of excessive drinking, smoking, taking drugs and engaging in risky sexual practices. In addition, religious faiths tend to encourage marriage, which in itself has been linked to longer life.

VISUALIZE LIFE AS YOU WANT IT   **27**

Tiger Woods once said he plays each golf hole in his head, seeing himself hitting a perfect shot, in preparation for the actual shot. Programming your brain with positive mental images can help reduce your stress. Life *is* as you picture it. The MacArthur Foundation Study findings suggest that longevity and successful aging are more mental than genetic.

TAKE UP TAI CHI   **28**

Tai chi, sometimes called "meditation in motion," is a Chinese martial art that improves physical function and promotes mental and spiritual well-being by lowering blood pressure, enhancing self-confidence and reducing levels of the stress hormone cortisol.

The highly disciplined movements and forms of tai chi help to unite the body and mind, thereby bringing harmony and balance to life. Unlike karate and other "external" martial arts, tai chi has an "internal" focus emphasizing complete relaxation. It is characterized by soft, slow, flowing, precisely executed movements.

Tai chi is a particularly good way to dissipate stress for people who prefer a physical basis for promoting a relaxation response. Says Dr. William Kaplindis of the Pacific College of Oriental Medicine, "We recommend that people go home and listen to a relaxing tape or do meditation, but many people are not going to do that. They want to do something physical for relaxation, and tai chi is perfect for them."

Because it is low-impact, tai chi has multiple advantages for elderly people who want to improve balance and prevent osteoporosis. One study found that when compared to nonstudents, tai chi students (average age, 76) went an average 48% longer before experiencing a first fall.

"People generally learn tai chi in a class, where beginners can learn the forms," says Dr. Kaplindis. "But ideally, they will incorporate tai chi into their daily practice, even doing it on days when there is no class, in order to get the maximum benefit." To find a qualified tai chi instructor in your area, consult your local alternative health association.

PRACTICE PMR

Progressive muscular relaxation (PMR) is one of the best ways to clear tension from the body. In this technique, you tense a group of muscles, hold them in their contracted state for a few seconds, then release and relax them. By concentrating on groups of muscles, you can imagine them relaxed, which in turn causes an actual relaxation to take place.

Begin by finding a quiet place where you can spend an uninterrupted half-hour. Lie on your back in a comfortable position with your arms at your sides and legs uncrossed. Loosen any restrictive clothing. Close your eyes and adjust your body position to be comfortable. Focus your attention on breathing. Notice the movement of air through your nostrils down into your lungs, filling them up, and then back out again. Breathing should be deep and easy, rhythmic and smooth. Bring attention to the muscles of your scalp and forehead; tune in to feelings of tension there. Tighten your scalp and forehead muscles. Squeeze and hold the tension, then release it, relaxing the area.

> ### JAW STRESS RELIEVER
>
> The Academy of General Dentistry suggests putting your tongue between your teeth or at the roof of your mouth toward the back during times of stress. This will keep your upper and lower teeth apart, thereby preventing your jaw from tightening and your teeth from grinding.

Repeat this cycle with all parts of your body, starting with your head and moving systematically through your arms, shoulders, abdomen, buttocks and legs down to your feet. Be aware of each area, tighten the area, then relax. Go slowly. Let go more and more until your whole body is in a state of deep relaxation. Allow the tension to flow out with each breath. After you've gone through these steps, you will feel very calm, refreshed and rejuvenated.

RELEASE STRESS NOW! 30

Don't wait until the end of the day to tackle stress. Whenever you're feeling uptight, frustrated, overwhelmed or mentally drained, ask yourself, "What can I do *right now* to relax and manage my stress burden?" Some good choices include changing your posture, listening to soft music, being kind to or doing something for someone, taking a short walk, soaking in a warm bath, having a drink of water, taking a relaxation break, making a change in your routine and taking a few moments to breathe deeply.

LAUGH 31

According to Dr. William F. Fry, Jr., of the Stanford School of Medicine, a good laugh—like a good workout—produces an overall sense of well-being. Laughter flexes the muscles of the chest and abdomen, including the diaphragm, and causes deep breathing to take place. By exercising the shoulders, neck and face, it releases tension in the muscles. And humor itself can help create a different perspective on life and its challenges. As cardiologist Dr. Steve Yarnall says, "Laughter is the shortest distance between two people."

Until recently, many health professionals discounted laughter's therapeutic effect. Now things are changing, in large part because of the groundbreaking work done by the late Norman Cousins, once editor of *Saturday Review* and subsequently a professor at the UCLA School of Medicine. In his book *Anatomy of an Illness*, he recounts how laughter helped to cure an unexplained sudden illness for which he had been hospitalized. After a period of time with no progress, he abandoned conventional thinking, stopped taking medication and ordered in reel upon reel of old Marx Brothers films. According to Mr. Cousins, his heavy, sustained laughter was the key to his recovery.

On average, adults laugh 15 times a day. If we can up that number, we can reduce the stress that underlies so many diseases. You can do that by cultivating friends and acquaintances who smile and joke, putting playfulness into your relationships and leaving work concerns at the office. Just remember the words of the late Milton Berle: "Laughter is an instant vacation."

32 PRACTICE YOGA

Yoga comes from the Sanskrit word *yuj*, meaning "to yoke," in this case to join or balance the mind, body and breath through the practice and mastering of three principles. First are the specific physical postures called asanas; held for an extended period of time, they are designed to relax and tone the muscles. Second are the pranayama, or breathing exercises, that slow breathing and increase the body's vital energy. And third is resting completely between postures.

Practiced for a thousand years, yoga's stretching, strengthening and meditative exercises encourage complete focusing on movement and the body parts involved. Yoga trains the mind and body to work together to create a healing environment.

There are few scientific studies regarding the health benefits of yoga, but participants report feeling better, more relaxed and centered, with fewer headaches, less back pain and less severe menstrual cramps. Yoga dissipates stress by increasing flexibility and reducing muscle tension and tightness, which the body interprets as a generalized reduction in tension and mental stress. It also teaches you to be more in touch with your breathing and to breathe more easily throughout the day to relieve tension. And finally, it can free your thoughts. Yoga teaches that your thoughts have the ability to affect your overall contentment and health. During the deep relaxation pose, every part of the body is systematically relaxed, serving as a kind of meditation to relieve stress.

Experts suggest that the best way to learn yoga is to take a class with a trained leader. Audiotapes and videotapes are available for practicing yoga at home, but most people make better progress with personal instruction. Classes are offered at private studios, health clubs and community recreation centers in many areas. Your instructor will be able to advise you on different moves and techniques to practice at home.

BE ASSERTIVE 33

For many people, feelings of stress arise from not knowing how to say no. These people feel put upon yet powerless to change the circumstances. Learning how to be more assertive, to make your own needs known to others in a forceful, honest and polite manner, can significantly reduce the level of stress.

If you don't express your feelings and needs when it's your right to do so, or if you discount your feelings as being unimportant or less worthy than someone else's feelings, emotions get bottled up and you feel miserable. On the other hand, aggression to the point of insults or criticisms fosters neither effective communication nor positive relationships.

Being assertive means stating your feelings and requesting appropriate change. If a meeting is scheduled for a time convenient for others but not for you, an assertive statement of feelings can avert later feelings of stress: "I'd really like to be at the meeting, but this isn't a good time for me." Follow up with a request for appropriate change: "I know we've tried to find a time good for everyone, but let's give it one more try."

Assertiveness is not rudeness. It's simply taking your own needs and desires into consideration, but often the mind has to overcome the heart in order to get there. Your mind knows you have a right to put yourself first sometimes, but your heart feels the familiar childhood programming that "nice people always put others first." Assertive thinking and action will place you in control.

34 TAKE A VACATION

Skipping vacations can have a devastating impact on cardiovascular health. Studies show that people who don't take an annual vacation are 21% more likely to die over the next nine years and 32% more likely to die of coronary heart disease than those who take time off each year. "This is either because vacations reduce heart problems or because people with heart problems don't take vacations," says Dr. Brooks Gump of the State University of New York at Oswego. "Either way, the more often you skip your vacation, the higher your risk of death. People need to start thinking of vacation as preventive medicine."

While no one is certain of the mechanism involved, evidence shows that the very qualities that lead us to bypass vacation also tend to promote heart disease. As Dr. Gene Ondrusek of the Scripps Center for Executive Health has observed, "Executives will say, 'Gosh, it's been years since I've had a vacation,' and it's almost said with pride, as evidence of their commitment and ambition. There's a driven quality there. There is also a cynical hostility, a paranoia: 'If I leave, someone working in the background is going to take my position.' Or they don't trust that whoever is filling in for them will do a good job.

SPEAKING FROM EXPERIENCE

As long as it relaxes you, any type of vacation can promote stress management. Obviously, touring 20 cities in Europe in 18 days is more stressful than lying on a beach in Maui for a week. But the real point of going on vacation is just to leave your normal life at home. If you bring your briefcase, cell phone and laptop, are you taking a break . . . or just setting up a new office location? One executive told me that on her last vacation she answered more than 100 e-mails a day! That, I think, is at odds with using vacation time to produce a relaxation response. —*J.P.*

Unfortunately, cynical hostility is linked to chronic stress and is known to promote heart disease." Equally unfortunate is the survey finding that many workers believe it will reflect positively on them if they don't take their allotted vacation time.

Some researchers believe that the scenic beauty encountered on many vacations can promote health; it focuses attention, helping people plan better and deflect distractions while lowering irritability. Others say that relaxation can be found in the escapism of reading on vacation (history or "trashy" novels, but not business books). And to Dr. Herbert Benson the benefit lies in the fact that vacations "break the train of everyday thought that often drives you up a wall, such as finances, family and deadlines."

"We don't know if it's just the absence of stress on vacations or some positive, restorative quality when you get away," says Dr. Gump. "But whatever it is, it works. Regular vacations help people handle stress and reduce the risk of heart disease."

STRETCH ㉟

In addition to decreasing the risk of injury, helping to relieve low-back pain and improving agility, regular stretching exercises promote a relaxation response. Stretching acts as an internal massage for the body.

There are many good books and videos to get you started. Health clubs and community recreation centers often offer instruction. Whether on your own or in a class, here are a few guidelines:

■ *A regular program is most effective.* Plan to stretch at least two to three times per week and more often if you're under chronic stress. Stick to a schedule.

■ *Muscles stretch best when they're warm.* Stretch after a cardiovascular routine, such as brisk walking, or after a hot bath or shower. If your muscles are "cold," jog in place before stretching.

■ *Don't bounce when you stretch.* View your stretching routine as a time for relaxation. Go slowly and gently.

■ *Avoid pain.* Stretch to the point of tension but not pain.

■ *Perform stretches in a slow, controlled manner.* Remember to breathe. Relax and exhale as you go into a stretch, then breathe normally and slowly.

■ *Never stretch injured or strained muscles.*

■ *Take your time.* Hold each stretch for 10 to 30 seconds, to the point of mild discomfort or where you "feel the stretch." Pause and then repeat the stretch at least three more times.

36 VOLUNTEER

People under chronic stress often make themselves the center of the universe. Almost everything in life—events, relationships, workloads—is seen in terms of how it impacts them. As a result, they are constantly vigilant and prone to anxiety.

Changing from an inward to an outward perspective can break this cycle. A great way to do this is by becoming a volunteer. Coach a youth soccer team. Read to elderly shut-ins. Man the information desk at the hospital. Get involved in a political campaign. Find an area of interest and give something of yourself to it. You'll forget your problems, widen your perspective and establish meaningful relationships. As cardiologist Dr. Fred Pashkow likes to tell his patients, "Volunteering helps to establish a realistic perspective and bring balance to your lives. Helping others simply makes it harder to dwell on your own troubles. And anytime you can put your own troubles aside, even temporarily, you reduce your stress."

37 GET A MASSAGE

Whether the method is Swedish, pressure-point, sports massage, shiatsu, acupressure, reflexology, deep-tissue or craniosacral, massage therapy is designed to improve health and well-being through the hands-on manipulation of muscles and other soft tissues of the body. It may also reduce heart rate, lower blood pressure, increase blood circulation, relax the muscles and improve range of motion. Many people use therapeutic massage as part of their regular health-care maintenance. As defined in the *Journal of the American Massage Therapy Association*, "Massage is to the human body what a tune-up is to a car."

But there are many positive results beyond physical benefits. Massage also:

- Fosters peace of mind and a sense of well-being.
- Promotes a relaxed state of mental alertness.
- Reduces levels of anxiety and helps to relieve mental stress.
- Improves the ability to monitor stress signals and respond appropriately.
- Enhances the capacity for calm thinking and creativity.
- Satisfies the need for caring/nurturing touch.
- Increases awareness of the mind-body connection.

The cost is typically $40 to $80 for a one-hour session. Be sure that your practitioner is licensed.

DON'T BE A STRANGER

The MacArthur Foundation's landmark study on successful aging identifies meaningful social relationships as being of equal importance to diet and exercise in a healthy life. Associate with people who share common interests, make you laugh and help you feel good about yourself. Stay in touch with friends and family. Talk things over. When tensions build up, discuss the problem with a close friend or with the people involved.

Positive social connections keep you from feeling that you're going through life alone. You have help and support.

BE REALISTIC

Set practical goals and expect to meet them. Don't overload yourself with more work or commitments than you can handle. Let go of perfectionism; your home doesn't have to be spotless, and you don't always have to be the last one to leave the office. And don't expect perfection from others, either.

Try to meet daily challenges in a logical manner. Even personal problems, if approached intelligently and systematically, have reasonable solutions. Focusing on one small part at a time will make each challenge seem less overwhelming.

GET A PET

This is not as offbeat as it may sound. Emerging scientific evidence suggests that those who keep pets are likely to benefit from improvements in physical and emotional well-being. Indeed, pets seem to be particularly therapeutic for people with or at risk of heart disease. Several years ago, researchers studied patients in a coronary-care unit at a major hospital. All had experienced a heart attack or had severe chest pain. In the one-year follow-up period, 28% of those who did not own pets had died, as compared with only 6% of pet owners. Critics said these findings might simply reflect an association; in other words, those who felt better had taken on the responsibility of caring for a pet. Yet even when other factors like physical health and severity of heart disease were accounted for, pet ownership remained an independent predictor of survival.

SPEAKING FROM EXPERIENCE

In my house it's impossible to walk past our dog Snickers without petting him or inviting him for a walk. When he's bad, he instinctively rolls over on his back so I can rub his stomach, and immediately my anger turns to laughter. I'm convinced that, of the two of us, I'm the one who benefits more from these interactions.

Surveys have shown that most people who keep house pets describe them as members of the family. And according to Dr. Redford Williams of Duke University, contact with animals helps to restore our bond with nature. —*B.F.*

People with pets seem to handle stress better and have lower blood pressure. In addition, many behavioral scientists contend that loneliness, isolation, depression and hostility—all powerful predictors of adverse health outcomes—may be partially alleviated by the companionship of pets. Some experts believe this may stem from active involvement in the daily care of pets and from the unconditional love and acceptance that the animals offer their owners.

And finally, dogs in particular have a positive effect on health because of a second factor: walking them is great exercise!

CONTROL YOUR ANGER AND HOSTILITY 41

Anger and hostility greatly increase cardiac risk. But you can learn to gain control:

- *Exercise regularly.* This can increase the natural painkillers called endorphins, which may help to reduce anxiety and frustration.

- *Accept conflict as a normal part of life.* Conflict is part of every relationship.

- *Find your triggers.* Keep a record of your "hot buttons" and what seems to trigger them. Then work to avoid them.

- *Don't insist that everyone agree with you.* Learn to disagree without being disagreeable.

- *Think before you speak.* Make sure your own attitude isn't the root cause of your anger. Don't assume people are out to get you or to insult you intentionally. Try to understand the other person's point of view.

- *Take time out.* Deep breathing, counting to 10 or removing yourself from an adverse situation can let you calm down and regain control.

- *Do more laughing.* Try to put some humor in the situation to defuse anger before it arises.

- *Practice positive self-talk.* Angry, negative words often cause a stress response from the body. Keep a positive perspective.

- *Don't blame others.* Take full responsibility for how you feel or for what happens to you.

THE DANGERS OF ANGER

Angry young medical students are apt to become angry old doctors with heart attacks, according to a long-term study conducted by the Johns Hopkins University School of Medicine. The study found that medical students who became angry quickly when under stress were three times more likely than normal to develop premature heart disease and five times more likely than their calmer colleagues to have an earlier heart attack. Said Dr. Patricia Chang, lead author of the study, "Our findings suggest that people who have a very high level of anger, in contrast to people with little anger or none in settings of stress, are at risk for premature cardiovascular disease, even when controlling for other risk factors like family history, hypertension and diabetes."

■ *Be forgiving and patient.* Remember that most people are doing the best they can.

If you can't control your anger, you may want to consult a psychiatrist or psychologist trained in cognitive behavior therapy. This can help you change the way you look at and react to situations. Medications are also available to help stabilize mood. Talk with your physician.

TURN OFF THE TV

Thanks to television, America is perhaps the most informed nation on earth. The morning news, the evening and late-night reports—these are staples of modern life. And if you're a real news junkie, you have all-day coverage on cable.

Unfortunately, what is presented on TV is often unbalanced, not necessarily in the "to the left or right" sense, but because TV news presents hyped-up versions of today's headlines that are invariably sensationalized and negative. Instead of producing clarity, it increases anxiety. Every day we are subjected to unforgettable images of violence and destruction; the more raw the footage (the shootings at Columbine or the destruction of the World Trade Center), the more we see it. "TV news is a fear factory," says Gavin de Becker, author of *Fear Less*. "It impersonates information when, in fact, most of the time it is delivering sensation."

When natural disasters—floods, tornadoes, earthquakes—cause terrible headlines, we feel sad for the people involved. But the events don't register as viscerally as when humans commit violent acts. These stories can fray the nerves and produce overwhelming uncertainty. "People can be vicariously traumatized," says Dr. Edward Hallowell of Harvard Medical School. "With the access we now have to bad news, you can be put into a worried state each night."

But you can always turn off your TV set and get more of your news from written reporting, which tends to provide a calmer, less-hyped account of events. It also helps to concentrate on immediate surroundings—family, work, friends and community. By being involved in "real life" events, you will feel less anxious and more in control.

Step 3
Make Exercise a Habit

The Exercise Advantage

"IF EXERCISE COULD BE PACKAGED into a pill," says Dr. Robert Butler, former director of the National Institute on Aging, "it would be the single most widely prescribed and beneficial medicine in the nation." With physical activity ranking so high on the list of smart things to do for your heart and health, you'd think most Americans would have gotten the message to exercise regularly. And if you judged us by our appearance—jogging shoes, biking pants, warm-up suits—you'd think the country was in the middle of a fitness boom.

Think again. Americans do not exercise. We just buy exercise stuff. According to government data, about half of the adult population admits to being completely inactive. "The interesting thing is that 97% of people place good health as their number one priority," says Joe Cirulli of the International Health, Racquet and Sportsclub Association. "But still a lot of people don't make the connection between exercise and health."

Of those who claim to exercise, fewer than 15% do it often enough or hard enough to produce benefits. Recent studies reveal that new members of health and fitness clubs typically use these facilities less than twice per month! Says Dr. Jeffrey Koplan, former director of the Centers for Disease Control and Prevention, "Physical inactivity, along with overweight, accounts for more than 300,000 premature deaths each year in the United States." Dr. Frank Booth of the University of Missouri echoes the thought: "The impact of inactivity-related diseases is so great that we've actually created a new category called sedentary death syndrome, or SeDS."

In truth, our grandparents didn't spend time jogging or working out at the gym, but there was a lot of physical activity built naturally into their lives. Then lifestyles changed radically with the advent of automation, labor-saving devices and all the electronic paraphernalia of the information age. "What occurred," says Dr. Michael Jensen of the Mayo Clinic, "was the culmination of a century of invention and industrial development. Technology took most people out of fields and factories and plopped them behind desks. As work became more sedentary, so did workers." The elimination of physical activity in the workplace is compounded by the fact that so many suburbanites commute to their jobs. As Dr. Gregory Heath of the Centers for Disease Control and Prevention has pointed out, "The average American rides about 22 miles a day in a car, bus or other form of motorized transportation."

> ## WHAT WERE THEY THINKING?
>
> In a recent CNN poll, 39% of men and 32% of women said they believe you can be sedentary and stay healthy.

Leisure-time activities have also shifted in the direction of non-physical pursuits. In past generations, families went to the park or out to the backyard after dinner to catch or kick a ball. Nowadays, we spend our free time in front of our computers or TV sets. (According to the Consumer Electronics Manufacturers Association, there are over 400 million TV remotes in use today, or about four for every household!) And if we've run out of time because of our harried, over-committed lifestyle, we use these precious hours for chores like grocery shopping or doing the laundry. All in all, physical activity has taken a back seat in modern America.

THE BENEFITS OF EXERCISE

Many people have come to think of exercise programs as synonymous with vigorous physical activity like jogging or running, but numerous health benefits can be derived at more moderate exercise intensities, including better management of coronary risk factors. Critical for weight loss, exercise also extends longevity and increases self-esteem.

The graph below shows the theoretical relationship between health and fitness from increasing doses of exercise. It is apparent that health benefits can occur at lower levels or intensities of exercise—amounts that may not necessarily improve aerobic fitness. Such programs, however, are usually associated with an increased exercise duration, frequency, or both.

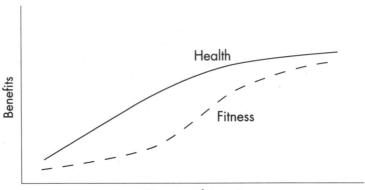

Exercise and the Heart

Exercise is particularly important because it both directly and indirectly influences all cardiac markers. Studies show that people who attain cardiovascular fitness through exercise reduce their risk of a heart attack by up to 50%—more than the best cholesterol-lowering drugs can accomplish. Conversely, physical inactivity is linked directly to an increase in cardiac risk. Says Dr. William Haskell of Stanford University Medical School, "Couch potatoes run nearly twice the risk of coronary heart disease as people who are physically active. . . . They are at the same risk for heart attacks as the obese and heavy smokers."

A number of studies have examined the relationship between regular exercise and the incidence of heart disease. One compared drivers with conductors on London's double-decker buses. While the drivers remained sedentary all day, the conductors went up and down stairs collecting tickets. The sedentary drivers had 30% more heart attacks than the active conductors. This finding was supported by a similar study at the University of Minnesota involving thousands of railroad engineers and switchmen.

Two landmark studies solidified the strong relationship between physical activity and protection from coronary heart disease. Dr. Ralph Paffenbarger and colleagues examined almost 17,000 Harvard alumni and found that the active men in the group had 35% fewer heart attacks and lived about two and a half years longer than their sedentary counterparts; moreover, fit persons who suffered heart attacks were more likely to survive. And Dr. Steven Blair of the Cooper Clinic showed that even a minimal improvement in fitness, which may be achieved by a half-hour walk daily, could reduce cardiac mortality substantially.

Newer results of the long-running Nurses' Health Study have shown that three hours of brisk walking each week or half that time spent in more vigorous exercise (such as jogging or aerobic dance) reduces the risk of heart disease by 35% to 40%. This study is important because 1) it's the first large study to look at women and exercise, and 2) it found that intensity matters, but moderate intensity can be as effective as vigorous intensity—it just takes more time. "Strolling won't do it, no matter how long you walk," says Dr. JoAnn Manson. "You have to stride out at three miles per hour or more, or 20 minutes or less per mile. But three hours of brisk walking and an hour and a half of vigorous exercise use the same amount of energy."

A program of regular exercise benefits the heart in a number of ways:

Strengthens cardiac muscle. All muscle responds to physical activity by increasing in size and strength. When exercised, cardiac muscle gets stronger and more efficient. Says Dr. Steven Blair, "If you exercise, what you get is a bigger, better, stronger pump. Exercising regularly promotes improvement in the heart's ability to transport and use oxygen. The more fit the cardiovascular system, the more oxygen the heart can deliver to the body's muscles and the more easily muscles can extract oxygen from the blood."

The ability to perform with less effort can greatly reduce strain on the heart because a strong heart can pump the same volume of blood in fewer strokes. This is how it works: an "average" resting pulse is 72 beats per minute, or 103,680 beats a day; however, if the heart becomes more efficient through regular exercise, the resting pulse might be reduced to 58 beats per minute, or just 83,520 beats

SPEAKING FROM EXPERIENCE

The Piscatella Protocol puts exercise before diet because it can positively influence what we call dietary compliance—the ability to make dietary changes once and for all. Anyone can eat healthfully for a week. The real challenge is to do it for a lifetime. Just look at the huge number of Americans who go on and off diets every year.

Starting and sticking to an exercise program is simply easier than making long-term dietary changes. Exercise is about doing something positive and enjoyable, whereas dieting is often seen as a negative experience centering on things you can't have. It's easier to establish a walking routine than it is to give up (or even cut back on) favorite foods.

But that isn't the only reason for this sequence. As the old axiom says, "Nothing breeds success like success." And success in establishing an exercise routine can provide a foundation for changing the way you eat. So, at this point in the protocol, I'd suggest putting questions of diet aside until you've learned to manage your stress and exercise regularly. Within a month or so, you can work up to walking 45 minutes, three to five times (or more) a week. Not only will this activity further help you to cope with chronic stress (which is often a trigger for mindless eating), but you'll have greater self-confidence and self-esteem. Once you feel better about yourself, you'll be ready to tackle your diet. —*J.P.*

a day. Even if a vigorous daily one-hour workout requires an increase of 5,000 heartbeats a day (as compared with rest), this still represents a net saving of 15,160 heartbeats each day.

Conditions the heart. Regular exercise can reduce the likelihood of extremely rapid heart rate resulting from physical or emotional stress. For instance, when the heart is called upon to beat faster because of a strenuous activity like shoveling snow, it may speed up to 180 beats a minute or more in an effort to supply blood to the muscles. This can strain the heart and cause plaque rupturing, which may lead to a heart attack, potentially fatal heart rhythm irregularities, or both. It's the same for emotional stress. We've all experienced near-misses with a car and that "heart in your throat" feeling. In a conditioned heart, the slowdown mechanism helps to keep racing heartbeats in check. But a deconditioned heart may refuse to slow down and instead speed up dangerously.

Boosts HDL cholesterol. High HDL is protective of cardiac health, while lower levels raise risk. Research conducted by Dr. William Haskell at Stanford University has added a regular program of exercise to that list. Some studies find that walking two miles a day, three times a week, can raise HDL by up to 10%. Greater increases may occur with more extensive exercise or in persons with low baseline values. However, you don't have to run marathons to get the HDL boost. Dr. Kenneth Cooper suggests that running no less than two miles four times a week, and no more than three miles five times a week, can have a profound impact on HDL, comparable to running even higher mileages. The key message is that moderate, regular exercise can provide optimal HDL benefit and positively influence cardiac health.

Protects the coronary arteries. The exact mechanism is not well understood, but exercise appears to reduce arterial inflammation. It may be that by helping to dissipate stress, exercise prevents hormones such as cortisol from injuring the artery wall. It may be because exercise helps to control high blood pressure, which is also a source of injury. And it may be that exercise improves the ability of the coronary arteries to dilate, increasing blood flow to the heart muscle.

Reduces blood clotting. Exercise is one of the best ways to lower your fibrinogen level and reduce the risk of easy platelet aggregation. In addition, people who exercise regularly have the ability to dissolve blood clots more easily.

Lowers blood pressure. A recent review of studies illustrated the effectiveness of exercise in reducing blood pressure, particularly in people with borderline hypertension. Approximately two-thirds of the subjects in these studies showed decreases in blood pressure, averaging about 11 and 9 points for systolic and diastolic blood pressure, respectively. Moderate-intensity training, like walking, seemed to be just as effective as higher-intensity training, and possibly even more so.

Exercise also promotes weight loss, which in turn reduces blood pressure. But exercise may trigger an independent blood-pressure-lowering mechanism as well. Studies at Boston University have found that regular exercise can cause blood vessels to dilate over time, thereby reducing resistance to flow.

Reduces stroke risk. Data from the Nurses' Health Study show that women who exercise regularly (five days a week) and moderately (30 to 60 minutes of brisk walking) have half the risk of stroke as their sedentary counterparts. Recently, this finding was echoed by researchers at the Cooper Clinic, who reported an inverse association between aerobic fitness and stroke mortality in men.

Exercise and Weight Loss

Can we say it often enough? Americans are getting fatter. As stated by Dr. William Haskell, "There has been an overemphasis on calories consumed, and too little emphasis on calories being burned. The major culprit in weight gain is lack of physical activity." This is echoed by the 1996 Surgeon General's Report on Physical Activity and Health, which cites physical inactivity as "a major cause of overweight and obesity."

According to Dr. James Hill, an internationally recognized expert on obesity, our increased reliance on technology has resulted in a positive energy balance (taking in more calories than we expend). Dr. Hill suggests that the most likely explanation for the current obesity epidemic among Americans is a continued decline in energy expenditure that has not been matched by an equivalent reduction in caloric intake.

This may surprise you, but many overweight people do not on average consume more calories than people of normal weight. Obviously, they consume sufficient calories to stay overweight, but they do not necessarily eat more than other people do. A study of San Francisco runners showed that the men consumed an average of 2,960 calories per day but weighed 20% less than inactive men their age who consumed only 2,360 calories per day; the women averaged 570 calories more per day but weighed 30% less than their inactive counterparts. Experts say that in about 70% of instances, being overweight is related to inactivity; in only about 30% is it linked primarily to increased food intake.

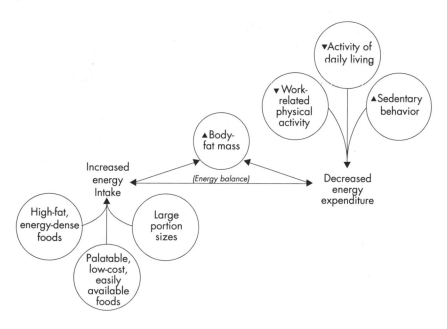

Many studies have demonstrated the effectiveness of exercise in promoting reductions in body weight and fatness. One study examined overweight women in three separate groups, each instructed to "lose" 500 calories a day. Participants in the first group, using diet alone, reduced their caloric intake by 500 calories a day but did not increase physical activity. The second group reduced calories by 250 a day but increased exercise by the same amount. The third group used exercise exclusively, leaving their eating pattern unchanged but increasing physical activity to burn 500 calories a day. The results showed that the two groups that exercised lost significantly more body fat than the group that only dieted. Moreover, the diet-only group was the only one that experienced an "unhealthy" loss of lean body mass (muscle tissue).

Your level of physical activity affects your weight for all of the following reasons:

Exercise burns calories. Walking for 30 to 45 minutes a day burns 200 to 300 calories in a 150-pound person. The chart below shows how long it would take that person to burn 250 calories in a variety of activities:

ACTIVITY	CALORIES PER HOUR	MINUTES TO BURN 250 CALORIES
Walking (4 mph)	355	42
Tennis (moderate)	425	35
Swimming (crawl, 45 yards per minute)	530	28
Downhill skiing	585	26
Handball/squash	600	25
Tennis (vigorous)	600	25
Jogging (5.5 mph)	650	23
Biking (in excess of 13 mph or up a steep hill)	850	18

Burning calories is essential to reducing body fat, which is simply a store of excess calories. When you take in more calories than are used, the excess is stored as body fat. It takes 3,500 extra calories to create a pound of body fat, and an energy expenditure of 3,500 to use up this pound of fat. Daily exercise can produce an energy deficit that requires the burning of body fat, which over time will lead to weight loss. Pretty simple, wouldn't you say?

Exercise raises metabolism. If burning calories directly were the only benefit, exercise would not be a very efficient way to lose weight. A 150-pound person has to walk for more than nine hours at a pace of four miles per hour to lose a pound. But regular exercise also raises metabolism, the *rate* at which the body burns calories, even after the activity stops. This means that even during rest the body needs to burn more calories.

How and why exercise increases metabolism is not clear, in part because metabolism is hard to measure and tends to vary greatly among people of the same weight, age and

> ### EXERCISE MAY MAKE YOU SMARTER
>
> Exercise may sharpen your ability to process information; consequently, you'll have enhanced learning capabilities. In particular, the left brain—which is responsible for logical reasoning and verbal and numerical skills—may become more efficient as a result of physical fitness.

sex. But studies show that those individuals who exercise vigorously experience a 7.5% to 28% increase in metabolic rate for up to four to eight hours after the activity is concluded. Dr. Jack Wilmore of Texas A&M University has translated this as follows: "If exercising regularly changes your metabolism even slightly, so that you burn an extra 100 calories a day, that small change can add up to 10 pounds of weight loss a year."

Exercise builds and maintains muscle. The body works like a car. The engine is muscle, which burns the fuel, which is fat. The more muscle you have, the bigger your engine, and the easier it is to burn fat. Studies show that every added pound of lean muscle burns an additional 30 to 50 calories each day.

DO IT FOR YOUR KIDS

Raised on fast food, television and computer games, kids today are more sedentary, overweight and out of shape than a generation ago. The number of seriously overweight children has more than doubled since 1980. One-third of kids have high cholesterol, two-thirds of teens fail basic fitness tests, less than 1% of children eat a balanced diet, and many, many of them are at greater risk for adult health problems at an earlier age.

Parents can change this dangerous trend by being active themselves and involving their children in physical activities. "Kids don't do what you tell them to do," says Paul F. Rosengard, director of the Sports, Play and Action Recreation for Kids (SPARK) program at San Diego State University. "They do what you do." Parents who work out regularly and who find daily physical activities to do with their children—play catch, take a walk or kick a ball—are sending a clear message: In this family, fitness and health matter.

Body fat, on the other hand, needs fewer calories to maintain itself; indeed, overweight people need one-third to one-half fewer calories to maintain their weight than do people of normal weight. This is why, of two people who eat the same amount of food, the fat person gets fatter and the lean person stays thin. "Diets can't build muscle tissue," says Georgia Kostas, a registered dietitian at the Cooper Clinic. "But exercise will." Aerobic exercise (walking, jogging, aerobics classes) combined with resistance training (light weight lifting, push-ups) will build and preserve muscle tissue.

Exercise reduces stress. People under pressure tend to overeat, binge or live on a diet of fast food and snacks. A calm, relaxed, de-stressed person is less likely to pig out on brownies or ice cream. A study at Case Western Reserve University of the dietary habits of sedentary versus physically active people clearly shows that active people choose to eat more healthful foods and fewer foods high in fat.

Exercise reduces food cravings. One reason that regular exercise leads to the intake of less high-fat foods may be that exercise promotes the production of endorphins. Acting as natural painkillers, endorphins generate a happy, self-satisfied attitude and are associated with feelings of increased self-esteem and control, which in themselves can reduce the desire for fatty foods.

Exercise and Aging

Regular physical activity is a characteristic shared by people all over the world who live long with good health. As Shay McKelvey of the American Council on Exercise says, "A good 70% of what we think of as normal aging is really a result of inactivity." In fact, large population studies found that moderate exercisers regularly lived two years longer than their inactive counterparts. "A simple rule of thumb is that, on average, for every hour of your life you spend exercising, you increase your life span by two hours," says Dr. Ralph Paffenbarger of the Stanford University School of Medicine.

A recent study of 6,000 men conducted by the VA Hospital in Palo Alto, California, found that the least fit were five times more likely to die within six years than their fitter counterparts. This led Dr. Kenneth Cooper to quip, "You're better off fat and fit than skinny and sedentary. I'm not promoting obesity. I'm just illustrating how important it is to become physically fit. Lack of exercise is deadly."

Specific age-related benefits of exercise include the following:

Strengthens bones. The aging process tends to leach minerals from bones, causing them to become so brittle and weak that even a moderate fall can produce a break or fracture. Osteoporosis is a particularly serious condition for older women. The first line of defense against this condition is to ensure an adequate intake of calcium. But exercise is also needed. Many studies show that bone, like muscle, tends to get thicker and stronger the more it is used. People who weight-train have thicker arm bones than joggers; joggers have thicker leg bones than swimmers. The critical point is that, without exercise, extra calcium in the diet may be useless in reducing the risk of osteoporosis. Taking this one step further, to keep bones strong and protect against osteoporosis, regular exercise is a necessary, even critical, need.

Maintains oxygen uptake. Our ability to process oxygen, called "maximal O_2 uptake," declines at a rate of about 1% a year after age 25, accelerating to 2% after age 55. Exercise can prevent or slow down this process.

In a study conducted at San Diego State University by Dr. Fred Kasch, participants in an adult fitness program had their oxygen-processing capabilities measured over 10 and 15 years. The study found that for those who exercised regularly, there was no difference in maximal oxygen uptake between ages 45 and 55. From the standpoint of cardiovascular performance, the two groups showed the same capabilities. In effect, exercise had retarded the aging process for the older group.

Maintains muscle strength. Other studies have demonstrated that the average person loses about 15% of muscle strength between ages 45 and 65. But a study by Dr. Herbert deVries at the University of Southern California found that this erosion was due to inactivity, not aging. People who continued to exercise in their senior years experienced no decrease in muscle strength through age 60.

EXERCISE CURES GRUMPINESS

In a review of 32 studies on elderly people, investigators found that regular exercise consistently promoted a positive outlook and mood. Says Dr. Shawn Arent of Arizona State University, "We've known that exercise fights disease. Now we know that activity makes older people just plain happy." Studies show that low-intensity exercise produces the greatest mood improvements and that the combination of aerobic exercise and strength training elevates mood to a greater extent than does aerobic exercise alone.

A BALANCED EXERCISE PROGRAM

While there has long been agreement that regular exercise is beneficial, questions arise about what types of exercise are most effective, how hard you need to work out and how often an exercise should be performed. Most experts recommend a balanced program that includes four components:

■ *Daily physical activity* as part of life's routine.

■ *Aerobic exercise* to promote cardiovascular endurance and fat burning.

■ *Weight training* for building strength and reducing demands on the heart.

■ *Flexibility exercises (stretching)* to prevent injury and allow aerobic exercise and weight training to be more enjoyable.

Daily Physical Activity

In 1996, the surgeon general issued guidelines to encourage people to be physically active every day, or on most days, for a minimum of 30 minutes. Regular moderate-intensity activities—walking up stairs, doing errands on foot, walking your dog, parking at the far end of the lot, gardening, raking leaves, washing the car and doing household chores—were suggested.

"In essence, the surgeon general said to look for opportunities in daily life to be physically active for a half-hour or more," says Dr. James Sallis of San Diego State University. "One big difference from past recommendations is that these activities do not have to be continuous. It can be 5 minutes here, 10 minutes there; as long as it adds up to at least 30 minutes and is of mild-to-moderate intensity, it meets the prescription." In other words, the deskbound executive who takes a lunch-hour jog three days a week may not be better off than the person who performs periodic moderate-intensity activity throughout the day on most days of the week.

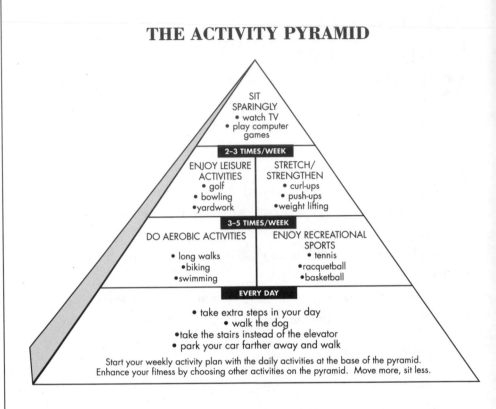

THE ACTIVITY PYRAMID

SIT
SPARINGLY
• watch TV
• play computer
games

2–3 TIMES/WEEK

ENJOY LEISURE
ACTIVITIES
• golf
• bowling
•yardwork

STRETCH/
STRENGTHEN
• curl-ups
• push-ups
•weight lifting

3–5 TIMES/WEEK

DO AEROBIC ACTIVITIES
• long walks
•biking
•swimming

ENJOY RECREATIONAL
SPORTS
• tennis
•racquetball
•basketball

EVERY DAY

• take extra steps in your day
• walk the dog
•take the stairs instead of the elevator
• park your car farther away and walk

Start your weekly activity plan with the daily activities at the base of the pyramid.
Enhance your fitness by choosing other activities on the pyramid. Move more, sit less.

Increased daily physical activity is *key* to cardiac health. Two recent studies in the *Journal of the American Medical Association* showed that doing moderate-intensity activities for 30 minutes daily is as effective in the long run at lowering body fat, improving blood pressure and boosting aerobic fitness in sedentary people as doing more traditional, structured exercise three to five days a week. Morever, such activities are great for dissipating daily stress. This is not to suggest that daily physical activity should replace more traditional workouts, but rather that it is a wonderful complement to any health and fitness program.

The Activity Pyramid above may help you visualize what we mean. Starting at the base of the pyramid, you'll see that you should accumulate at least 30 minutes of moderate-intensity activity on most and preferably all days of the week. The next tier of the pyramid represents structured aerobic activities and/or recreational sports, which you should be doing three to five days each week. Complementary leisure-time activities, such as playing golf, bowling or working in the yard, as well as calisthenics and weight training, are recommended in the third tier, at the lesser frequency of two to three days a week.

Collectively, the activities listed in the first three tiers should reduce the amount of non-exercise time at the top of the pyramid, that is, time spent on sedentary activities such as watching television or playing computer games.

Aerobic Exercise

As illustrated in the pyramid on page 168, vigorous, longer-lasting exercise—three or more sessions per week of aerobic activity—is required in order to attain cardiovascular fitness. Indeed, according to Dr. Paul Williams, an exercise expert at the Lawrence Berkeley Laboratory, increased fitness has nearly twice the impact on reducing your risk of heart disease as does merely increasing your daily physical activity.

Aerobic exercise, involving continuous, rhythmic movement of the large muscle groups, conditions your heart, lungs and vascular system, and promotes your body's ability to burn fat by causing your heart and lungs to process oxygen at a steady rate over a sufficient period of time. Some of the best examples of aerobic activities are listed below:

Brisk (power) walking	Jogging
Cycling (stationary and spinning)	Running in place
Skipping rope	Swimming
Aerobic dancing (high-impact, step)	Cross-country skiing (indoor)
Rowing (indoor)	Stair stepping
Stair climbing	Elliptical exercise

Other activities can be considered aerobic if they're done at a vigorous pace and continuously maintained for the proper duration. These include:

Basketball	Handball/squash/racquetball
Hiking	Skating (ice/roller/in-line)
Soccer	Rowing (outdoor)
Tennis (singles)	Aerobic dancing (medium-
Jumping rope	impact)
Cycling (outdoor)	Cross-country skiing (outdoor)

In order to be classified as aerobic, an activity must meet the F.I.T. criterion: *frequency, intensity* and *time.* How often, how hard, how long—these are the three critical elements.

F = Frequency. Most health professionals recommend an aerobic program of at least three or four days a week. This takes into account the guidelines of the American College of Sports Medicine:

- Fitness is *improved* if you exercise more than three days a week.
- Fitness is *maintained* if you exercise three days a week.
- Fitness is *lost* if you exercise less than three days a week.

Exercising every other day is very effective for cardiovascular conditioning. (People who need to lose weight may need to exercise daily.) However, anyone who exercises more than four days a week should be certain to alternate high-impact activities with non-jarring ones such as brisk walking and swimming, to minimize strain and other injuries.

People who exercise vigorously but infrequently have an increased risk of heart attack. One study found that almost 50% of heart attack deaths while exercising occurred among people who exercised once a week or less. Dr. Gerald Fletcher of the Mayo Clinic in Jacksonville, Florida, warns, "You can't 'catch up' with exercise by cramming a week's worth of exertion into one day."

I = Intensity. "Intensity plays a role in making people fitter and healthier," says Dr. Miriam Nelson, author of *Strong Women Stay Slim.*

"How hard you exercise is important because of the relationship between intensity on one hand, and cardiovascular fitness and weight control on the other." Echoes YMCA exercise expert Carol Rhodes, "You can enjoy light exercise such as golf and casual walking; just don't confuse these activities with those designed for cardiovascular benefit. Light exercise simply doesn't stress the heart muscle sufficiently to improve cardiac fitness, and it doesn't necessarily lead to weight loss. In fact, that's one of the prime reasons people give up. They exercise at too low an intensity, don't get the results, and quit. You have to raise your heart rate to get benefits."

Research shows that the most effective exercise is done at a sustained moderate-to-vigorous pace. If you're walking, make certain that you keep up a "brisk walk"—that your stride is aggressive, your arms are pumping and you may even break a sweat on your upper lip. Brisk walking means covering three and a half to four miles in an hour, certainly not a leisurely pace.

> ### MYTH ALERT! SWEATING DOES *NOT* GET YOU IN SHAPE
>
> There is no downside to being comfortably cool while you're working out; in fact, it's an absolute disadvantage to be uncomfortably warm. Sweating merely provides a way to get rid of body heat. It does nothing to improve your fitness.

While matching your pace to an effective level of intensity, do not subscribe to the "no pain, no gain" school of exercise. Unless you're a competitive athlete, "going for the burn" may cause you to exercise too hard or too fast, which can lead to injury or exhaustion. Either way, you get nowhere.

But how to know what's the best pace for you—that "in between" place we call the training zone? One way depends on monitoring your heart rate during the activity by checking your pulse. (Physicians have traditionally measured heart rate by timing the pulse at the wrist, on the thumb side. The neck pulse is easier to find, but you have to remember not to press too hard, as this may produce a marked slowing of the heart rate and an underestimation of the true exercise intensity.)

Practice taking your pulse when you're not exercising. If you have difficulty finding it, try putting your hand over your heart and counting the beats. Once you've found your pulse, count it for 10 seconds. Be sure to count the first beat as zero. Then multiply the count by six to calculate your pulse for one minute.

Once you're comfortable taking your pulse, you should determine your maximal heart rate, a limit on how fast the heart is capable of beating during exercising to exhaustion. Ideally, it should be measured during a medically supervised exercise stress test; however, a widely accepted formula is also used:

$$220 - \text{your age in years} = \text{maximal heart rate}$$

THE TALK TEST

If your forehead feels dewed but you can still carry on a conversation with a fellow exerciser, your pace is probably just about right. If you can't exercise and carry on a conversation at the same time, you're probably exercising too strenuously.

Maximal heart rate is largely determined by age as opposed to physical fitness. This means a fit 40-year-old will have an estimated maximal heart rate of 180, while that of a sedentary 24-year-old will be 196. The 40-year-old may be more fit, but being older he'll have a lower maximal heart rate.

You never want to exercise at your maximal heart rate, so the next step is figuring out what your actual training zone should be. The American Heart Association defines it as being between 70% and 85% of maximal heart rate. The estimated target heart rate zone for a 50-year-old, for instance, is between 119 (70%) and 145 (85%) beats per minute.

The table on page 173 offers a quick way to estimate maximal heart rate and target heart rate zone by age group. Because of the variability in maximal heart rate, individual ranges may differ from 10 to 20 beats per minute, or more. An exercise stress test determines your true maximal heart rate—another good reason to see your doctor before starting an exercise program.

HEARTBEATS PER MINUTE

AGE	ESTIMATED MAXIMAL HEART RATE	ESTIMATED TRAINING HEART RATE ZONE
20	200	140 to 170
25	195	137 to 166
30	190	133 to 162
35	185	130 to 157
40	180	126 to 153
45	175	123 to 149
50	170	119 to 145
55	165	116 to 140
60	160	112 to 136
65	155	109 to 132
70	150	105 to 128
75	145	102 to 123
80	140	98 to 119

Once you've determined the parameters of your training zone, use them as a guideline for how hard you should be exercising. Wait until you're 5 or 10 minutes into the exercise, then stop and locate your pulse on the side of your neck or on the thumb side of your wrist. If your pulse rate is below the lower training heart rate limit, you probably need to increase effort; if it's above, you can ease off a bit. An alternative way to determine your exercise heart rate is to use an accurate heart rate monitor to track exercise intensity.

There is no magic to being at the upper end of the zone. In fact, musculoskeletal and cardiovascular complications are more likely to occur at such intensities. Research shows that less intensive activities such as low-impact aerobics are highly effective. Also, remember that your training heart rate, which is geared to age, does not change as you lose weight and get in better shape. What will change is the amount of effort needed to reach the zone. People who are overweight and out of shape have an easier time reaching it than those who are slimmer and in shape. As level of fitness improves, the pace or work-load may have to be increased for the activity to achieve the appropriate heart rate range.

The disadvantage of this approach to estimating your training zone is that the formula doesn't always reflect how hard you are working aerobically. There are variations in age-predicted maximal heart rate, usually plus or minus 10 beats per minute. In addition, other factors such as extremes in environmental conditions (e.g., hot, humid weather) or caffeine consumption can throw off results. Even greater errors in estimation can occur in persons with heart disease (all of whom should check with their doctor about an appropriate exercise heart rate), or in those taking certain cardiac medications (such as beta-blockers).

How Much Is Enough?

Dr. Barbara Ainsworth, an exercise researcher at the University of South Carolina, suggests thinking of exercise in terms of a U-shaped curve. The worst place to be is at the start of the curve, doing nothing. As you begin exercising, you move down the curve and start getting some of the health benefits. The base of the curve represents a wide range of physical activity, and added health benefits can come from increased activity. But doing too much exercise does not produce extra benefits. Indeed, as you move back up the curve on the opposite side, too much exercise can be harmful. Here's a quick guide:

■ Cardiovascular benefits are apparent once you expend more than 500 calories a week in exercise.

■ Optimal improvements generally occur when you expend between 2,000 and 3,500 calories a week.

■ When more than 3,500 calories a week are burned in exercise, benefits may taper off and the incidence of injury may increase disproportionately.

An alternative way to monitor your exercise intensity is to use the Rating of Perceived Exertion scale, or the Borg RPE scale. Based on the simple concept that the mind is an excellent judge of how much work the body is doing, the RPE scale grades exercise levels based on the individual's overall feeling of effort and physical fatigue, from rest (6) to maximal exertion (20). These ratings correspond well with certain metabolic responses to exercise, such as heart rate and oxygen consumption.

BORG RPE SCALE	
6	No exertion at all
7	Extremely light
8	
9	Very light
10	
11	Light
12	
13	Somewhat hard
14	
15	Hard (heavy)
16	
17	Very hard
18	
19	Extremely hard
20	

Here's how to use it. After you've been exercising for 5 or 10 minutes, ask yourself the question "How hard am I working?" If it feels "extremely light" or "very light," the intensity is probably too low to be effective. You'll need to increase the level of intensity to reach your training zone. Conversely, if your response is "very hard" or "extremely hard," you are probably working too vigorously. Your breathing is labored and you have difficulty sustaining the activity. You should back off a bit on your effort. The training zone is generally described as a perception of intensity somewhere between "light" and "hard"—ideally, "somewhat hard." At this level of intensity you are neither breathing too easily nor out of breath. Instead, your oxygen consumption matches the activity, allowing you to sustain it over a period of time.

T = Time. You need to exercise vigorously in your training zone for a minimum of 20 continuous minutes in order to promote cardiovascular health and weight control. *This is only a minimum* and may not be a long enough time for you to achieve your cardiovascular goals. An ideal duration would be 30 to 45 minutes, depending on the type of activity.

According to the American College of Sports Medicine, moderate-intensity exercise in 10-minute increments can provide appreciable benefit for general health as long as it adds up to at least 30 minutes per day of physical activity. The Nurses' Health Study as well as other studies found that shorter exercise bouts provide some cardiovascular benefit as well; however, most cardiac experts still recommend a continuous session of vigorous exercise for at least 20 minutes for cardiovascular benefit.

MYTH ALERT! SUGAR DOES *NOT* RAISE YOUR ENERGY LEVEL

Eating sugar before physical activity can actually do more harm than good, driving the body's sugar into storage. Extra sugar doesn't give extra energy. Think of it as filling up your gas tank to drive your car around the block. It's just not necessary.

Time spent exercising is particularly important for weight control. Nonstop exercise for at least 20 minutes helps to rev up metabolism and increase fat-burning. During the first few minutes of exercise, glucose is the primary fuel. As the activity continues past that point, utilization of body fat increases, especially at mild to moderate intensities. Thus, the more time spent in continuous aerobic exercise, the greater the opportunity to burn body fat.

Also, be sure to leave enough time in your schedule for warm-up and cool-down, such as stretching or the same aerobic activity done at a lower intensity. For example, if you use brisk walking during the endurance phase, you should conclude the warm-up period with slow walking. Similarly, brisk walking serves as an ideal warm-up for jogging. These warm-up and cool-down activities are *not* part of the 20-minute duration.

Weight Training

For years, the American Heart Association counseled people with heart disease to stay away from weight training (also called resistance exercise). No longer. The AHA now acknowledges that weight training builds and tones muscles, increases the ability to burn body fat and strengthens bones. It reduces the heart rate and blood pressure responses to manual labor, thus decreasing the demands on the heart during daily activities such as carrying groceries or lifting moderate-to-heavy objects. It helps to maintain or increase lean body mass, which means that the body burns more calories throughout the day. It increases resting metabolic rate (particularly in men), which also allows muscles to burn extra calories all day. (Some studies suggest that you can increase your metabolic rate by at least 7% after six months of weight training. For a person consuming 2,000 calories a day, that represents an additional 140 calories burned each day. At that rate, you would lose over seven pounds of fat in six months.)

Before you start a weight training program, get an O.K. from your doctor. This is particularly important if you have coronary heart disease, high blood pressure, heart valve problems, congestive heart failure, a weight problem or a strong family history of heart disease.

A good weight training program includes exercises for every major muscle group, including arms, chest, back, legs and abdomen. Free weights, machines, rubber tubing and calisthenics are effective. Do not overlook your own body for resistance. Push-ups and leg raises are excellent.

Be sure to get good instruction before you start your program. Look for an instructor who has been certified by the American College of Sports Medicine, the American Council on Exercise or the National Strength and Conditioning Association.

> ## MYTH ALERT! EVEN MARATHON RUNNERS ARE NOT IMMUNE TO HEART DISEASE
>
> One sad but notable example: the author and distance runner Jim Fixx, who died of a heart attack while jogging one cold winter morning in Vermont. Still, physically active people are at a lower overall risk. Above all, exercise needs to be balanced with healthy eating, stress management and no smoking to create a lifestyle package more likely to ward off, stabilize and possibly even reverse coronary disease.

SAFETY FIRST

Compared with risk at other times, the risk of cardiovascular complications appears to increase transiently during vigorous physical exertion. This seems to be particularly true among infrequent exercisers or occasional weekend athletes with known or hidden heart disease who exercise too strenuously. On the other hand, the *net effect* of regular physical activity is a lower overall risk of dying from cardiovascular disease.

■ Regular exercise seems to reduce the risk of an exertion-related fatal cardiovascular event, such as a heart attack while jogging.

■ If you're an infrequent exerciser, stick with a moderate-intensity activity such as walking.

■ Novice exercisers should consider appropriate medical screening before starting. This is critical for those with major coronary risk factors, signs or symptoms of heart disease, or people with known heart, lung or metabolic disease.

Recommendations to reduce the incidence of strains, sprains and cardiovascular complications during exercise programs include:

■ *Obtain good supervision.* Competent exercise professionals can reduce the rate of exercise-related injuries or complications.

■ *Warm up and cool down.* Avoid sudden strenuous exertion and abrupt cessation of vigorous exercise.

■ *Start gradually.* If you plan to take up jogging, start with a brisk walking program and gradually progress to slow jogging over several weeks. Give yourself time to build up a tolerance to exercise. Don't expect to walk briskly for an hour your first day out.

■ *Exercise regularly.* Don't try to cram all your exercise into one day per week.

■ *Avoid high-intensity activity.* As a general rule, exercise should feel no more than "somewhat hard." Remember, if you can't carry on a conversation during exercise, you're probably working too hard.

The instructor should know your goals and personalize the program based on your needs. It is also important to learn how to perform the exercises effectively. Form is critical to your success, as is proper breathing (exhale when you lift).

Progress in strength training depends on the number of times a week you train, the amount of weight you lift and the number of times you lift it. Although the traditional routine involved performing each exercise three times (three sets of 10 repetitions per set), a recent review has shown that one set provides nearly the same improvement in muscular strength and endurance. Consequently, for the average person beginning a strength training regimen, single-set programs performed a minimum of two times per week are recommended over multiple-set programs.

Such regimens should include 8 to 10 different exercises at a load that permits 8 to 12 repetitions per set for healthy, sedentary adults or 10 to 15 repetitions per set for cardiac patients and for healthy individuals who are older than 50 years of age. The American College of Sports Medicine recommends biceps curls, triceps extensions, chest presses, shoulder presses, pull-downs, abdominal crunches, lower-back extensions, quadriceps extensions, leg curls and calf raises.

Flexibility Exercises

Stretching, the fourth component of a balanced exercise program, is essential for maintaining (or improving) your joint range of motion and function and for enhancing muscular performance. Without a specific program to maintain flexibility, many middle-aged and older adults become hampered by stiffness in the hamstrings, shoulders and back.

It's simple to do: starting slowly, gently stretch the muscles of each major muscle group for about 10 to 30 seconds to the point of mild discomfort. At least four repetitions per muscle group should be performed a minimum of two to three days per week. Be sure to keep your breathing rhythmic and steady. Make certain not to bounce. At no time should you feel pain.

Stretching (as well as activities that incorporate stretching, such as yoga and tai chi) is a great way to get your muscles ready for more strenuous exercise. But it has other benefits as well. Over time, stretching can keep you from losing flexibility (a consequence of aging) and may even make you more flexible. Increased flexibility reduces the risk of musculoskeletal injury from varied activities and can help you to perform exercise more efficiently.

Many good books, audiotapes and videotapes are available on stretching, yoga and tai chi. In addition, classes are often offered at YM/YWCAs and other community centers.

IT'S NEVER TOO LATE

A provocative study by Dr. Benjamin Levine and associates at the University of Texas Southwestern Medical Center suggests that cardiovascular fitness can be reclaimed. Doctors worked with a small group of men who were originally studied 30 years ago. At that time, these men demonstrated an above-average level of cardiovascular fitness. But, not surprisingly, the men became less physically active over time. Their cardiovascular fitness eroded and their body fatness increased.

For six months, researchers had them exercise in a training routine that included walking, jogging and cycling. By the end of the study, they were exercising pretty rigorously for about 4.5 hours a week. Measurement of their aerobic capacity showed that 100% of the cardiovascular decline that had taken place over 30 years had been reversed. The men returned to the same level of cardiovascular fitness they had three decades earlier!

"The message is that no matter what your age, it's your current fitness level, not your past fitness level, that really dictates how fit you are," says Miriam Nelson, Ph.D., an exercise physiologist at Tufts University.

How to Burn 150 Extra Calories a Day*

ACTIVITY	MINUTES
Washing/waxing car	45 to 60
Washing windows/floors	45 to 60
Volleyball	45
Touch football	30 to 45
Gardening	30 to 45
Walking 1¾ miles (20 minutes/mile)	35
Bicycling 5 miles	30
Dancing (fast)	30
Pushing a stroller 1.5 miles	30
Raking leaves	30
Walking 2 miles (15 minutes/mile)	30
Water aerobics	30
Swimming laps	20
Basketball	15 to 20
Jumping rope	15
Running 1.5 miles (10 minutes/mile)	15
Shoveling snow	15
Stair walking	15

*These values are estimates for a 154-pound person.

Time for Action

HARVARD RESEARCHER DR. JOANN MANSON once observed, "If there were a magic potion that could make you feel great and could cut your risk of getting heart disease, cancer and diabetes in half, people would be willing to spend hundreds, even thousands, of dollars for it." And then she dropped the other shoe: "But it's already available and virtually free—regular physical activity." The fact is, most of us know that exercise is good for us. If you want proof, just look at the soaring sales of exercise equipment and gym memberships every January. So why is it that, according to Dr. William C. Roberts, editor of the *American Journal of Cardiology*, New Year's commitments to lose weight and get in shape begin to waver after only two weeks?

Some of the reasons are understandable. An exercise program is voluntary and time-consuming. Additionally, not all the health benefits of exercise are readily apparent: a definite demotivator. But somehow—and this is the fact we ought to be focusing on— almost half the people who start an exercise program stick with it. What's their secret? Well, it's not just willpower, which is why we devote the rest of this section to tips for incorporating physical activity into your daily routine and making it an integral part of your lifestyle. Pick the Heart Savers that make the most sense for you, and then stick with them for 90 days.

Just three months: that's all you'll need to get hooked on exercise for a lifetime.

43 DON'T WAIT TILL WEDNESDAY

Right about now you're probably muttering, "How in the world do they ever expect me to fit all these 'things' into my day?" And it's true—finding the time for relaxation, meditation, exercise and eating right may feel like an insurmountable task all by itself. Part of the solution is a sense of perspective. Think about this: there are plenty of people who had no time to exercise on Monday, had a heart attack on Tuesday and found time to exercise on Wednesday.

■ *Imagine yourself healthy and fit.* Becoming healthy is a journey, not a one-time experience. Set the tone for your journey before you pack your bag. Take the time to think about the benefits of change. We know one woman who lost 100 pounds—20 pounds five different times! She had resolve, that's for sure, but she didn't have a clear picture of what it would mean to change her bad habits *forever.* "When I saw losing weight as a problem, I failed," she recalls. "Then one day my

> ## Q & A
>
> Exercise critics often ask the question "Fitness for what, exactly?"
> Exercise enthusiasts respond, "Fitness for life!"

daughter said she was afraid my weight would make me get sick and die. That's when I saw weight loss as an opportunity for better health, with a real benefit for both of us." Next time out she lost 20 pounds and kept them off.

■ *Define your goals.* Do you want to be less anxious? Lose weight? Increase your stamina? Remember, this is a journey. If you don't know where you're going, you won't know if you're on the right road, let alone if you've arrived. Likewise, be specific—"I'm going to lose 20 pounds," not "I'm going to lose some weight"—and realistic about how long it will take to reach your destination. If you expect to lose 20 pounds in two weeks, you won't get there.

■ *Slow down.* The problem for most people is that they want to make all the healthy changes at once. Right now. That's overwhelming and a recipe for failure. The fact is that you *do* have to devote a lot of time to staying healthy, but when you think of the change as evolutionary rather than revolutionary, your chances for success go way up. Walk slowly today and know that tomorrow you can walk more briskly.

■ *Plan for progress.* Take at least a week to think about your program *before you do anything.* Perhaps you need to manage stress. Choose a handful of stress-management Heart Savers—maybe keeping a journal, practicing deep breathing, doing yoga. Outline your plan. Will you set aside 10 minutes for journaling before you go to bed at night? Five minutes right after lunch for deep breathing? A yoga class that meets twice a week? Put your plan into action for two or three weeks before deciding how to refine your stress management program.

Meanwhile, you can start planning your exercise routine. Read through the exercise Heart Savers and outline a plan: get up earlier so you can walk with a friend for 30 minutes three mornings a week; take the stairs at work; make an appointment to work with a weight-training instructor. When you're ready, put the plan into action, again taking the time to live with it before you figure out how to refine it.

You get the picture. Strive for balance. Focus on successes—and be proud of yourself.

 ## TAKE THE MIRROR TEST

Think about your present activity level for just a moment. Then think about how it would feel (and may have felt in the past) to be strong and flexible, to have endurance, to be confident in your physical abilities. As one physical therapist counsels, "Forget the sophisticated tests. Just take off your clothes and stand in front of a mirror. Don't judge and don't feel guilty. Simply make an honest assessment of where you are now."

Are you carrying a few more pounds than you should? Have you lost muscle tone? Now visualize yourself as you would like to be: stronger, leaner, healthier. Seeing where you are today can lead to a fitness vision of where you want to be in the future.

JUST DO IT!

A program of regular exercise starts with a conscious decision. Make the decision now to "just do it." Commit it to paper: write down what you want to accomplish, which exercises you plan on doing to meet your goal and when you'll do them.

The form of exercise is not important. Do something you enjoy—walk, bike, swim, go to an aerobics class or use an exercise machine. As Confucius taught, "It does not matter how slowly you go, so long as you do not stop."

GET AN O.K. FROM YOUR DOCTOR

Too often people use a concern about a medical condition as an excuse not to exercise. If you're a man over 45 or a woman over 55, ask your doctor for a checkup, including an exercise stress test. This is particularly important for people at increased risk for heart disease (those with symptoms of heart disease and/or two or more major risk markers, such as high blood pressure, elevated cholesterol, cigarette smoking, overweight or sedentary lifestyle) and those with known heart, lung or metabolic disease, especially when vigorous exercise is contemplated. Your doctor can help you decide which exercise is best for you and monitor your progress over time.

START SLOW AND STEADY

Don't expect to go overnight from reclining in a BarcaLounger to running road races. It takes a minimum of six to eight weeks, depending on age and condition, to begin to notice a difference. Another good rule of thumb according to Dr. Steve Van Camp, a cardiologist in San Diego and a past president of the American College of Sports Medicine, is that it takes about one month to get in shape for every year you've been out of shape.

If you push yourself too hard at the beginning, you can injure yourself. And nothing takes the steam out of an exercise program faster than muscle soreness and stiffness, strains and sprains. Start by picking an exercise of light-to-moderate intensity such as walking. A pace of two to four miles per hour works fine. Begin to integrate two or three 15-minute workout intervals into your day. Once your body gets used to this routine, gradually increase your workout time. Build slowly and steadily to a 45-minute walk, four or five times a week.

Always pay attention to how you feel. Be alert to chest pain, unusual shortness of breath, heart palpitations (irregular or racing pulse rate) and lightheadedness. If any such symptoms occur, discontinue training and seek medical attention.

48 HAVE FUN

The best exercise is one you'll keep doing. There are hundreds of activities to try—ballroom dancing, rowing, martial arts, skating, handball, volleyball . . . even playing Frisbee. Select an activity that's enjoyable, not a punishment. Think about your personality: are you an extrovert who loves group activities or an introvert who needs time alone to recharge your batteries? Or you may be an introvert who wants to socialize more or an extrovert who needs more time alone. Do whatever sport or exercise you love. Don't force yourself to jog if you dread it. Advises Dr. Carl Foster of the University of Wisconsin at La Crosse, "Try different forms of exercise until you find something you like well enough that you'd do it even if it weren't for your health."

49 WORK TOWARD A GOAL

If cardiovascular fitness is your goal, an aerobic workout three or four times a week is generally effective. But if weight loss is your primary aim, it takes more. Plan to do some type of aerobic exercise—walking, jogging, stationary bike, aerobic dancing—on a daily basis. Then look for ways to incorporate a little "extra" into your days: shooting hoops with your kids, dancing to the radio, taking the stairs or parking the car farther away from the store when shopping.

50 TAKE TIME TO STRETCH

Stretching may not be as flashy as aerobics or strength training, but it's an important part of a complete exercise program. By stretching major muscle groups, especially those involved in whatever exercise you're doing, you'll maintain flexibility while preventing injuries.

Until recently, exercise experts recommended stretching before and after a workout. But that's changed. Instead of doing a warm-up stretch when your muscles are cold, the experts now say you should simply ease into your exercise gradually. If you're going to take a run or a brisk walk, start slowly and gently, increasing your pace only after your muscles are warmed up. It still makes good sense to stretch *after* your workout, when your muscles are warm, to reduce the risk of injury.

But stretching does more than end a workout; it keeps you flexible. After age 30, the body's connective tissues—the muscles, tendons and ligaments—start to shorten, tighten and lose elasticity. Stretching can help you stay limber and improve your range of motion by actually lengthening muscles and tendons. As a result, it can offset age-related stiffness, improve athletic performance and optimize functional movement in daily life. Stretching makes everything easier, from bending to tie your shoes to getting out of a chair or car to pulling up a zipper in the back of a dress.

The American College of Sports Medicine recommends making flexibility training a priority in your exercise program. While brief stretching bouts are better than nothing, to get maximum flexibility benefits you'll have to stretch the major muscle groups two to three days a week.

JOIN A GROUP

A commitment to others strengthens resolve. Let's suppose you've made a decision to walk at seven A.M. If you're doing it by yourself, you might just turn over when the alarm goes off, grab some extra sleep and miss your walk. But if you've made a pact to walk with two friends, chances are you'll get up in time to meet them. Joining an aerobic dance class or doing weight training with a friend can also be more fun than going it alone. And you'll find that social interaction often provides the incentive needed for those times when your interest sags.

52 MAKE A CONTRACT

Commit yourself *in writing* to exercise for six weeks—not an eternity but just long enough to see some results. Plan your activities a week or two in advance. What exercises will you do? Where and with whom? Then mark your schedule on a calendar as if it were a doctor's appointment. Try to exercise at the same time each day so that you develop a routine.

Be careful not to procrastinate by searching for the "right" time. In fact, any time you can and will exercise is the right time—it's up to you, your schedule, your interests and, some would say, your biorhythms. If you're a "morning person" who can't wait to get going, there are many advantages to early morning exercise: it makes you more alert, provides a sense of control that lasts all day and is usually easier to schedule. But not everyone is a morning person. Some people prefer to do their exercise at noon because it helps them dissipate morning stress and control luncheon appetite. People who exercise before dinner often like the feeling of tension release.

SPEAKING FROM EXPERIENCE

The act of writing something down makes it real. After my bypass surgery, when I got started on a program of exercise, it was a bit hit-and-miss. Some days I'd have the time and do it. Some days I wouldn't. But exercise was too important to my rehabilitation to treat so casually. I needed to make it a priority. What I did was take my calendar and write at the top of it, "I will exercise every morning." That was a contract with myself. Then I marked out one hour a day in the morning as a meeting with "Mr. Nike." Everything else in my life worked around that appointment, those hours of blocked time. Thanks to "Mr. Nike," I was able to develop the exercise habit. But it started with a written contract with myself. —*J.P.*

KEEP AN EXERCISE JOURNAL 53

Positive feedback reinforces behavior, which is why keeping an exercise journal (or a computer record) is so valuable. As you watch your minutes and miles build, you'll feel enormously satisfied. A notebook will also keep you honest; in the absence of a written record, people often take credit for more exercise than they actually do.

SAMPLE EXERCISE LOG

GOAL: Exercise 4 days a week

DATE	TYPE OF EXERCISE	HOW LONG?	HOW FAR?
4/1	Walking	45 minutes	3 miles
4/3	Aerobics class	45 minutes	
4/4	Walking	45 minutes	3 miles
4/6	Spinning class	45 minutes	
4/7	Walking	45 minutes	3 miles

Pick a goal for yourself. Write it down so that you see it every day. Perhaps it's walking a cumulative 50 miles in a month. As you get closer to your goal, you'll feel a renewed commitment. When you reach it, reward yourself with theater tickets or a new pair of exercise shoes. Then create a new goal and go after it.

DON'T BE A FOOL FOR FRAUDS 54

Sales of quick-fix weight-loss gadgets and gimmicks have skyrocketed, while sales of diet pills and supplements rose from $168 million in 1996 to $782 million in 2000. Don't be a sucker, particularly when so many of these products are potentially dangerous.

■ *Spot reducing.* Basing their claims on the false notion that it's possible to "burn off" fat from a particular part of the body, deceptive advertisers promise that you can "take inches off your waist, thighs or buttocks without vigorous exercise or dieting and in just minutes a day." Think about it: if spot reducing worked, people who chew gum would have skinny faces!

■ *Effortless exercise.* Several years ago, researchers examined the weight-reducing claims made for mechanical vibrating belts. One study showed that the average caloric cost of a 15-minute period of abdominal vibration was 11 calories more than an equivalent period of seated rest (or about $\frac{1}{23}$ of an ounce of fat). The investigators concluded, "The vibrator is not to be taken seriously as a device to assist in fat reduction or shifting of fat deposits within the body."

■ *Weight-reducing clothing.* Special weight-reducing garments rely on dehydration and tissue compression. Measurements may be temporarily reduced, but these losses are exclusively water weight.

■ *Electrical muscle stimulators.* Ads for some electric muscle stimulators say they provide the same effects as "3,000 sit-ups or 10 miles of jogging while lying flat on your back." Some of these units have a legitimate purpose in physical therapy; nonetheless, the Food and Drug Administration considers muscle stimulators that are promoted or used for "body shaping and contouring" to be misbranded and fraudulent. In addition, these devices have been known to burn the skin and deliver electric shocks. They can be especially hazardous to pregnant women, heart patients with pacemakers and people who have epilepsy.

55 WALK BRISKLY

Brisk walking, also called "power walking," is one of the easiest and most effective aerobic activities. It can be done anywhere, virtually by anyone, and takes no great expertise. In addition, the chance of injury is low. Walking does not jar joints or strain muscles as much as jogging does. And if you allow for gradual conditioning, walking is especially appropriate for novice exercisers and overweight people.

A generally accepted standard for cardiovascular and weight-control benefits is 12 miles of brisk walking per week. This equates to four 45-minute walks per week of three miles each. If you need to lose a great deal of weight, you might consider a more frequent schedule.

GET THE MOST OUT OF WALKING

■ *Keep up a good pace.* Every minute you shave off your time helps. A 150-pound person, walking for one hour at a brisk pace of four miles per hour four days a week, will, when compared with someone walking at a moderate pace of three miles per hour, burn enough extra calories to lose an extra six pounds in a year.

■ *Use good technique.* Bend your arms at a 90° angle and swing them back and forth, not side to side. The palms of your hands should not swing lower than your hips or higher than your sternum. Arms should stay close to the torso. Pumping your arms to chest level with each stride has the effect of propelling your body forward (rather than side to side), elevating your heart rate and making the pace aerobic. It's not necessary or even wise to hold or swing hand weights, which can cause arm or shoulder soreness or injury, but your arms should be fully engaged if you want to lose weight and attain cardiovascular fitness.

■ *Practice interval training.* Walk at your normal brisk pace for five minutes, then push it a little harder for the next five, then revert to your normal pace. Or walk using telephone poles (or blocks or fire hydrants) as your guide—go faster from one pole to the next, then ease up to the following pole, then go faster again.

■ *Consider using rubber-tipped walking poles.* Not only do they help reduce stress on the joints, but they also work upper body muscles that normal walking doesn't. And that means you'll burn more energy. Researchers at the University of Wisconsin at La Crosse estimate that if you normally burn 400 calories walking, you can burn 500 calories using walking poles—without walking any faster.

Intensity counts. Brisk walking is just that—brisk! It's not a casual stroll. Practice good form. Walk with a straight spine and a high center of gravity. Don't lean forward too much. Keep your chin up, shoulders back. With your arms swinging upward to shoulder level, your stride should be purposeful. Think of the pace as one you would use if you were late for a doctor's appointment. And that may be faster than you think. As University of Florida research associate Dr. Glen Duncan explains, "Studies show that most people think they're pushing themselves harder than they really are when walking for exercise. So it's important to concentrate on keeping your heart rate up for maximum benefit."

Although you don't need any special gear, make certain you have a pair of comfortable, sturdy shoes that have arch supports and that elevate the heel one-half to three-quarters of an inch above the sole of the foot. Clothing should not be binding.

Start by picking a pleasant place to walk (outdoors in good weather; inside at a YM/YWCA, health club or mall in bad weather). Begin by walking slowly as a warm-up, then increase your pace over a 5-to-10-minute period and gradually swing your arms faster. This action forces your legs to keep pace with your arms. Pumping your arms frees your hips for longer, faster steps. After about 10 minutes, you should be walking in full stride at your aerobic pace. You should feel "dewed," but your breath should be steady. You should never feel breathless. Keep up this pace for 45 minutes, then cool down by gradually slowing your pace over an additional 5 to 10 minutes.

TAKE ONE STEP AND THEN TEN THOUSAND

If walking is a good form of exercise for you, consider buying a pedometer. These instruments are easy to use and can be worn on your belt. The basic models just count steps, but the newer electronic versions (costing about $25 to $35) convert steps to miles and calories burned and include a built-in stopwatch.

Use the pedometer to gauge the level of your normal activity. Inactive people take between 2,000 and 4,000 steps per day; moderately active people, between 5,000 and 7,000 steps per day; active people, at least 10,000 steps per day (roughly 5 miles or 500 calories). Or, as one dedicated walker explained, "Ten thousand steps a day keep the doctor away."

Set a goal: 5,000 steps, 7,000 steps, whatever's right for you. You'll find that the pedometer can provide the motivation needed to go for that extra walk when you're short of your goal.

RUN WHEN YOU COULD HAVE WALKED

Jogging and its faster cousin running are two of the best calorie- and fat-burning exercises, and a top-notch cardiovascular workout. They require no particular skill and they're convenient, practical indoors or out. People without orthopedic problems or medical conditions such as overweight or high blood pressure should give running a try, though no one should jog or run without clearance from a physician.

In addition, runners should be aware that pavement pounding can lead to overuse injuries. According to the Centers for Disease Control and Prevention, one-third of people who run at least six miles per week are injured—usually in their knees, ankles and shins. The running surface should be soft—a dirt track, a park trail, the grass next to the sidewalk.

One benefit of jogging or running is speed: it takes less time than walking to accomplish cardiovascular and weight benefits. The accepted minimum for cardiovascular fitness is 9 miles spread over

GET THE MOST OUT OF
RUNNING AND JOGGING

- Relax your upper body and let your arms swing slightly.
- Keep your back straight; don't hunch over.
- Run or jog with a relaxed stride. Overstriding can cause injuries and strains.
- Make sure your weight is on your heel, not your toes, when your foot hits the ground.

four days per week. Greater cardiovascular and weight control benefits accrue with more mileage, perhaps 12 to 15 miles per week.

Essential exercise gear is minimal, but what you use must be of good quality. A bad pair of shoes can ruin a good pair of legs. They must be specifically designed for jogging or running with firm support for your arches and heels. The heel area should have about one inch of padding to cushion the shock of your foot hitting the ground. Clothing should be comfortable—which means no rubberized or plastic clothing, ever—and offer protection from the weather. Dress for warmth in the winter by wearing several layers of light clothing rather than one or two heavy layers. The extra layers trap heat, and it's easy to shed clothes if you get too warm. Make sure the layer closest to your skin is made of a synthetic material (or silk) designed to wick away moisture and keep you dry. In cold weather, wear gloves and, very importantly, a hat: a great deal of body heat escapes from your head.

If you're new to running, it's a good idea to alternate walking with very slow jogging, and to slow to a walk whenever you become breathless. This will give you time to get your legs into shape. Gradual progress is the key to success. Over time, increase the ratio of jogging to walking until you're jogging on a nonstop basis. Once you reach the physical condition needed for jogging or running, begin your workout with a brisk walk for 5 to 10 minutes. As you begin to jog, slowly increase your pace. Remember, cardiovascular and weight benefits are a function of time and intensity. Stay in your training zone for a minimum of 20 minutes nonstop; longer is better. Pay attention to how you feel: if the activity is too hard or too easy, it will not produce the benefits you desire. When you're finished with the aerobic portion of your routine, spend another 10 minutes cooling down. Wind down to a slow jog, then a brisk walk, then a slower walk.

LOCATION, LOCATION, LOCATION

When looking for a health club, one of the most important considerations is location. If the club isn't convenient, you won't use it.

TRY SNOWSHOEING

If you live in a northern climate or can get to the mountains, snowshoeing is a terrific way to have fun and improve your fitness. It takes you into beautiful, serene settings that calm your mind while exercising your body. And it's easy.

Start by renting or buying snowshoes; they retail for about $75 to $300 a pair. You may also want to rent or buy poles; they'll help your balance and ensure a good upper-body workout as well. Wear warm socks and waterproof boots; wearing gaiters over your shoes will keep snow from getting in. If you're just learning, start out by walking on level ground. (Many areas set aside for snowshoeing have marked trails.) Once you feel sure of yourself, you can go anywhere—up the mountain, into the woods, around the lake.

There are two things that need your attention when snowshoeing. First, drink plenty of water. Staying hydrated will keep your energy up, which is essential for an activity that burns 400 to 600 calories an hour, depending on your speed. Second, if you get off the trail, pay attention to direction so that you can find your way back. An easy way, of course, is to retrace your steps.

BE A ROAD WARRIOR 58

If you travel as part of your job, you know that airport lines, unfamiliar hotel rooms, meetings, eating on the run and time changes (to say nothing of the business at hand) make it easy to forget your exercise habits. After a hard day, it's also easy to relax in a bar or with HBO and skip your workout. But that won't help you with your fitness goals or with your stress. These days, its fairly easy to get a workout at your hotel if you have the resolve to do it. Find out from your travel agent if your hotel has a workout facility or a pool; if so, be sure to pack your exercise clothes or swimsuit. If the hotel doesn't have an exercise room, find out if it's affiliated with a local gym or health club where you can get a one-day pass for free or for a small fee.

If you're strapped for time or no workout room is available, most hotel rooms have enough floor space to allow you to do some basic exercises—stretching, push-ups, sit-ups—before starting your day. (Packing a jump rope is a great idea.) Many hotels also have VCR or DVD machines in the room, a perfect way to use a favorite exercise video.

SPEAKING FROM EXPERIENCE

My lectures take me out on the road a lot, so I choose hotels with exercise facilities and make sure I use them. It takes a certain amount of discipline to climb off an airplane and onto an exercise bike, but I find that sticking to my routine refreshes me and de-stresses my day. If it's good weather, I might just go out for a walk. It's a great way to see a new area, particularly in a big city. You can cover a lot of ground in New York or Chicago with a 45-minute walk, and it's great fun to people-watch, window-shop and be a tourist on the move.

—J.P.

BANISH NEGATIVITY

Here are some things you should never say to yourself:

■ *"It's too hard."* If you exercise at the right pace, you won't get tired, sore and out of breath. Starting out slowly and attaining fitness over time takes the "work" out of exercise.

■ *"I don't have the time."* An effective daily exercise session takes no more than 45 to 60 minutes, including warm-up and cool-down. The American College of Sports Medicine recommends 30 minutes or more of moderate-intensity activity and 20 minutes or more of vigorous activity. It's certainly possible to find that time just from the hours spent in front of the TV set and/or the computer. Recognize that the effects of exercise are cumulative: three 10-minute moderate-intensity exercise bouts confer the same benefits as one 30-minute session. (Although two separate 10-minute sessions of vigorous activity are acceptable, most experts recommend one continuous session lasting at least 20 minutes.) It might be helpful to think about physical activity in terms of banking. You don't have to put a dollar bill in your piggy (exercise) bank each time. Four quarters deposited over time add up to the same amount.

> **A Motto to Live By**
>
> Over time, even ordinary effort can yield extraordinary results.

- *"I'm too tired."* Low aerobic fitness often leads to chronic fatigue. When fitness improves, muscles can extract more oxygen from the bloodstream, thus providing a boost to your energy. Gardening, for example, requires a relatively constant supply of oxygen. People who are not aerobically fit may use their entire aerobic capacity, while those who are aerobically fit may use the same amount of oxygen but have a greater "energy reserve."

Here's what you *should* say:
- *"Exercise will help me lose weight and keep it off."*
- *"My muscles will have shape and tone."*
- *"I'll feel more confident."*
- *"I'll meet new people with similar interests."*
- *"My cholesterol and blood pressure will improve."*
- *"I'll feel less stress."*
- *"My heart will get stronger."*

DRINK UP 60

Be sure to drink water before, during and after each workout. Studies suggest that being properly hydrated before an exercise session can boost your performance and reduce the likelihood of exertional heat stroke, a medical emergency characterized by a markedly elevated body temperature, dry skin, nausea and even unconsciousness. Heat stroke can also be lethal, as it was for Korey Stringer, an All-Pro tackle with the Minnesota Vikings who died after working out in withering heat.

SPRING FOR A LESSON

Exercising with good form and technique maximizes effectiveness and minimizes injury. Check with your local YM/YWCA, community center or gym, or with university- or hospital-affiliated exercise programs to find an exercise professional or personal trainer who has a college degree in physical education and/or is certified by one or more of the prominent organizations in the health/fitness industry: the American College of Sports Medicine, the Cooper Institute, the American Council on Exercise and the National Strength & Conditioning Association. Each has established rigorous knowledge and proficiency standards for exercise professionals, as well as certification programs.

Don't hesitate to ask about the credentials of your exercise instructor or personal trainer.

MAKE EXERCISE A FAMILY AFFAIR

One widely cited study showed that a male participant's adherence to an exercise program is directly related to his wife's attitude toward it. Of those men whose spouses had a positive attitude toward the exercise program, 80% demonstrated good to excellent adherence; in contrast, when the spouse was neutral or negative, only 40% showed good to excellent adherence.

Let family members know what you want to accomplish, how you intend to use exercise as a means to that goal and how they can contribute by providing support. Ask for a commitment from them to match that of your own.

TAKE A SEAT

Both outdoor and indoor biking strengthen the muscles of the back, abdomen and legs, tone the buttocks and thighs, and provide cardiovascular conditioning if done at a sufficient pace or intensity. You can burn a significant number of calories, depending on the terrain, exercise duration and how fast you ride—without the joint and muscle stress often incurred by running or jogging. (People with neck and/or back conditions, however, may find that biking aggravates their problem.)

Outdoor biking can provide cardiovascular benefit, as can indoor biking; either activity can elevate your heart rate into the training zone. To achieve cardiovascular fitness, you'll have to bike outdoors for an estimated 24 miles a week at an aerobic pace (more if you want to lose weight). Start at a slow pace for 5 to 10 minutes to warm up the leg muscles, then progressively increase your speed until you find a comfortable, rhythmic pace within your training zone. Stay in the zone for at least 20 minutes, then pedal slowly for 5 to 10 minutes to cool down.

Aerobic exercise should be continuous, so stoplights and coasting can be problematic. Look for a bike path or a straight stretch of road that will allow you to keep pedaling. And never ride without a protective helmet.

Indoor biking lets you exercise at a steady pace while simultaneously reading, watching TV or listening to music. It's a particularly good activity if you need to squeeze exercise into a busy day—and you won't get wet or too hot or cold. On an indoor bike, the way to elevate your heart rate into the training zone is to increase tension (resistance), speed, or both. One problem is that too much tension can take too much out of your legs, which may lead you to give up on biking altogether. Some indoor bikes require a simultaneous pumping action of the arms, thereby providing better aerobic benefits than pedaling alone.

According to Dr. Thomas Dickson, Jr., an orthopedic surgeon who specializes in sports medicine, it's a mistake to think that if you pedal in a harder gear, you'll give yourself a better aerobic workout. Increased resistance will make it harder to pump (not good for the knees), but will also reduce the number of revolutions per minute. A greater benefit is derived from riding in a gear that allows for 60 to 100 rpm.

GET THE MOST OUT OF BIKING

If you want the most bang for your buck in the shortest amount of time, take a spinning class. Like aerobic dance, spinning is performed in a group setting with an instructor and music. Everyone uses a stationary bike. The instructor takes the class through a workout/ride at a variety of intensities—sprint, ease-up and added resistance to simulate hills.

The instructor calls for changes in resistance that generally provide nonstop pedaling in your training zone for a minimum of 20 minutes. (Most classes provide about 30 minutes of aerobic work in a 45-to-50-minute class.) Group dynamics, upbeat music and the challenge to keep pace with your instructor combine to increase the intensity and therefore the effectiveness of this biking exercise.

At the same time, you get to control resistance on the wheel of your bike. When the instructor says, "Go to medium resistance," the response is different for each participant. For newcomers, it might mean a setting of 3 or 4; for veterans, it will be closer to 8 or 9. So, go at whatever pace is right for you to achieve your training zone.

Indoor bikers should follow the same basic program as outdoor bikers. Pedal slowly with low-tension resistance to warm up. After 5 to 10 minutes, increase the tension slightly until the training zone is reached. A cool-down period should follow at least 20 minutes of continuous cycling at an aerobic pace.

PLAN A FITNESS VACATION

Why not get your heart pumping by going skiing, backpacking, hiking, kayaking or scuba diving? Bike the San Juan Islands, hike the English coast, dive in Maui, or spend a week exercising and eating right at a health spa. The choice is yours to make. It doesn't have to be expensive or exotic to be fun and effective. The important thing is to get yourself out of your daily routine. A vacation that challenges you both physically and mentally will increase your physical fitness, relax your mind, reduce your stress and open your heart to your place in nature.

LIFT THOSE WEIGHTS! 65

First off, have a certified professional develop a program tailored to your needs. This should include the following:

- Establishing goals.
- Determining how much weight you should lift.
- Teaching you the correct technique, using free weights, machines, or resistance tubing and bands.
- Set up a program that covers all muscle groups, including abdominal muscles.

The key is to build muscle gradually. Start with relatively light weights that you use 20 minutes twice a week. Don't worry about getting through your entire routine. Add weight gradually over time and adjust the load until you can perform the entire routine. The traditional recommendation is 8 to 12 repetitions of each exercise, three sets of repetitions each. But recent research has shown that one set of each exercise can be nearly as effective for most people. This is great news for nonathletes who want increased muscular strength and endurance but don't want to spend a great deal of time on this type of training.

Don't be afraid to start slow. Numerous studies have shown that a three-month weight training program in previously sedentary adults can increase strength by 25% to 100% or more.

USE YOUR GROCERIES

Make weights out of empty plastic bottles filled with sand or rice, or do a few reps with some big cans of soup.

> ## TRY PILATES
>
> Designed to engage the core muscle groups (abdominal, back and inner thigh) in precise movements that stretch and strengthen the body, Pilates exercises (named after Joseph Pilate, who developed the technique in the 1920s) are performed on a mat or on specialized equipment using springs as resistance. Deborah Schneider, senior program director for the YMCA in Tacoma, Washington, explains the increased popularity of Pilates nationwide: "People go to Pilates for strength," she says. "They use it as an alternative to the more traditional jumping up and down of aerobic exercises."

DISGUISE YOUR EXERCISE

Not everyone is comfortable with high-tech gym equipment, and many of us are simply unable to make it to a weekly aerobics class. But we can still exercise. Here's how:

■ *Stop circling!* Forget about driving around in search of the "closest" possible spot to the shopping mall, movie theater or doctor's office. Park your car at the farthest end of the parking lot and walk to your destination.

■ *Find the stairs!* Forget about the elevator or escalator and move from floor to floor the old-fashioned way, burning calories and building strong leg muscles while you do. One study at an at-work stair-climbing program showed it to be a feasible method of increasing aerobic fitness.

■ *Get up!* Conveniences such as TV remotes and drive-through windows allow us to stay glued to our seats for hours on end. Try "losing" the remote control. Eliminate unnecessary extension phones in your home. Walk the dog more often. Walk the golf course instead of riding in a cart. Use a bike for short trips.

■ *One at a time!* Unloading grocery bags from the car is another way to burn calories and maintain muscular fitness. To get added exercise out of your groceries, bring the bags in from the car one at a time.

▪ *Clean up!* Vacuuming, dusting, mopping the floor and gardening are not only ways to keep your house in shape, but also a great opportunity for you to increase activity in daily living.

BUY SHOES THAT FIT 68

Wait until the end of the day (when your feet are largest) to fit your shoes. Be sure to wear athletic socks, since they can move you into another size. Check that the soles are firm and the arch support good. And women: If the shoes seem too narrow, move to the men's or boys' department.

DON'T NEGLECT YOUR ARMS 69

So you're walking, jogging or bicycling three or four times a week and you think your exercise program is ideal. Think again. You aren't achieving "total fitness" or "fitness for life." You need aerobic exercise for the upper body as well.

Why arm exercise? The benefits of exercise are largely specific to the muscles that have been trained; in other words, lower extremity training, like walking or jogging, results in improved fitness for your legs but not your arms.

Specially designed bicycles called arm ergometers (they have "levers" instead of handlebars), rowing machines, wall pulleys and light dumbbells are all good for conditioning the upper extremities. Several commercially available devices are noteworthy because they combine arm and leg exercise. One ergometer offers a workout for the arms, using only the bicycle's arm levers; for the legs, using only the pedals; or for both, using the levers and pedals simultaneously. Simulated cross-country skiing machines also provide total body conditioning.

Remember, real-life activities seldom involve jogging in circles or foot pedaling for extended periods. If you'd like to improve your golf drive or tennis slam, or perform household chores or manual tasks without breathlessness or fatigue, include arm training in your personal exercise program.

FEEL THE BEAT

Here's one that demands no prior knowledge or experience, as long as you're willing to just jump in and try (and perhaps feel a little silly until you get the moves down). Aerobic dancing is easy, fun, upbeat— and a great way to burn calories, exercise the whole body and, when done three to four times a week, achieve cardiovascular benefits. You can take a class that includes steps (or not), at either high- or low-impact levels. Normally, a class will last 45 to 60 minutes with stretching and slow movements to warm up and cool down, sandwiched around at least 20 minutes of nonstop aerobic activity.

A word to men: aerobic dancing is not just for women. A study in *The Physician and Sportsmedicine* reported on a group of men aged 33 to 72 who attended aerobic dancing classes three times a week for 45 minutes each session. After six weeks, they had lost weight, lowered resting heart rate and reduced blood cholesterol levels.

Like any aerobic activity, aerobic dance must be done with some intensity and for a long enough period of time to be effective.

GET THE MOST OUT OF AEROBIC DANCING

If you're looking to increase intensity, take a step aerobics class. Stair climbing can increase fitness, burn additional calories and increase metabolism (as well as reduce cardiac risk), and all of that holds true for dancing that uses 6-to-8-inch steps. Some of these classes are high impact; if you're just starting out, pick a class that is appropriate for your physical condition. But the increase in effectiveness can be enormous. A 150-pound person will burn up about 280 calories in a 45-minute aerobics class. That same person will burn almost 450 calories in a 45-minute step class.

But effectiveness also rests on the talent of the instructor and the value of the routines. When selecting a class, be sure to find out from the sponsoring agency whether or not the instructor is properly qualified. Sit in on a class before joining. Make certain that warm-up, dancing and cool-down are part of every session and that the proposed intensity matches your ability to perform. Also, check out the floor. Stay away from concrete (and linoleum or hardwood over concrete), which has no "give." The best floor is cushioned hardwood.

And finally, wear loose clothing and shoes specifically designed to offer support during side-to-side movement. Aerobic dancing shoes absorb shock, stabilize the foot and minimize twisting. Never use worn-out shoes or exercise barefoot.

> ### JUMP IN THE WATER
>
> Don't overlook water aerobics, especially if you need a workout that's gentle on the joints. "Water exercise is a legitimate form of exercise," says Yvette Corsey, swim supervisor for the Baylor–Tom Landry Fitness Center in Dallas. "It offers resistance training, burns calories and works core muscles."

SWITCH GEARS TO BOOST METABOLISM

Sustained exercise at a relatively constant intensity enhances endurance, but interval training with its work-rest periods, varied exercise intensities or both may be especially well suited to novice exercisers and heart patients.

Whichever type you do is fine; however, if weight loss is one of your fitness goals, interval training may be more effective in boosting total calories burned because it transiently increases metabolic rate over several exercise bouts. Instead of walking for 45 minutes at a steady pace, walk for 10 minutes at your normal pace, then walk or jog at a higher level of intensity for another 5 minutes. Follow this alternating pattern for an additional 30 minutes. Some walkers and joggers make a music tape, alternating fast and slower songs to match various speeds.

VISIT THE MALL

Exercise indoors when temperatures are extreme—freezing cold or blistering heat—or anytime the weather is simply unpleasant. Being miserable is not part of an exercise routine. If you don't belong to a gym, walk at your local shopping mall. Many malls open their doors early just for this purpose.

 MIX IT UP

Nothing saps exercise resolve faster than boredom, unless it's injury. To avoid both, cross-train. Someone who only runs, for instance, will have strong calves and hamstrings but may have relatively weak abdominal muscles, limited strength in the upper extremities, and weak quads and shins. To avoid injuries such as shin splints or pulled hamstrings, vary your routine. Likewise, if all you do is walk, there will come a time, no matter how much you love it, when walking will feel like a job. Instead, sign up for new classes, try different exercises and experience the enthusiasm and success of a more challenging routine.

SPEAKING FROM EXPERIENCE

Patients often ask me if just walking and jogging is enough. I vividly recall the response of the late Dr. Herman K. Hellerstein to a similar question. "There are very few occupations that require sustained walking or jogging," he replied. "Examples included mail carriers, protective service personnel, police officers and their fugitives." Most exercise programs are improperly designed to enhance a person's capacity to perform activities required for daily living. The inclusion of dynamic arm exercise, resistance training and stretching in a physical fitness program should serve to maximize the training benefits to real-life situations. —*B.F.*

MAKE MACHINES WORK FOR YOU   **74**

First things first. Get instruction so that you know how to perform the exercise effectively without hurting yourself.

Next, be sure to vary the machines you use so that you don't overtrain and strain certain muscles. As you get stronger, try to devote more time—30 to 45 minutes for an effective workout.

And finally, take a look at how you can subtly increase the intensity of your exercise. If you program a treadmill, for example, to a 5% grade, you will burn an extra 150 calories at a pace of three miles per hour in 60 minutes.

- The *treadmill*, a fine alternative to walking or jogging (particularly in inclement weather) allows you to exercise while on an incline, thus increasing the workload and aerobic effect. A study published in the *Journal of the American Medical Association* compared calories burned at a given level of perceived exertion for six different indoor exercise machines. The treadmill evoked the highest caloric expenditure as compared with the other machines.

- The *indoor cross-country skiing machine* is another excellent calorie-burning machine, although it's harder to master unless you're already familiar with cross-country skiing. If you're not, go easy and just take your time.

- *Stair climbers* and *stair steppers* allow for a great workout in a short period of time. They're good calorie burners and generally carry a low risk for injury, although some people with back problems may find that these machines worsen their condition.

- The *elliptical exercise trainer* provides a combination of jogging and stair stepping, and may include (on newer models) arm levers as well. This machine can give you a low-stress but highly aerobic workout.

- *Indoor rowing machines* strengthen arms and legs and provide cardiovascular fitness. They're great calorie-burners, particularly for women, although people with neck and back conditions should be very careful on them.

EXERCISE TIPS FOR DIABETICS

Numerous studies have shown that aerobic exercise programs improve blood sugar control; however, insulin-dependent diabetics should take the following precautionary measures:

■ *Obtain proper medical clearance.* Before starting an exercise program, individuals over 35 who have had Type 1 diabetes for more than 15 years should have a medical exam, possibly including an exercise stress test, and be closely screened for complications such as eye problems, kidney disease, poor nerve function, small-vessel disease or heart disease.

■ *Wear proper footwear and practice good foot hygiene.* Diabetics, especially those with impaired nerve conduction in their feet, should use cushioned shoes (gel or air soles). It's crucial to look closely before and after exercise for blisters and persistent foot infections that could progress to gangrene.

■ *Monitor blood glucose* when starting an exercise program. Diabetics who take insulin or oral medications should check their blood glucose before, during and after exercise if taking insulin or oral medications.

■ *Exercise at about the same time each day.* Strenuous or unplanned activity may cause blood glucose levels to drop too low. Exercising late in the evening also increases the risk of hypoglycemia (low blood sugar). Because exercise has an insulin-like effect, exercise-induced hypoglycemia is the most common problem experienced by exercising diabetics who take insulin (and, to a lesser extent, oral hypoglycemic medications).

■ *Inject insulin in body areas not affected by exercise.* Injecting insulin into active working muscles increases the likelihood of hypoglycemia. To alleviate this potential problem, an inactive injection area like the abdomen should be used before walking, jogging or bicycling.

■ *Avoid exercising when insulin is reaching its peak effect.*
Glucose levels may decrease markedly during peak insulin action.
Thus, the action of various insulin preparations should be discussed
with a physician in relation to exercise timing.

A particularly good time to work out is 15 to 45 minutes after
meals, when glucose levels are relatively high, rather than before
meals, when blood sugar level may be low.

■ *Consider ingesting 20 to 30 grams of additional carbohydrate before exercise if glucose level is below 100 mg/dl.*
A carbohydrate-rich snack—for example, 6 to 12 ounces of fruit
juice or 6 to 8 saltines—should do the trick.

■ *Avoid exercise when diabetes control is poor.* Guidelines from
the American College of Sports Medicine suggest that exercise
should be avoided if the glucose level is greater than 300 mg/dl
or greater than 240 mg/dl if ketones are present in the urine.

■ *Know the signs and symptoms of hypoglycemia.* Diabetics
who have heart palpitations or who feel confused, unusually weak,
tired, shaky, anxious, visually disturbed, or dizzy during or after
exercise should *immediately* eat or drink some simple form of sugar.
Unrecognized and untreated, these symptoms could lead to unconsciousness or convulsions. To reduce the likelihood of hypoglycemia,
a decrease in your insulin dosage or an increase in carbohydrate
intake may be necessary before or after exercise. As an additional
precaution, exercising with a partner is recommended.

■ *Watch for high blood sugar (hyperglycemia),* which can
lead to ketoacidosis, commonly called diabetic coma. Symptoms
such as excessive thirst, frequent urination, blurred vision, weakness, itchy, dry skin or a fruity odor or breath may result from taking
too little insulin, extreme inactivity, overeating, infection or emotional upset. Urine or blood glucose levels should be checked on a
regular basis.

Step 4
Balance Your Diet

Know What You Eat

FROM THANKSGIVING DINNERS TO SUPER BOWL SNACKS, food embodies pleasure, home, love, tradition and entertainment. It can also have an enormous influence on our physical well-being: eating a balanced diet is one of the smartest things we can do to manage cardiac markers, ward off disease and maximize good health.

Unfortunately, the American diet has become progressively unbalanced. We're eating more animal foods, fast foods, convenience foods and restaurant meals, all of which have made for a diet too rich in fat, sugar, salt and calories. At the same time, we're eating fewer fruits, vegetables, beans and whole grains—foods rich in complex carbohydrates, fiber and antioxidants. And to top it off, we're eating more, *period*. The increase in portion size of common foods is a main contributor to overeating and the current obesity epidemic. As characterized by Harvard economist John Kenneth Galbraith, these trends have made America one of the "most overfed and undernourished" countries in the world. Just look at what is eaten in a typical day in the United States:

- 13 pizzas the size of the Roman Coliseum
- 47 million hot dogs
- 3 million gallons of ice cream
- 1.2 million gallons of hard liquor
- 6 million pounds of chocolate

Of course, there is no one American diet. Anyone who has enjoyed crab cakes in Baltimore, tacos in Los Angeles or prime rib in Kansas City knows that favorite foods differ from one end of the country to the other, reflecting regional preferences and ethnic traditions. But there is a common American diet pattern. From Boston to San Diego, Seattle to Miami and every place in between, the basic diet is sweet, salty and full of fat.

According to the Centers for Disease Control and Prevention, almost two-thirds of our calories come from fat, sugar and alcohol, with the remaining calories left to meet our major nutritional needs. This is a poor ratio. What business or sports team could succeed with only one-third of its people pulling the oars for everyone?

As the Surgeon General's Report on Nutrition and Health says, Americans are "gobbling their way to the grave." The report identifies a causal link between the typical American diet and 5 of the 10 leading causes of death—coronary heart disease, cancer, high blood pressure, stroke and cirrhosis of the liver—and the nation's leading ailment, obesity. It also links diet to the less threatening but serious problems of gout, osteoarthritis and gallbladder disease.

Says former surgeon general C. Everett Koop, "As diseases of nutritional deficiency have diminished, they have been replaced by diseases of dietary excess and imbalance—problems that now rank among the leading causes of illness and death in the United States. After smoking, food choices can influence long-term health prospects more than any other factor."

A DIETARY SNAPSHOT

Health experts consider the contemporary American diet to be seriously out of balance. But it wasn't always that way. A comparison of foods consumed in 1910, when the Department of Agriculture first started to keep figures on the food supply, with those consumed today shows a dramatic shift.

■ Early in the last century, dietary fat made up just 27% of calories eaten. Today, because of our reliance on meat, dairy products, fried foods, snack foods and fast foods, that figure has risen to almost 35%, with the average family of four consuming an estimated 400 pounds of fat per year. The predominance of animal foods has led to a high consumption of saturated fats, a leading factor in the development of heart disease. Moreover, the prevalence of foods containing trans fats—mainly margarine, commercially baked goods, chips, crackers and fast food—has contributed to higher levels of cholesterol.

- In 1910, the average adult consumed some 70 pounds of refined sugar. Today that figure has risen to 150 pounds, or more than one-third of a pound of sugar each day. It's even worse for children and adolescents. They consume, on average, about 275 pounds of sugar a year. "America's sweet tooth is out of control," says dietitian Bonnie Liebman of the Center for Science in the Public Interest. "Sugar now accounts for about 24% of calories eaten in the American diet." This dramatic increase bears much responsibility for a steady rise in the number of overweight Americans, and for those with elevated triglycerides and Syndrome X.

- Americans consume an estimated two to four teaspoons of salt daily—about 15 pounds a year! About 75% comes from packaged foods and foods eaten away from home, whereas 25% comes from the salt shaker. According to the American Heart Association, the recommended level is about one-half to one teaspoon. The overeating of salt and sodium has helped to make high blood pressure a cardiac marker for over 63 million people.

- Today, Americans eat about 150 more calories per day than they did 20 years ago. These extra calories could add up to a 15-pound weight gain in one year. It's easy to overeat when cookies are the size of pancakes, muffins are bigger than baseballs, and sodas are large enough to drown in. Even *The Joy of Cooking* has given in to the trend; recipes that used to feed six now feed only four. According to the latest National Health and Nutrition Examination Survey (NHANES), which periodically reviews American eating habits, even those who are choosing healthy foods and avoiding high-fat, high-sugar items are still "super-sizing" their selections. A good example is pasta, a healthy food choice. In Italy, it comes in a moderate serving. But in the United States, one person often eats enough for a family of three!

■ With the rise in affluence over the last 100 years, animal foods and refined foods have been systematically substituted for fruits, whole grains, beans and vegetables. It is estimated that 25% of adults do not consume even one serving a day of vegetables. And for those who eat vegetables, French fries constitute one-quarter of all vegetables eaten. Since complex carbohydrates are critical to successful weight control, their waning popularity has worsened the national obesity problem.

Why Do We Eat This Way?

Clearly, most people understand that the modern American diet can be hazardous to cardiovascular health. But only 34% of American adults describe themselves as being "health-conscious" in terms of their eating habits. Why, then, do so many of us eat so poorly?

While a number of factors influence food choices, none is as important as our contemporary way of life. Modern society is stress-

---

A DAY IN THE LIFE OF AN AMERICAN TEEN

Dr. Theresa Kicklas, director of dietary studies for the ongoing Bogalusa Study, recorded the dietary intake of one 17-year-old boy over a 24-hour period: "For breakfast, he had a fast-food egg-and-bacon sandwich and orange juice on the bus to school. Many of his friends left the school campus for lunch at a fast-food place, but he ate lunch at school: chicken nuggets, baked potato with butter and cheese, two rolls, a canned pear and whole milk. His other choices were pepperoni pizza or a cheeseburger with fries. His afternoon snack took place at a deli: a chicken sandwich globbed with mayonnaise, and a bag of potato chips. Dinner at home was two fried pork chops, another baked potato and two slices of bread. The fact that he didn't eat a single green vegetable in a 24-hour period, and only a little fruit, doesn't surprise us. Unfortunately, this today is more the rule than the exception."

ful and pressure-packed, often driving us to choose on the spur of the moment and without thought to health. "And when you add in what choices are available, the problem is compounded," according to Dr. Kelly Brownell, an obesity expert at Yale University. "Modern society is a toxic environment for making healthy food choices," he states. "Everywhere you turn there is an opportunity to eat poorly, backed up by an advertising industry that encourages overeating. In the lab, if you take a rat and toss food from the 7-Eleven into its cage, if you throw in candy bars, throw in Chee-tos, throw in marshmallows, things like that, you duplicate such a toxic environment, and as a result you'll get an enormously obese rat."

Eating competes with many other activities in our fragmented schedules. Says registered dietitian Evelyn Tribole, "People are no longer inclined to shop, cook or make food choices based on good nutrition. They often eat on the run and settle for what is available, quickly, from restaurants, take-outs and food stores. Many have simply traded nutrition for convenience." At four P.M. on any given day, 70% of Americans do not know what they'll be having for dinner that night. But it starts with breakfast: in about 50% of families, one or more persons skip breakfast regularly. Nancy Clark, a sports nutritionist, says, "People tell me they don't have time for breakfast. What they don't realize is that by skipping this meal, they can become ravenous later in the day, make all the wrong food choices and overeat." Almost 50% of people in a Gallup survey stated that on a typical night they depend on frozen, packaged or take-out meals for dinner. According to the American Restaurant Association, Americans eat out about 3.5 times a week and spend over 40% of their food budget on restaurant fare. Unfortunately, fast-food meals typically average 1,050 calories, 41 grams of fat, 2,150 milligrams of sodium and virtually no complex carbohydrate foods.

With family meals diminishing, the consumption of junk and snack foods is on the rise. The typical person consumes over 22 pounds of snack foods each year. To put that into perspective, consider this:

TOO MUCH OF A GOOD THING

America has an abundance of food. It's available everywhere, and for the most part, it's cheap. Until the middle of the last century, cyclical food shortages resulting from bad weather and crop failures were a way of life. Refrigeration and rapid transportation of food products had not yet been perfected. As a result, people often didn't get enough to eat. (Indeed, records show that many men who enlisted in World War II were so undernourished that they had to be fed for a period of time before starting basic training.) Diseases of insufficient nutrition such as rickets and scurvy were not unusual.

Today, most of us can eat what we want when we want it. But abundant food does not equate to a healthy diet. Eating too often and too much subjects the average American to diseases of excess.

we pay about $2 billion a year for every sports ticket in the country . . . pro, college and high school. But we spend the same amount on just five candy products: M&M's, Snickers, Reese's peanut butter cups, Milky Ways and Hershey's Kisses. In addition, our portions dwarf those of past generations, with "supersizing" (for a few pennies more) in fast-food restaurants, pizza promotions (two for the price of one), and all the "giant" candy bars, oversize bagels (4 to 7 ounces) and jumbo soft drinks (32 to 64 ounces) that are currently available. Restaurant servings of 22-to-38-ounce steaks and fish are now commonplace. In some movie theaters, a "medium" popcorn now contains 16 cups—and many people order it buttered.

Time for a Change

Dietary habits are a significant factor in managing cardiac markers—particularly lipids, weight, blood pressure and diabetes—but what most of us choose to eat bears little resemblance to what we should eat for good health. Rather than choosing foods for their nutritional value, we base our dietary decisions on convenience, advertising, taste and cravings. Says Laura Shapiro of *Newsweek*, "We've handed over our appetites to the food companies. Our relationship to food is not based on anything that makes sense. It's not based on our bodies, it's not based on family life and the family sitting down to the table, it's not based on what is good for the planet. There's no relationship with the body and the soul and the heart."

WHAT WERE THEY THINKING?

According to a recent CNN poll, 33% of men and 23% of women said they believe you can eat badly and stay healthy.

"The diet we eat today was not planned or developed for any particular purpose," echoes Dr. Mark Hegsted, former director of the Human Nutrition Center of the Department of Agriculture. "It is a happenstance related to the productivity of our farmers, the marketing activities of our food industry, particularly fast food, and the pace of life."

The evidence is clear: the modern American diet is linked to an imposing list of chronic diseases and debilitating conditions. That's why over 17 major health organizations and initiatives, including the American Heart Association, the National Cancer Institute and the National Cholesterol Education Program, have called for changes in the way we eat. As Dr. Hegsted states, "The risks associated with eating the American diet are demonstrably large. The question to be asked, therefore, is not why we should change our diet, but why not?"

The indictment of the American diet is serious, valid and understood, but this has not moved people to take action. For most of us, the chronic stress of everyday life keeps us eating too much, too often and too many harmful foods—particularly fast food, junk food and snacks. The Piscatella Protocol uses stress management techniques (including exercise) as a vehicle for dietary compliance. People who handle stress effectively are less responsive to anxiety, depression, anger and "the blues" as eating cues. People who exercise regularly feel better about themselves and expect success in making healthy eating changes.

WHAT DOES AND DOESN'T MAKE A HEART-HEALTHY DIET?

A healthy, balanced diet can improve virtually all cardiac markers, while a poor, unhealthy diet can turn those same markers into significant coronary risks. This section will provide you with key concepts on which to build a diet geared for life rather than for quick and easy weight loss. Numerous ways to put this knowledge into action can be found among the Heart Savers that follow.

Complex Carbohydrates

Experts recommend that foods rich in complex carbohydrates—fruits, vegetables, whole grains, beans, nuts and legumes—should make up at least 55% of total calories. The National Research Council's Committee on Diet and Health advises all Americans to "every day eat five or more servings of vegetables and fruits, especially green and yellow vegetables and citrus fruits, and eat at least six or more servings of a combination of whole-grain breads, cereals, pasta, rice and legumes."

While this might sound like a lot of food, in reality it's not. One serving from the grains group is one slice of bread, or half a cup of cooked cereal, rice or pasta, or one cup of cold cereal. A serving from the fruit and vegetable group is one medium piece of fruit, half a cup of cooked or canned fruits/vegetables or one cup of leafy vegetables. Meeting these recommendations is not that hard, and it's important to do so. Studies throughout the world suggest that people who habitually consume a diet rich in plant food have a low risk of coronary heart disease both because of what they do consume (antioxidants, soluble fiber, unsaturated oils, fiber and other nutrients) and because of what they do *not* consume (a lot of saturated fat from animal foods and trans fats from convenience foods).

This is not exactly news. In the 1940s and '50s, pioneer researcher Dr. Ancel Keys of the University of Minnesota conducted a classic study involving three groups of Japanese subjects, each residing in a different environment and eating a different diet. The first group lived in Japan and ate a traditional Asian diet: lots of vegetables, fruit, legumes, soy products, rice and fish, and little meat. They had a low incidence of heart attacks. The second group lived in Hawaii and ate a mixture of Asian and American foods, which meant less fruits, vegetables and grains, and more meat and butter. They had a greater incidence of heart attacks. The third group lived in Los Angeles and ate a totally Americanized diet, from steaks to ice cream. Their intake of fruits, vegetables and grains decreased substantially, and these individuals had the highest incidence of heart attacks.

More recent studies have reaffirmed the benefits of plant foods. The Harvard Nurses' Health Study found that those participants who ate at least five servings a day of fruits and vegetables lowered their risk of heart attack by 25%. The Harvard Physicians' Health Study came to the same conclusion: unrefined foods high in complex carbohydrates and fiber are cardioprotective and can help to control blood pressure and weight.

WHAT WE KNOW VS. HOW WE LIVE

Despte all the relevant published studies and a general awareness on the part of the public, only one in five Americans eats the recommended five servings a day of fruits and vegetables. Some 20% eat no fruit at all, and 15% rarely eat a vegetable other than potatoes. Amazingly, according to the American Medical Association, doctors do no better when it comes to fruit and vegetables.

In addition, the deeper the color of the food, the more effective the protection against heart disease, cancer and other chronic diseases. This is because deeply colored fruits and vegetables, especially green, red and yellow ones, have the most vitamins and minerals, and the plant pigments themselves are high in antioxidants. This doesn't mean you should quit eating light green grapes or white potatoes. But experts recommend including some "darks"—such as spinach, prunes, red grapes, kale, cherries, raisins, carrots and oranges—every day.

Plant foods also contain mass, which is useful in filling you up, not out. Foods that need a lot of chewing, like apples or carrots, take a long time to eat and therefore provide sufficient time (about 20 minutes) for satiety to be attained. These foods also absorb water in the digestive system, thereby helping to create a feeling of fullness and satisfaction that keeps you from overeating.

And finally, since excessive animal protein in the diet leaches calcium from the bones, relying more on fruits, whole grains, vegetables, beans and soy products can decrease the risk of osteoporosis.

Dietary Fats

Like cholesterol, dietary fat plays an important role in promoting good health. It is used in the transportation of important fat-soluble vitamins in the body. And polyunsaturated fats (mostly vegetable oils) supply the body with linolenic acid, an essential fatty acid. Without fat in the diet, we wouldn't be able to absorb vitamins A, D, E and K. Fat also provides the body with a concentrated source of energy. At nine calories per gram, fat packs more than two times as many calories as the same amount of protein and carbohydrates.

It's clear: fat is fine when consumed in the proper amount. From a nutritional standpoint, the daily requirement for fat can be fully satisfied by consuming one tablespoon of vegetable oil. The average American, however, eats eight times that amount: between 800 and 1,000 calories in fat every day, the equivalent of one full stick of butter. It is this overconsumption of fat that constitutes a health issue.

NOT ALL CARBOHYDRATES ARE CREATED EQUAL

*C*omplex carbohydrates such as fruits, vegetables and whole grains are highly recommended for heart health. Not so for *simple carbohydrates,* found in cake, sugar and white flour. High in calories and low in fiber, simple carbohydrates cause blood sugar to increase rapidly, resulting in more insulin production and the ready conversion of calories into body fat. Experts now place complex carbohydrates at the base of the food pyramid; simple carbohydrates at the "eat sparingly" pinnacle.

For years, "eat low-fat" has been the dietary mantra of the American Heart Association. "Eat a diet with no more 30% of calories from fat," they said. And some doctors went farther, calling for maximum fat levels of just 10%. But there has been a change in thinking. "It's a myth that one low-fat diet is best for everyone," says Dr. Wayne Calloway of George Washington University. "In fact, research shows that for some, cutting fat too much could reduce protective HDL cholesterol and even increase their risk of heart disease." This thinking is reflected in new American Heart Association guidelines that allow for up to 35% of calories from fat, as long as you restrict saturated and trans fats, and eat an otherwise healthful diet of fruits, vegetables, legumes, whole grains, fish, nuts and low-fat dairy products.

■ *Reduce saturated fat for cholesterol control.* The fact that saturated fat causes a rise in both total and LDL cholesterol is not news. In the Seven Country Study (Finland, Greece, Italy, Japan, the Netherlands, the United States and Yugoslavia), Dr. Ancel Keys observed some 12,000 men in the 40-to-49 age range and found that cultures in which saturated fat made up a high percentage of calories demonstrated elevated cholesterol and a high incidence of coronary heart disease. Thus, the Finns, who ate 20% of their calories as saturated fat, had cholesterol levels that averaged 265. The Japanese ate only 5% of their calories as saturated fat and had correspondingly low levels of cholesterol, averaging just 165. A key finding was that the heart attack rate for Finnish men in the study was six times greater than for Japanese men of the same age.

A further study divided the continent of Europe into two distinct geographic areas based on diet patterns. "High-fat Europe," comprising the British Isles, Germany, Holland, Scandinavia, northern France, Belgium and northern Switzerland, was categorized as a "beer and butter" culture with a diet pattern uniformly rich in saturated fat and a population plagued by elevated levels of cholesterol and a high rate of heart attack. At odds with this area was "low-fat Europe," comprising Spain, Italy, southern France, southern Switzerland and Greece, which exhibited a diet pattern where much of the fat consumed came in the form of mono- and polyunsaturated oils; categorized as a "wine and oil" culture, this group had much lower levels of cholesterol and a lower incidence of heart attack. The study illustrated that cholesterol levels and incidence of coronary heart disease cut across geographic and ethnic boundaries where similarities in diet patterns did the same.

More recently, the Framingham Heart Study, the MRFIT Trial and the NIH Cholesterol Study, among others, have found that reducing saturated fat lowers cholesterol, especially LDL cholesterol. Says Dr. Virgil Brown, a past president of the American Heart Association, "The goal for saturated fat intake is about 7% of calories, no more. What we'd really like is for saturated fat and trans fat together to constitute no more than 10% of all calories. Unfortunately, most people consume about 13% to 18% of calories as saturated fat, and for some as much as one-third of total calories eaten. That's a big reason why heart disease is still our number one killer."

> ### A RULE OF THUMB
>
> Saturated fat is the fatty part of food that generally stays hard at room temperature. Both mono- and polyunsaturated oils tend to stay liquid at the same temperature.

Animal foods are a primary source of saturated fat—the visible fat on red meat, poultry skin, bacon drippings, cheese, lard and butter. A second source of saturated fats is "tropical oils"—palm oil, palm kernel oil and coconut oil. Studies show that diets rich in these saturated oils elevate LDL cholesterol and increase the risk of heart attack. Unfortunately, tropical oils are used freely in processed foods because they're relatively cheap. They're found in nondairy creamers, soups, potato chips, salad dressings and crackers—in so many processed foods that on average each American consumes over seven pounds of tropical oils annually.

■ *Avoid cholesterol-raising trans fat.* When polyunsaturated oils are hardened or stiffened into a solid or semisolid state in a process called hydrogenation, a chemical change takes place that produces trans fatty acids, or trans fat. There is much evidence that trans fat can raise total and LDL cholesterol and also reduce HDL cholesterol. In the Nurses' Health Study, women who ate lots of foods rich in trans fat had a 66% higher risk of heart disease than those who did not.

Margarine is a good example of how hydrogenation can alter the health characteristics of a food product. As a healthful alternative to cholesterol-raising butter, margarine seems ideal; it's made from polyunsaturated oil (usually corn or safflower oil), which lowers cholesterol. And that holds true as long as the oil remains liquid, in the form of soft, tub-type margarines, spray and squeeze-type margarines, or "diet" margarines.

But when hydrogenated into stick form, margarine can raise blood cholesterol. So, if you're concerned enough about your cholesterol to avoid butter and other saturated fats, it makes sense to also avoid stick margarine and other hydrogenated food products. Watch out for solid shortening, crackers, potato chips and other processed foods, commercially prepared baked goods (cookies, muffins, pies and cakes) and fried fast-foods such as chicken nuggets and French fries. Trans fat may soon be on nutrition labels, which will be helpful in identifying foods to be avoided.

■ *Reduce total fat for weight control.* Too much fat in the diet can produce an overabundance of calories leading to overweight and obesity. Unfortunately, high-calorie fatty foods—processed meats, baked goods, fast foods, snack foods such as potato chips and chocolate bars, salad oils, whole milk products, and packaged foods and meals—are central to the American diet. Frying is a favorite method of cooking, while fatty sauces and gravies are routinely used as flavor enhancers.

For most of us, gaining weight takes place over a period of time. A few more calories taken in, a few less expended, cause body fat to accumulate. As few as 50 extra calories a day—a single chocolate-chip cookie—can add 350 calories a week. That doesn't sound like much, but it equates to a gain of 5 pounds in a year, or 52 pounds in a decade.

Because of the caloric density of fatty foods, a high-fat diet produces a lot of calories. Fat contains more than twice as many calories as the same amount of protein or carbohydrate: one gram of fat has 9 calories; one gram of protein or carbohydrate has 4 calories. That's why a small package (1.74 ounces) of M&M peanut candies contains 250 calories, while an entire pound of apples has just 240 calories.

■ *When you choose to eat fat, make it the good kind.* If you need to lose weight, you should reduce the total fat in your diet; however, if managing blood lipids is your goal, concentrate on including healthy oils and excluding cholesterol-raising fats. The key is that when you choose to eat fat, make it a heart-healthy one. Like carbohydrates, fats can be divided into good and bad. The best choices are monounsaturated and polyunsaturated oils, as they can help to lower LDL and total cholesterol when used in place of saturated and trans fats. Monounsaturated fats include olive oil and canola oil (the two "best" oils of the group), olives, peanuts, peanut butter, avocados, almonds, cashews and almond oil. Studies in the United States and Canada indicate that these oils reduce LDL and total cholesterol, reduce the risk of blood clot formation and minimize decreases in protective HDL cholesterol. The next best choice is polyunsaturated oils, which are effective in reducing cholesterol when

---

CALORIE FOR CALORIE, FAT IS MORE FATTENING

There are marked differences in the body's metabolic response to fats as opposed to carbohydrates or proteins. Some of the calories we consume are utilized immediately as fuel. Those not used right away are converted to body fat for future use; this requires energy, and some of the calories being converted are burned in the process. But not all foods call upon the same amount of energy for calorie conversion. Studies at the University of Massachusetts Medical School found that 23% of the calories in carbohydrates are burned off when converted to body fat. So, if you eat 100 calories of potato, 77 calories are available to be stored as body fat. But dietary fat burns just 3% of calories in the conversion process. Eat 100 calories of butter and 97 of them are available to become body fat!

substituted for saturated fats. Polyunsaturated vegetable oils, in order of preference for heart health, include safflower oil, soybean oil, sunflower oil, corn oil, cottonseed oil and sesame oil.

New research suggests that the oil in flaxseed is rich in omega-3 fatty acids, which reduce blood clotting and thereby lessen the chance of a heart attack. (Other sources of omega-3s include fish, leafy green vegetables, tofu, almonds and hazelnuts.) The Family Heart Study, a long-term study of 4,600 people, found that a relatively small increase in omega-3s greatly reduced coronary risk.

While most of the emphasis on healthy fats has centered on vegetable oils, new research has shown that the unsaturated fat in nuts—particularly peanuts, walnuts, hazelnuts and almonds—provides similar cardiac benefits. A study at Hershey Medical Center, affiliated with Pennsylvania State University, suggests that when included as part of a balanced diet, nuts can reduce LDL cholesterol and lessen coagulation, potentially helping to reduce cardiac risk.

Dr. Walter Willett of the Harvard School of Public Health suggests that good fats—those from vegetables and fish—should go at the base of the food pyramid, along with complex carbohydrates. Bad fats—saturated and trans fats—should join simple carbohydrates at the top of the pyramid.

■ *Eat more fish and seafood.* "Fish is very hard to beat as a food item," says Dr. William Castelli, former director of the Framingham Heart Study. "There's something special about fish and fish oil that is extremely beneficial and protects against cardiac disease. In fact, I think people who have had a heart attack or know they have a cholesterol problem would be crazy not to eat fish at least twice a week."

Fish oil is a great source of omega-3 fatty acids and therefore instrumental in reducing the risk of heart attack by lowering cholesterol. It also reduces triglycerides, prevents clotting and promotes the health of coronary artery walls. In its latest dietary guidelines the American Heart Association recommends that everyone eat at least two three-ounce servings of fatty fish (salmon, mackerel, sardines, pompano and tuna) each week. One major study, published in the *New England Journal of Medicine*, concluded that eating "as little as two fish dishes a week, about 7.5 ounces of fish total, may cut the risk of dying from heart attack in half."

The relationship between fish consumption and cardiovascular protection was first noticed in Greenland, where between 1950 and 1974 only three heart attacks occurred in an Inuit population of 1,800 people. Among a similar American population, over 100 people would have had heart attacks. This finding initially confused the researchers, who were familiar with the link between a high-fat diet and coronary heart disease. After all, the Inuit eat a lot of fat—in the form of walrus and seal meat, cold-water fish and whale blubber—yet their incidence of heart attack was low. At first it was assumed that they received cardiac protection from their substitution of fish for red meat, which cut down on cholesterol-raising saturated fat. It soon became evident, however, that their lower risk derived from marine fat containing beneficial oils.

> ### OMEGA-3S ARE A-1
>
> Although our bodies do not manufacture omega-3s, we're fortunate in our ability to get them from food. Besides fish, leafy green vegetables, nuts, flaxseeds, canola oil and tofu can provide us with hese heart-healthy fatty acids.

This same finding came out of a Dutch study started in 1960 at the University of Leiden. Researchers monitored the diets of 1,088 middle-aged men for 20 years. They found that those who ate no fish had two times the risk of heart attack as compared with those who ate just seven ounces of fish per week.

More recently a study at Brigham and Women's Hospital in Boston found that men who eat oily fish regularly are greatly protected from heart attacks and in particular from sudden cardiac death. New results from the Nurses' Health Study found this to be true for women also. As reported in the *Journal of the American Medical Association*, "the more frequently a woman ate fish, the less likely she was to suffer a heart attack or die of any cardiac cause."

THE CAPSULE CONTROVERSY

What about fish oil capsules as an easy way to get omega-3s? The American Heart Association's dietary guidelines state that "the limited information available at present does not justify specific quantitative recommendations." In other words, as of this writing, we have no idea what constitutes an optimal and safe dosage of fish oil from capsules.

Fiber

Often called roughage, bulk or bran, fiber is a nondigestible component of plant foods. (Think in terms of whole fruits, raw vegetables, whole grains and cereals, beans and high-fiber snacks such as nuts.) Fiber aids in weight control because it passes through the digestive system intact, which means that not all calories consumed stay with the body.

The typical American diet is too low in fiber, providing only about 11 grams of fiber per day per person, far short of the American Dietetic Association's recommendation of 20 to 35 grams per day. For an idea of how much this is, remember that 28 grams equals one ounce, so the total amount of fiber in your daily food does not have to be unreasonably large. But you can overdo a good thing. Eating more than 50 or 60 grams of fiber a day may decrease the amount of vitamins and minerals your body absorbs.

Research shows that *soluble* fiber can reduce total and LDL cholesterol. As it moves through the digestive system, soluble fiber forms a gel that interferes with the absorption of cholesterol and is particularly effective in reducing cholesterol in people with levels over 200. Soluble fiber is found in oat bran, oatmeal, barley, rice bran, fruits (apples, oranges, strawberries, prunes), vegetables (carrots, corn, broccoli), and beans and peas (lentils, navy and pinto beans). Psyllium, sold commercially as Metamucil, also contains soluble fiber.

Studies conducted by Dr. James Anderson at the University of Kentucky showed that participants reduced their cholesterol by 13% to 19% by consuming one cup of oat bran, or about three bowls cooked, per day. (Eating three bowls of oat bran is not a dietary recommendation. It's important to get soluble fiber from a variety of foods.) Similar results were reported in a study at Louisiana State University. This is important information in light of evidence that a 1% reduction in cholesterol produces a 2% to 3% lowering of heart attack risk.

Soluble fiber is not a magic pill. (One woman reportedly sprinkled oat bran on ice cream, thinking it canceled out the fat.) Instead, understand that maximum benefits occur when foods rich in soluble fiber become part of an eating plan that is healthful overall. How much soluble fiber do you need? Experts are not certain, but the consensus is that consuming three grams a day—about the amount in one and a half cups of cooked oat bran—is sufficient to elicit a cholesterol-lowering response.

Soy Protein

Rich in protein and isoflavones, soy products such as soybeans, soy milk and tofu have a positive impact on cardiac health. (Some soy foods, tofu among them, are rich in protective omega-3 fatty acids as well.) The cholesterol-lowering properties of soy were first seen in early studies on Asian populations who exhibited lower cholesterol and far less heart disease than western populations. It was initially thought that the fat content of the respective diets—low among Asians, high for westerners—was the key factor. But upon further investigation researchers found that what Asians were eating—rice, vegetables, whole grains and particularly soy—was just as important as the fat they were not eating.

Subsequent studies have confirmed soy's effectiveness. An analysis of 38 clinical studies demonstrated that substituting soy products for animal foods could lower LDL cholesterol by as much as 8%. In addition, soy protein can lower triglyceride levels, raise

HDL cholesterol levels, inhibit cholesterol oxidation (which can damage coronary arteries and cause inflammation) and reduce the risk of blood clotting.

For most people, then, eating more soy protein is a smart move to protect the health of your heart. Says Dr. John W. Erdman, Jr., professor of nutrition at the University of Illinois, "Substituting soy products such as tofu for meat as well as other foods containing animal protein makes sense for everyone. But people with high cholesterol in particular should consume soy protein daily as a part of a healthy diet."

The evidence of soy's efficacy is so compelling that the Food and Drug Administration suggests that "25 grams of soy protein a day, as part of a diet low in saturated fat and cholesterol, may reduce the risk of heart disease." The link between soy protein and heart-disease protection is strong enough that the FDA allows foods with at least 6.25 grams per serving to carry a health claim on their label. It would require up to four servings of such products to yield the cholesterol-lowering benefit.

Two things are becoming clearer as the result of soy research. First, the more soy you eat, the greater the cholesterol benefit. A study at Wake Forest University Medical Center found that participants with a daily intake of 37 milligrams of isoflavones (about 1.5 cups of soy milk) lowered their total cholesterol by 8%. On the other hand, participants who took in 27 milligrams of isoflavones showed no cholesterol-lowering benefit. Secondly, the greatest benefit from soy products goes to those with the highest cholesterol. According to a study published in the *New England Journal of Medicine*, eating 47 grams of soy protein daily dropped cholesterol by 24% in people with levels above 335, but only by 8% in those with cholesterol under 200.

While it is clear that soy lowers cholesterol, other health claims are more tenuous. Some studies suggest that soy protects against hormone-related cancers; others do not. Some studies have found soy to protect against osteoporosis; others have not. Some researchers claim that soy relieves the hot flashes from menopause; others say soy is ineffective. At this point, there is solid scientific consensus only on the heart-health benefits of soy.

Alcohol

Moderate alcohol consumption, such as a glass of red wine with dinner, is associated with a reduced risk of heart disease and stroke. Says Dr. R. Curtis Ellison at the Boston University School of Medicine, "It's now commonly accepted in the medical community that alcohol can reduce the risk of atherosclerosis, the gradual 'silting up' of arteries that can lead to a heart attack or stroke." Even the American Heart Association acknowledges that moderate alcohol consumption may be cardioprotective.

Alcohol works to improve cardiovascular health by causing HDL to increase and LDL to decrease. Anytime you can get that movement—HDL going up, LDL coming down—it's good for your cardiac health. Alcohol also decreases the blood's propensity to clot and aids in dissolving clots that have already formed.

Many alcoholic beverages, including red wine and beer, contain powerful antioxidants that are even more potent than the antioxidants found in citrus fruits, soy foods or black tea. (Antioxidants comprise a broad array of naturally occurring compounds that aid in protecting cells against inflammation by reducing the damaging effects of oxidation.)

And finally, recent studies have found that people who drink moderately show signs of less arterial inflammation when compared with nondrinkers and heavy drinkers. In particular, moderate

> ## YES OR NO?
>
> Should everyone drink alcohol? Of course not. But if you do drink alcohol, moderate intake can be beneficial in terms of cardiovascular health. Excessive alcohol consumption, on the other hand, is linked to overweight, high blood pressure, accidents and liver disease.
>
> Most doctors advise abstinence from alcohol during pregnancy.

231

drinkers have significantly lower levels of C-reactive protein, a marker of inflammation.

Dr. Arthur Klatsky, a cardiologist with Kaiser Permanente in Oakland, California, conducted some of the early research on alcohol in the 1970s. Using the computerized health records of more than 100,000 people, Dr. Klatsky looked for factors that significantly affected the risk of heart disease. "We found that moderate drinkers, those who consume from one to three drinks per day, have a lower risk of dying from heart disease than either those who abstain altogether or those who drink heavily," he says. "In fact, nondrinkers and heavy drinkers seem to have heart attacks at the same rate. Light drinkers, on the other hand, have a decreased rate."

Subsequent population studies by the World Health Organization, the American Cancer Society and Oxford University in 21 countries validated Dr. Klatsky's findings. But until recently it was not known whether or not a reduction in stroke risk also occurred in moderate drinkers. As reported in the *New England Journal of Medicine*, a study of more than 22,000 men found that just a single glass of wine or beer a week was associated with a 20% reduction in the risk of ischemic stroke, which is caused by clots that reduce blood flow to the brain. Of interest is the fact that men who had only one drink a week had the same risk reduction as men who had one drink a day.

Does the type of alcohol make a difference? This question first came up in response to the so-called French Paradox: why it is that the French seem to be able to consume large amounts of food high in fat and cholesterol, and still have one of the industrial world's lowest rates for cardiovascular disease? Was red wine the key to health? Actually, while some experts believe red wine to be superior to white wine and spirits, studies on beer and whiskey show that it is alcohol, and not a particular type of alcohol, that provides increased heart attack and stroke protection. Says Dr. John Trevithick of the University of Western Ontario, "Our study found that beers have as many antioxidants as red or white wine, which ties in with other studies. The key, of course, is consuming beer in moderation."

Antioxidants

While the research on how antioxidants—beta-carotene, vitamin C and vitamin E—may reduce cardiovascular risk is still incomplete, experts agree that antioxidants definitely counteract oxidation, which plays an important role in atherosclerosis. During normal biological activities, the body produces small amounts of unstable substances called free radicals. (Free radicals are also generated upon exposure to environmental insults such as infectious agents, pollution and UV light.) Free radicals can potentially damage everything they come in contact with—including the cells that produce them.

Most free radicals are neutralized by "balancing" antidotes found in our cells, but if the generation of free radicals exceeds the body's capacity to neutralize them, an excess of harmful radicals can cause great damage. For example, free radicals can oxidize LDL cholesterol, resulting in its rapid absorption by the cells of artery

A NEW ANTIOXIDANT: LUTEIN

Researchers are finding lutein to be a power-packed anti-oxidant, potentially more beneficial than beta-carotene in preventing the thickening of blood vessel walls. An 18-month study by Dr. James Dwyer at the University of Southern California found that participants with the lowest blood lutein had carotid arteries four times thicker than those with the highest levels. The working theory is that lutein prevents LDL cholesterol from sticking to artery walls.

While its effects are still being investigated, early indications are that lutein may also protect eyesight, reduce cancer risk and combat arthritis. Good sources include kale, collard greens, spinach, broccoli, brussels sprouts and corn.

walls. This can start the buildup of plaque, promote inflammation and lead to coronary heart disease.

Some studies suggest that antioxidant vitamins may neutralize free radicals. According to Dr. Ishwarlal Jialal of the University of Texas Southwestern Medical Center in Dallas, "Antioxidants scavenge free radicals and neutralize them, thereby blocking LDL oxidation and curbing the earliest stages of plaque formation." Studies have also found that a high intake of antioxidants correlates with elevated HDL and lower blood pressure.

Dr. JoAnn Manson of Harvard Medical School agrees: "The evidence is mounting that foods rich in antioxidants really protect against cardiovascular events." The key antioxidants for cardiac health are vitamin E, beta-carotene (a precursor of vitamin A) and vitamin C. In the Nurses' Health Study, Dr. Manson found that women who ate at least five servings a day of deeply colored fruits and vegetables lowered their risk of heart attack by 33% and their risk of stroke by 71%. These reductions are among the largest gained by any means of intervention, including other lifestyle changes and prescription drugs.

While experts agree on the efficacy of antioxidants from food, the same does not hold true for supplements. Early studies, among them the Cambridge Heart Antioxidant Study, found that the risk of a heart attack among individuals who took vitamin E supplements was 77% lower compared with patients in the group who did not take vitamin E. Moreover, two important large-scale studies, one on men and one on women, showed that taking vitamin E was associated with a significantly decreased risk of coronary artery disease.

More recent studies, however, have found just the opposite. The Heart Outcomes Prevention Evaluation (HOPE) Study found that vitamin E supplements did not affect cardiovascular outcomes in patients at high risk for cardiovascular events. Other studies suggest there is even less evidence to support the efficacy of vitamin C and beta-carotene. In addition, work by Dr. Greg Brown at the University of Washington indicates that antioxidant supplements may blunt the benefits of statin drugs and niacin, used to lower LDL and raise HDL in heart patients.

Should you rely on antioxidant supplements for cardiovascular protection?

- If you're a heart patient, or if you have a high risk of heart attack or stroke, don't rely on antioxidant supplements alone for protection.

- If you take statin drugs and high doses of niacin, recognize that the cardioprotective benefits may actually be reduced by taking antioxidant supplements.

- If you don't have heart disease, taking antioxidant supplements for prevention probably won't hurt and may be beneficial, particularly if your diet is poor. But until more studies are completed, there's no way to tell.

- The most prudent and scientifically based recommendation for the general population should be to consume a balanced diet with emphasis on antioxidant-rich fruits, vegetables and whole grains rather than supplements.

- Always consult with your doctor.

Sugar

The American sweet tooth is getting bigger. In the early 1800s, each person consumed about two pounds of sugar a year. Today, the average adult eats and drinks more than 600 calories a day from sugar, or about 150 pounds a year. We eat it by the spoonful from the sugar bowl, and we get huge amounts more from soft drinks, cookies, cereals, salad dressings and candy. Sugar now accounts for 24% of calories consumed by Americans.

Consider the following points:

- A diet with too much sugar can elevate triglycerides and promote Syndrome X, increasing the cardiac risk of these important markers.

■ When consumed in excessive amounts, refined sugars such as table sugar, honey and corn syrup can contribute to overweight and obesity.

■ Foods that are rich in refined sugar contain "empty calories" with little or no nutritional value. They take up space in your diet that could otherwise be filled with nutritious foods rich in vitamins, minerals and fiber.

DRINKING SUGAR

About 65% of young girls and 74% of young boys consume sugar-sweetened drinks each day. These drinks are the leading source of added sugars in the diets of today's American kids. Overconsumption may increase the likelihood of childhood obesity.

■ We consume most of our sugar, which by itself is not so fattening (16 calories per teaspoon), in high-calorie processed foods. A 12-ounce can of orange soda, for example, has almost 12 teaspoons of sugar and 175 calories. Many sugary foods such as candy bars are also rich in fat (and thus high in calories), producing a double whammy on weight-control efforts.

■ Most sugary foods provide little fiber and mass, so there's no signal that you've had enough to eat. You can consume virtually an unlimited number of cookies (and a large number of calories) without feeling full.

B Vitamins

Get your B vitamins. One of the most effective ways to control homocysteine is to consume an adequate amount of three B vitamins—folate (called folic acid when it is used in a supplement or to fortify foods), B_6 and B_{12}.

In a study of over 80,000 female nurses, women who consumed more than twice the USRDA of these three vitamins reduced their risk of a heart attack by more than 45%. A study of 1,500 men and women in Europe found that those who took supplements of these vitamins cut their heart attack risk substantially. In an editorial in the *Journal of the American Medical Association*, Dr. Kilmer S.

McCully wrote that "consuming an adequate amount of folate, B_6 and B_{12} is as important to reducing coronary risk as quitting smoking, lowering high cholesterol and controlling blood pressure."

Doctors are also finding that people who undergo angioplasty have a much better chance of avoiding restenosis, or the closing up of opened arteries, when they get an adequate supply of these B vitamins.

But how much is enough? The USRDA currently suggests that adults should consume 400 micrograms of folate, 1.3 milligrams (women) and 1.7 milligrams (men) of B_6 and 2.4 micrograms of B_{12} daily. However, these levels may be inadequate to provide maximum protection against heart disease. "Everyone should be at two to three times the current USRDA for folate, B_6 and B_{12} to achieve the maximum reduction in risk," says Dr. Eric B. Rimm of the Harvard School of Public Health.

Fortunately, B vitamins are readily found in common foods. Fruits, vegetables and whole grains are good sources of folate and B_6. Vitamin B_{12} presents more of a challenge because it's found in meat, organ meats and dairy products—foods that tend to be high in saturated fat. Look for lower-fat sources such as fortified cereals, lean meat, and low-fat and nonfat milk.

■ Good sources of folate include whole grains, orange juice, leafy green vegetables, broccoli, beans, wheat germ, fortified oatmeal and cooked spinach. A cup of cooked oatmeal, for instance, has 199 micrograms of folate.

■ Good sources of vitamin B_6 include whole grains, bananas, beans, fish, potatoes, meat and poultry. A banana has almost .7 milligrams of vitamin B_6.

■ Good sources of vitamin B_{12} include meat, liver, poultry, eggs, dairy foods, fish and fortified cereals. A three-ounce serving of lean beef has two micrograms of B_{12}.

You may also want to consider using supplements. There is evidence that a multivitamin with B vitamins provides nutrition insurance for keeping artery-damaging homocysteine in check. Talk with your doctor about their appropriateness for you.

Salt and Sodium

It's dinnertime, and somewhere between grace and the first forkful of food comes the hallmark phrase of American table conversation: *Please pass the salt.* For most Americans, salt is something you sprinkle on your food even before you've tasted it—and that quantity is modest when compared with the amount of salt we eat in processed foods. Thirty-five percent of our daily sodium is consumed in condiment form, but fully 50% comes from processed and restaurant foods. Indeed, the average American snacks on about 21 pounds of potato chips, pretzels, popcorn, nuts and other "salty" foods every year. The problem is, sodium in excessive amounts has been directly linked to high blood pressure, stroke, kidney and thyroid disease, and edema.

And eating too much sodium is easy. A teaspoon of salt contains 2,300 milligrams of sodium; the appropriate consumption should be limited to no more than 2,400 milligrams a day. For the estimated 10% to 30% of the population with a predisposition to salt sensitivity, this may be problematic. Because there are no tests for sodium sensitivity, it's just prudent to err on the conservative side and moderate salt and sodium intake.

Water

Even with all the so-called "designer" water being carried around, Americans are still drinking nowhere near the recommended six to eight glasses (two quarts) of water a day. In fact, most of us are dehydrated.

An adequate intake of water is necessary for good overall health. But if weight control is a goal, there are a number of reasons to drink more water:

■ *It contains no calories.* You can drink water all day long and not have it contribute extra calories to your diet. But reach too frequently for a cola (144 calories), a beer (regular, 150 calories; light, 90 calories) or a glass of apple juice (120 calories), and those liquid calories will add up.

■ *It's filling.* In analyzing why many people are not successful in restricting calories to lose weight, experts found that dieters weren't getting enough food to feel satiety. They felt deprived and dissatisfied, and soon reverted to their old way of eating. Water (along with complex carbohydrates) helps to maintain satisfaction without adding calories. An adequate intake not only keeps the stomach full, but actually decreases hunger pangs.

> ## HOW MUCH WATER DO YOU NEED?
>
> To answer this question, some experts advise calculating your fluid needs by taking your weight in pounds and dividing it in half. This number in ounces is your recommended daily water intake. Thus, a 160-pound man would require 80 ounces of water each day, equivalent to 10 8-ounce glasses.

■ *It can help you to cut down on snacking.* When you're dehydrated, your brain receives a message that your body needs more water. But this message may be interpreted as a hunger cue. So instead of having a glass of water, you might have a snack. Surveys of American eating habits show that as water has been replaced as the drink of choice by diet soda, iced teas and specialty coffees, snacking habits have skyrocketed. But staying hydrated, experts say, often prevents snacking and overeating.

SPEAKING FROM EXPERIENCE

After writing and lecturing on healthy eating for more than two decades, I've learned that putting a cardioprotective diet together involves more than reading the latest data in the field of nutritional science. We cut sugar out of our diets, only to find that it's a minor player compared with fat. We threw out the salt shaker, only to learn that salt's major danger is to sodium-sensitive people. And we overreacted to oat bran, treating it like arterial Drano. Single-idea messages don't work. We need a sense of perspective and balance.

There is no such thing as a bad food. All foods are good, including chocolate, Brie, ice cream and Oreos—as long as they're part of a balanced diet. Eating well is about enjoyment and health. This is where my recommendations depart from low-fat and high-fat extremes. Some experts feel that a diet extremely low in fat—no more than 10% of calories from fat—provides optimal cardiovascular protection. But while that may be so, I found such a diet to be very restrictive—it proposes no meat, poultry or fish, and just one cup of nonfat milk a day. Also, I was constantly worried about my next meal: finding the right ingredients, using correct cooking methods, requesting changes when ordering in a restaurant. And, because the diet is so low in fat, I was constantly hungry.

The other extreme, of course, is the theory of high-protein, low-carbohydrate eating. Centering food choices on increased meat and whole-milk dairy products and eliminating pasta, bread, fruits and most vegetables is supposed to help with weight loss. And for some people it may (although their weight loss is likely of fluids, not body fat). But for others, such a diet may simply provide a means of eating fewer calories. Remember, what proponents of this style of eating call "high-protein"—a bacon cheeseburger, for example—most nutritionists call "high-fat." And fat satisfies. Suppose you're trying to eat no more than 1,000 calories a day to lose weight. If you ate all those calories as fruits and vegetables, chances are you'd be hungry all day and might end up eating more than your calorie goal. But if your 1,000 calories came mostly from meat, the fat content of these foods would probably keep you satisfied longer, helping you get through the day without eating more than your calorie goal. The result would be a diet higher in fat but lower in total calories.

This style of eating makes little sense to me and other people concerned with heart health. Many of the recommended foods are rich in saturated fat, which increases harmful LDL cholesterol. And while the diet rightly counsels the reduction of *simple carbohydrates* (commercially baked goods, for example, usually rich in sugar and white flour), it also calls for a reduction or elimination of *complex carbohydrates*—fruits, vegetables and whole grains. Where, then, am I to get cardioprotective fiber, soluble fiber and antioxidants?

My advice is to base your diet on foods high in complex carbohydrates and fiber, particularly vegetables, fruits, whole grains and beans. Eat lean meat and poultry, and be sure to eat fish at least twice a week. Watch portion control. Be sure to get a good supply of antioxidants and B vitamins. Attempt to fit more soy products into your diet. When you eat fats, olive and canola oils should be the first choices. Stay away from stick margarine and food products with trans fat. Use nonfat and low-fat dairy products. Enjoy alcohol in moderation. Drink plenty of water.

But most important, give yourself time to make permanent changes. That's where stress management and regular exercise can help as precursors of dietary change. Remember, the process is evolutionary, not revolutionary.   —*J.P*

Time for Action

THE TRADITIONAL APPROACH TO MANAGING DIET was based on exclusion. It concentrated on what you couldn't have, such as high-fat foods that might cause cholesterol to rise. Many doctors even provided patients with a listing of so-called "bad" foods. Red meat, chocolate, ice cream . . . all were banned.

While deprivation might work initially, the pendulum eventually swings to bingeing. Anyone who has attempted to give up ice cream knows the scenario. The craving hits and you eat a peach, then another, and then another. But the ice cream craving is still there, stronger than ever. So you have a little taste. Now you feel like a total failure. You've eaten forbidden food! You're just a weak-willed wimp

SPEAKING FROM EXPERIENCE

People often ask whether they need to be vegetarians to have healthy diets, but not everyone can manage a vegetarian diet correctly. Some young women, for example, proclaim themselves to be vegetarians and then eat cereal three times a day. That's a terrible idea. Other vegetarians have a diet rich in cheese and simple sugars. That's no good, either. Certainly, a vegetarian diet rich in complex carbohydrates can have a very positive effect on cardiac health, but there is evidence that eating some lean protein can make you feel full longer and keep you from overeating a high-carbohydrate meal.

The secret is not necessarily to eliminate animal foods, but to eat these foods less often. Basically, we need to rethink meat and potatoes. In the traditional American meal, meat has been the star of the show and whole grains, vegetables and fruit have been the bit players. It's time to reverse the roles.   —J.P.

(one patient exclaimed, "I have the backbone of a chocolate éclair!"), so you eat more ice cream—and often give up the hope that you'll ever be able to eat "right."

It's time for a fresh approach to diet based on inclusion, focused on foods that you *should* eat, particularly plant foods.

GIVE UP DIETING

The most common New Year's resolution is to lose weight. Things usually start out well: an orange stands in for a candy bar, whole-grain cereal for a doughnut, a turkey sandwich for a double cheeseburger. But by January 15 most dieters have started to settle back into their old eating patterns. This is a tough lesson to learn: if you want ongoing success, you must first get rid of the concept of "dieting"— a short-term weight reduction program during which you shed excess pounds rapidly by decreasing caloric intake. In this context, there is often no relationship between diet and habit.

You'll form a habit only when you make permanent changes to your diet pattern over the long run. That's why the question is not "How do I want to eat for the next week?" The question to ask is "How do I want to eat for the rest of my life?" It's not as scary as it sounds, if you base your decisions on the following time-tested standards:

■ *Sound nutritional science.* Contrary to the claims of infomercials and full-page ads for pills, powders, magic drinks, the latest crash-diet book or "effortless" exercise equipment,

> ### DIETING IS . . .
>
> ". . . the all-consuming obsession with the food you shouldn't have eaten yesterday, but did; the food you have eaten today, but shouldn't have; and the food you shouldn't eat tomorrow, but probably will."—Sandra Bergeson, *I Hate to Diet Dictionary*

there are no slimming supplements or quick-fix solutions for losing weight. Remember the line from *Jerry Maguire*: "Show me the money!" Apply that to your health decisions and say, "Show me the science!"

■ *Moderate and realistic expectations.* If your new diet forbids favorite foods and indulgences, depends on your spending long hours in the kitchen and involves complicated record-keeping, it will not work. It's about moderation, not undue sacrifice.

■ *A reasonable timetable.* Take time to institute important changes. There is no need to do everything at once. If you're drinking whole milk, for instance, and want to move to skim milk, don't think it will happen overnight. Take five or six weeks to move gradually from whole to 2% milk, then to 1% and finally to fat-free. The gradual reduction of fat will allow your taste buds to adapt.

76 DECIDE TO LOSE FAT, NOT POUNDS

Most people rely on the bathroom scale as an arbiter of weight. Up a few pounds and it's like a little death. Down a few and its better than winning the lottery. But a scale can tell you only what you weigh, not how much of that weight is fat-free muscle and bone, and how much is body fat. Suppose two people each weigh 150 pounds. One person is 140 pounds of muscle and 10 pounds of fat, while the other is 100 pounds of muscle and 50 pounds of fat. Do you need more proof that not all weight is created equal?

The real goal, then, is to lose body fat. A good starting point is an estimate of your own body fatness. This can be determined in most fitness centers, many sports medicine clinics and universities, and some physicians' offices, using one or more of the following methods:

■ *Water immersion.* This technique, in which you're weighed on a hanging scale immersed in water, is based on the principle that bone and muscle tissue are denser than water, whereas fat tissue is less dense. Therefore, a person with higher body fat weighs less in water than a person of the same weight who has more lean body mass.

■ *Skinfold measurements.* Popular in health clubs, this technique uses calipers to pinch folds of tissue in areas such as your stomach above the waistline, your hips and the backs of your arms. Since the amount of subcutaneous fat is proportional to the overall amount of body fat, the sum of the skinfold measurements can be plugged into a formula to estimate relative body fatness. The technique doesn't meas-

---

YO-YO DIETING

The late Erma Bombeck once wrote, "One-third of the country is on a diet. Another third just fell off a diet. And the remaining third is going on one next Monday." Statistics say she was right, but data also suggest that about 97% of crash dieters not only regain the lost weight within one year but actually put on extra weight. This is particularly true when caloric intake falls to under 1,200 calories a day for men and 900 for women.

Large weight losses do occur with fasting or on near-starvation diets, but approximately 60% of the loss can come from the body's "lean" weight (water, muscle and organ tissue). This happens with the so-called "high-protein/high-fat, low-carbohydrate" diets. By eliminating carbohydrates, which retain fluids, these diets merely act as short-term diuretics. Scale weight goes down because of fluid loss.

But scale weight and fluids will reappear. To make matters worse, some of these diets are so low in calories that they may result in the utilization of muscle tissue as fuel. Since muscle is an effective calorie burner, this may make efforts at weight reduction even more difficult.

---

ure fat embedded between muscle fibers, however, and the formulas are population-specific, accurate only when the subject is matched to the correct equation, based on age, gender and ethnicity.

■ *Electronic impedance.* This test involves passing a small electrical current through the body and measuring the impedance, or opposition to current flow. Since fat-free tissue is a good conductor of electric current, whereas fat is not, the greater the resistance to current flow, the higher the proportion of fat tissue. Similarly, infrared beams, which travel faster through muscle than through fat, can be used to assess body composition.

■ *Dual energy X-ray absorptiometry.* Clinical settings commonly use this method (sometimes referred to as DXA or DEXA), which not only measures body composition but also detects osteoporosis.

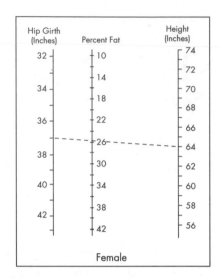

If you don't want to bother with the foregoing tests, you can estimate your body fat at home using the charts above, developed by Dr. Jack Wilmore for his book *Sensible Fitness*. Men should measure their waist (at belly-button level) and then line up that number on the body weight scale. Draw a line from girth to weight. Note where the line crosses the percent body fat line. In this example, we have a 180-pound man with a 35-inch waist. His body fat content is about 18%. Women should measure their hips at the widest point, then line up that number on the height scale. In this example, a woman with 37-inch hips who stands five feet four inches (64 inches) has just under 26% body fat.

Now that you know your body-fat percentage, compare it with the following guidelines for age and gender. Remember, it's not the loss of pounds that makes a difference, it's the reduction of body fat.

RECOMMENDED BODY-FAT PERCENTAGE

AGE	MALES	FEMALES
20 to 29	12	19
30 to 39	16	20
40 to 49	18	23
50 to 59	19	26
60 and over	20	27

Now that you know how much body fat you need to lose (translated into inches off your waist or hips), you can set realistic and attainable goals. Don't expect to lose 50 pounds or drop two collar or dress sizes in 30 days. It took months, perhaps years, to gain the extra weight, so you can't expect to lose it overnight. Instead, set short-term goals: the challenge of trimming 5 pounds seems more doable than losing 25. And finally, always keep the "why" behind your goals in mind. If you're overweight, you're more likely to reduce your body fat if you focus on health benefits such as lowering blood pressure and raising HDL rather than on simple poundage.

KEEP A FOOD JOURNAL

To change the way you eat, you have to know what, when, where and how much you're eating right now. The problem is, we often forget (or choose to forget) what we eat. As one chronic dieter said, "I count calories whenever I sit down to eat. But the food I eat when I'm walking through a mall or clearing the dinner dishes, those are *standing calories*—and standing calories don't count!"

Before you start any sort of diet plan, you should write down everything you put in your mouth for at least three days; a five- or seven-day record is better. And that means *everything*: the half an orange left over from breakfast, the handful of gumdrops on your way out the door, the bite of your friend's dessert. Be sure to include salad dressings, coffee creamers and other easily forgotten foods. Use one of the popular calorie-counters available at most bookstores to estimate calories and, if you wish, fat.

It's important not to change anything during this time. Don't try to be "good." Just record everything you eat, when you eat it and, above all, *why*. Were you truly hungry or were you eating simply as a response to emotional stress, anxiety or boredom?

If this sounds like a drag, consider the research by Dr. Daniel Kirschenbaum of Northwestern University Medical School, who tracked 38 dieters from two weeks before Thanksgiving to two weeks

247

SAMPLE FOOD JOURNAL

Day of Week: Tuesday

WHEN/ WHERE?	WHY?	WITH WHOM?	FOOD EATEN	CALORIES	FAT-GRAMS
7:30 A.M. Kitchen	Very hungry	Family	½ cup orange juice	55	0
			Jelly doughnut	225	9
			Coffee w/ 2 tbsp. half-and-half	40	4
10:00 A.M. Cafeteria	Not very hungry; ate for social reasons	Coworkers	Large mocha coffee	390	25
			Cinnamon bagel	195	1
Noon Office	Moderately hungry; worried about presentation	Alone	Tuna sandwich	585	28
			French fries, regular	230	13
			8 oz. 2% milk	120	5
2:00 P.M. Meeting room	Not hungry; anxious about presentation	Managers	Bag of jelly beans	250	0
6:30 P.M. Kitchen	Hungry	Family	5 oz. London broil	300	22
			Baked potato	145	0
			w/ 2 tbsp. sour cream	50	6
			Green salad	15	0
			w/ 2 tbsp. blue cheese dressing	155	16
			Glass of white wine	70	0
8:30 P.M. TV room	Not hungry; social eating	Kids	1 cup corn nuts	375	12
9:15 P.M. TV room	Not hungry; feeling lonely	Alone	½ cup French vanilla ice cream	265	17
Total				3,465	158

after New Year's. The participants who wrote down everything they ate managed to lose an average of seven pounds during the holidays, while those who didn't gained three pounds on average. "After a week of writing down foods, most people have a good idea how many calories are in about 75% of what they eat," he says. "Keeping a food diary works so well because it focuses you. It makes what you're doing real, reminds you forcefully of your goal and helps you feel more in control."

At the left is an example of a page from a food journal. Keep to the format we've shown here, or modify it to work specifically for you. You'll be surprised how fast the numbers can add up—the totals in our sample journal represent nearly two to three times the recommended daily values for calories and fat. But when you take the time each day to record your intake, the journal will become a tool for managing your diet.

DEVELOP A HYDRATION PLAN

Water regulates body temperature, transports nutrients and oxygen, carries away waste, helps to detoxify the kidneys and liver, and dissolves vitamins and minerals. It also helps in maintaining a balanced diet, not overeating, and exercising more effectively. And while milk, juices and soft drinks may do the trick, experts recommend an increase in the intake of water, plain H_2O, to meet daily fluid needs. This may seem like a simple suggestion, but evidence indicates that you may not be drinking enough water on your own. You need a plan:

■ Spread out your consumption over the entire day. Don't wait until you're thirsty.

■ Drink before you get the urge. If you wait for the signal that you are thirsty, you may already be slightly dehydrated.

■ Drink one glass of water with each meal.

■ Drink one glass before you exercise and another two glasses afterwards.

249

■ Drink a glass of water when you brush your teeth as part of your morning ritual.

■ Keep a pitcher of water laced with fresh lemons in the refrigerator. It's a satisfying alternative to soda pop.

■ Carry a water bottle around with you and sip from it steadily throughout the day. Experiment with different-size bottles. A 32-ounce water bottle might seem more overwhelming to finish than two 16-ounce bottles.

■ Try different temperatures of water. Some people like their water room-temperature, while others like theirs icy cold. Know what you like.

 ## MAKE A DAILY FAT BUDGET

Reducing dietary fat is great in theory but difficult in practice. Establishing a daily fat budget, as odd as that may sound, will really help you get on the right track. The money analogy works: you have to know how much you can spend before you decide how you're going to spend it. You can calculate your fat budget with the three simple steps that follow.

First, estimate your ideal weight. Unfortunately, most height-weight charts simply allow for too much weight, whether you're a man or a woman. A more accurate way to determine ideal weight is to use the following formula developed by Dr. Richard Freeman at the University of Wisconsin Medical School:

■ *Women* get 100 pounds for their first five feet of height. Every additional inch is plus five pounds. Thus, a five-foot-five woman has an ideal weight of 125 pounds.

■ *Men* get 105 pounds for the first five feet of height. Every additional inch is plus six pounds. Accordingly, a man of six feet has an ideal weight of 177 pounds.

These recommendations apply only if you have a "medium"-size frame. To find out whether your frame is medium, large or small, measure your wrist just below your wrist bone (toward your hand) with a cloth measuring tape, then use the table below to determine your frame size in inches:

FRAME SIZE	SMALL	MEDIUM	LARGE
Men	Under 7	7	Over 7
Women	Under 6	6	Over 6

If you have a medium frame, the Freeman formula predicts your ideal weight. For a large frame, add 10% to the ideal weight; for a small frame, subtract 10%. Experts like the Freeman formula because it represents an ideal weight that corresponds to a healthy body-fat percentage (see page 246). If your scale weight and your ideal weight are the same, then your body-fat percentage is also in line.

Second, you need to know how many calories you can consume each day to sustain your ideal weight. (Remember, if you weigh 180 pounds but your ideal weight is 150 pounds, you need to eat for 150 pounds, not 180.) According to the American College of Sports Medicine and the American Dietetic Association, you can estimate your daily caloric needs as follows:

LEVEL OF ACTIVITY	CALORIES NEEDED PER POUND PER DAY
Extremely inactive, or sedentary (*Example*: No aerobic exercise in the course of a week)	11
Moderately active, or light activity (*Example*: Aerobic exercise 2 to 3 times a week)	13
Active, moderate exercise and/or work (*Example*: Aerobic exercise 4 to 5 times a week)	15
Extremely active, heavy exercise and/ or work (*Example*: Aerobic exercise 6 to 7 times a week)	18

Your level of activity: _____

Multiplying your ideal weight by appropriate calories provides you with the number of calories you need for the day. For example, if your ideal weight is 125 pounds and you are "moderately active," you need 1,625 calories on a daily basis to sustain that weight and activity level.

The third step is to convert daily calories into grams of fat—your fat budget. If you want to lose weight, no more than 25% of your daily calories should come from fat.

GRAMS OF TOTAL FAT PER DAY

TOTAL CALORIES PER DAY	20%	25%	30%
1,000	22	27	33
1,100	24	30	36
1,200	27	33	40
1,300	29	36	43
1,400	31	39	47
1,500	33	42	50
1,600	36	44	53
1,700	38	47	57
1,800	40	50	60
1,900	42	53	63
2,000	44	56	67
2,100	47	58	70
2,200	49	61	73
2,300	51	64	77
2,400	53	67	80
2,500	56	69	83
2,600	58	72	87
2,700	60	75	90
2,800	62	77	93
2,900	64	80	96
3,000	66	83	100

Remember, your budget is a maximum for the day. Unless you're extremely active (you run 10 miles a day) or work outdoors in very cold climates, there's no reason to go above 60 grams of fat per day. On the other hand, most health professionals counsel not to go lower than 15 fat-grams daily.

NOW KEEP TO YOUR BUDGET! 80

Start each day with your fat budget number in an "account." As you make food choices throughout the day, the key is to stay within the maximum number of fat-grams—and to use fewer than your maximum if you want to lose weight. Let's use an example of a woman who eats 1,800 calories a day. On a 25%-fat diet, she can have a maximum of 50 fat-grams. She's home for breakfast and dinner, but often eats lunch in a restaurant. Here's how she can use her budget to make smarter choices, with commentary from registered dietitian Bev Utt:

SAMPLE FAT BUDGET

FOOD CHOICES	FAT -GRAMS
Starting Balance	50
Breakfast	
Oatmeal, ½ cup	1
Banana, 1 medium	1
Nonfat milk, 1 cup	1
Whole-wheat toast, 1 slice w/	1
strawberry jam	0
Coffee w/ whole milk, 2 tbsp.	1

What Bev Utt has to say: "Breakfast should provide good nutrition without a lot of extra calories or fat. Spending only five grams of fat to get good taste and nutrition makes great sense. By comparison, if she had two scrambled eggs with hash browns, toast and margarine, it would have eaten up 26 fat-grams—over half her budget for the entire day."

Midmorning Snack

Apple	1.0
Large cappuccino w/ nonfat milk	.5

What Bev Utt has to say: "A low-fat breakfast often leaves you a little hungry in the mid-morning, so a snack can be a good thing. She has made a smart choice. The apple is filling and contains fiber, and the cappuccino with nonfat milk provides calcium. Compare this selection with the more typical American morning snack of a cinnamon roll at 9 grams of fat and a large mocha made with whole milk at 25 grams of fat. It's easy to see how high-fat snacking has contributed to America's weight problem."

Lunch

McDonald's Chicken McGrill Sandwich (no mayonnaise)	6
Side Salad	1
w/ nonfat vinaigrette dressing, 1 packet	0
1% low-fat milk, 8 oz.	2.5

What Bev Utt has to say: "Up to lunchtime, she's in great shape for the day . . . only 6.5 grams of fat 'spent.' But like a lot of people, she has little time for lunch. McDonald's will have to do. The key, then, is making smarter choices in a fast-food environment. She has eaten a fast-food meal with only 9.5 grams of fat. Compare her choices with a Big Mac at 34 grams, a chocolate shake at 17 grams and a large order of French fries at 26 grams."

Dinner

Grilled salmon fillet, 4 oz.	12
Wild rice, 1 cup	4
Stir-fried vegetables, 2 cups	1
Pear, fresh, sliced	1
Wine, 4.5 oz.	0
Coffee w/ whole milk, 2 tbsp.	1

What Bev Utt has to say: "Going into dinner, she has spent only 17 grams of fat—less than half of her budget. And that's good because Americans usually have dinner as their big meal of the day. She has a tasty, healthy dinner and it's only 19 grams of fat. Plus, much of that fat came from heart-healthy fish oil. Again, when you decide to eat fat, make it a healthy choice."

Evening Snack
Microwave low-fat popcorn, 2 cups	1

What Bev Utt has to say: "This compares nicely with a cup of cheese combos at 21 fat-grams or potato chips at 10 grams."

Total fat-grams spent
	36

Bev Utt's final comments: "The above example illustrates how to manage fat and calories, yet eat satisfying food—even including lunch in a fast-food restaurant. No one would go hungry on such a day, yet total fat was contained. Do you have to go through life with a fork in one hand and a calculator in the other? No. But remember, if you want to develop the low-fat habit, you must practice it successfully in real-life situations, like eating on the run. Having—and using—a daily fat budget makes it easier."

GET YOUR CALORIES EARLY IN THE DAY 81

Many people skip breakfast and lunch altogether. And those who do eat these meals often have a Danish for breakfast and fast food for lunch. When these people get home in the evening and relax, they tend to become ravenous and eat much more at dinner than they need. The American Dietary Association estimates that over half of overweight women eat 70% of their daily calories after seven P.M. A better way is to take in the majority of calories at breakfast and lunch so they can be burned during the course of the day. *New York*

HOW MANY CALORIES SHOULD YOU EAT?

According to new guidelines from the American College of Sports Medicine, the optimal approach to weight loss combines mild caloric restriction (no fewer than 1,200 calories a day) and an exercise program that promotes a daily energy expenditure of more than 300 calories.

Here's another way to think about it. If you want to lose an average of one pound per week (and if you have fewer than 25 pounds to lose), multiply your current weight in pounds by 10. That's roughly your daily calorie level, though it obviously depends on your level of physical activity.

Times columnist Jane Brody offers her perspective: "If you're driving from New York to Los Angeles, does it make more sense to fill the gas tank after you've arrived in Los Angeles or before you leave New York?"

Numerous studies suggest that timing affects caloric utilization. In one study, each of two groups of women ate 2,000 calories a day. The only difference was that the first group received all their calories at breakfast and the second group ate all 2,000 calories at dinner. The results: every person in the breakfast group lost weight, and every person in the dinner group gained weight. The expert advice: "Eat like a king at breakfast, a prince at lunch and a pauper at dinner."

82 BE CAUTIOUS ABOUT DIETARY CHOLESTEROL

It's frustrating and disillusioning when experts lift the ban on something they once condemned. And for many people, this is a good excuse to stop trying to eat right. In the 1960s and '70s, eliminating foods rich in dietary cholesterol—eggs, liver, shrimp and organ meats—was touted as a means of controlling blood cholesterol. But science marched on, and current research shows that dietary cholesterol has much less impact on blood cholesterol than dietary fat. This means that the fat you cook your egg in may be more significant than the egg itself. "I'd rather eat a poached egg from time to time," says dietitian Bev Utt, "than have an Egg Beaters omelet fried in butter." This advice is echoed by Dr. Ernst J. Schaefer of Tufts University: "Reducing saturated fat consumption by 50% may lower blood cholesterol twice as much as a similar drop in dietary cholesterol."

Still, it's important to moderate your intake of dietary cholesterol: no more than 300 milligrams per day, and no more than 200 milligrams if you have heart disease, according to the American Heart Association. The best way to do that is to reduce the amount of all animal foods in your diet. Keep in mind that simply replacing large portions of beef with large portions of chicken won't do any good, since the flesh of all animals contains similar amounts of cholesterol—about 100 milligrams per three-ounce portion.

ROUGH UP YOUR DIET 83

We should all be eating 20 to 35 grams of fiber a day, with at least 3 grams as soluble fiber. But most of us don't even come close. A good step in the right direction is to learn which foods are fiber-rich. Be sure to read labels on packaged foods; they'll tell you the amount of dietary fiber in each serving.

Now figure out how to incorporate high-fiber foods into your diet. Center your meals on plant foods rather than animal foods. Serve reasonable portions of meat, poultry or fish, and surround them with larger servings of vegetables, beans, peas, potatoes, rice and fruits. Plan for a cooked vegetable and a salad at dinner.

■ *Have a high-fiber breakfast.* It's easy to get fiber at breakfast: oatbran cereal, oatmeal, other bran cereals and low-fat bran muffins. Or you can find a whole-grain cereal that contains at least five grams of fiber per serving (or mix it with your regular brand). Top it with wheat bran, wheat germ, oat bran, raisins, bananas or berries, all of which are good sources of fiber. It always makes sense to start your day with oats, which, because of their soluble fiber, are allowed to bear a heart-healthy claim. But don't try to get all of your soluble fiber at breakfast. It takes about 1.5 cups of cooked oatmeal or 3 cups of dry oat cereals to get enough fiber to have a cholesterol-lowering effect.

■ *Go for fruits and vegetables.* Choose whole fruits with skin. Eat a baked potato with the skin on. Instead of iceberg lettuce, choose romaine or spinach for your salad. Serve hummus, made from chickpeas, instead of sour-cream dips. Eat raw fruits and vegetables whenever possible. Keep fresh and dried fruit on hand for snacks.

■ *Eat beans.* Studies have suggested that just four ounces of cooked beans a day can significantly reduce your levels of total and LDL cholesterol.

■ *Choose whole, unprocessed grains.* Try barley (excellent in hearty soups and as a side dish), bulgur (great to replace rice in recipes and a main ingredient in tabbouleh), triticale (a hybrid of wheat and rye that can also be cooked as a breakfast cereal or as a substitute for rice), whole-wheat couscous, millet, quinoa, amaranth, buckwheat (kasha) and whole-wheat or whole-rye berries.

■ *Buy whole-grain breads and crackers.* Look for those made from stone-ground flour. The next best choice is 100% whole-wheat or other whole-grain bread such as rye or pumpernickel.

SPEAKING FROM EXPERIENCE

Decreasing fat is important, but increasing fiber is also critical to a healthy diet. A recent study of 13,000 middle-aged men from seven countries suggests that fiber, not fat, determined how successful they were at managing weight. In fact, the leanest men ate a whopping 40% of calories from fat, far more than is recommended, but they consumed 41 grams of fiber a day. The study concluded that a high-fiber diet can go a long way in canceling out the effect of fat calories, at least in relation to body weight.   —*J.P.*

COMMON SOURCES OF FIBER

FOODS	AMOUNT	GRAMS OF FIBER	GRAMS OF SOLUBLE FIBER
Fruits			
Apple, w/ skin	1 medium	3.5	1.0
Apple, w/o skin	1 medium	2.5	1.0
Banana	1 medium	3.0	0.5
Blackberries	½ cup	4.0	1.0
Dates, dried	½ cup	4.4	1.2
Figs, dried	½ cup	8.2	4.0
Orange	1 medium	3.0	2.0
Peach	1 medium	2.0	1.0
Pear, Bartlett	1 medium	4.0	2.0
Prunes, dried	½ cup	6.6	3.8
Raisins, dried, seedless	½ cup	2.3	1.1
Vegetables			
Asparagus	½ cup	1.0	0.4
Beets	½ cup	1.3	0.6
Broccoli	½ cup	1.5	0.5
Brussels sprouts	½ cup	4.5	3.0
Cauliflower, cooked	½ cup	2.0	0.5
Carrots	½ cup	2.0	1.0
Collard greens, cooked	1 cup	5.5	3.0
Green beans	½ cup	2.0	1.0
Potato, with skin	1 medium	3.0	1.0
Soybeans, green, cooked	½ cup	4.0	1.5
Spinach	½ cup	1.8	0.6
Squash, winter, cooked	½ cup	1.5	0.5
Sweet potato, w/ skin	1 medium	4.0	1.5
Tomato, fresh	½ cup	1.0	0.0

COMMON SOURCES OF FIBER (*continued*)

FOODS	AMOUNT	GRAMS OF FIBER	GRAMS OF SOLUBLE FIBER
Beans, Peas and Legumes			
Baked beans, plain or vegetarian, canned	½ cup	6.5	2.0
Black beans, cooked	½ cup	5.5	2.0
Black-eyed peas, cooked	½ cup	5.5	1.0
Chickpeas, cooked	½ cup	6.0	1.0
Green peas, cooked	½ cup	4.5	1.5
Kidney beans, cooked	½ cup	6.0	3.0
Lentils, cooked	½ cup	8.0	1.0
Lima beans, cooked	½ cup	6.5	3.5
Navy beans, cooked	½ cup	6.0	2.0
Northern beans, cooked	½ cup	5.5	1.5
Pinto beans, cooked	½ cup	7.0	2.0
Breads, Grains and Pasta			
Barley	½ cup	4.0	1.0
Rice, brown	½ cup	2.0	0.0
Rice, white	½ cup	0.5	0.0
Rice, wild	½ cup	1.5	0.0
Rye bread	1 slice	1.5	1.0
Spaghetti	½ cup	1.0	0.5
Spaghetti, whole wheat	½ cup	2.0	0.5
White bread	1 slice	0.5	0.0
Whole-wheat bread	1 slice	2.0	0.5
Breakfast Cereals			
All-Bran	¾ cup	19.0	3.0
Bran Buds	¾ cup	4.6	1.5
Bran flakes	¾ cup	5.5	1.5
Oat bran	¾ cup	4.5	1.5
Oatmeal	¾ cup	3.0	1.5
Raisin bran	¾ cup	4.8	0.8
Shredded wheat	¾ cup	3.5	0.5

COMMON SOURCES OF FIBER (*continued*)

FOODS	AMOUNT	GRAMS OF FIBER	GRAMS OF SOLUBLE FIBER
Nuts and Seeds			
Almonds	1 oz.	3.0	0.0
Brazil nuts	1 oz.	1.5	0.0
Cashews	1 oz.	1.0	0.0
Peanuts, dry-roasted	1 oz.	2.5	0.0
Pecans	1 oz.	2.0	0.0
Pistachios	1 oz.	3.0	0.0
Sunflower seeds	¼ cup	3.5	0.5
Walnuts, English	1 oz.	1.5	0.0

PUT MORE FISH IN YOUR DIET 84

Because of the protective omega-3 fatty acids found in fish oil, the American Heart Association recommends eating fatty fish at least two times a week. Some types of fish are richer in omega-3 fatty acids than other types. Highest on the list is Atlantic mackerel, with 2.5 grams of omega-3s per three ounces. The figures for three-ounce portions of other fish are shown below:

TYPE OF FISH	OMEGA-3s (Grams)
Herring	1.7
Lake trout	1.6
Salmon	1.2
Tuna	0.5
Pacific halibut	0.4
Channel catfish	0.3
Shrimp	0.3
Dungeness crab	0.3
Swordfish	0.2
Red snapper	0.2
Sole	0.1

DON'T DROWN YOUR FISH IN FAT

It's very easy to dilute the benefits of fish-eating in a sea of high fat. But that doesn't have to happen:

■ *Be smart about tuna.* Picking up a four-ounce can of tuna packed in water instead of oil can save you 20 grams of fat, or about 180 calories. And if you're making tuna salad, remember that three tablespoons of mayonnaise will add about 300 calories to a sandwich.

■ *Use heart-healthy cooking methods* such as grilling, broiling, poaching, barbecuing and microwaving. Avoid frying or deep-fat frying, which can add more than a gram of fat per ounce of fish. If you do fry, use a grill pan or a nonstick pan with a little cooking spray.

■ *Skip fatty condiments* such as butter, butter sauce, mayonnaise and tartar sauce, particularly if weight control is your goal. A tablespoon of melted butter is 100 calories; the same amount of tartar sauce is 90 calories. Better choices include fresh lemon and lime, horseradish, tomato salsa, low-sodium soy sauce, flavored vinegars, vinaigrettes, wine and oil-free dressings.

■ *Read labels.* Be sure the fish in a frozen meal is not breaded, deep-fried and/or drowned in a fatty sauce.

■ *Order smart in a restaurant.* In a sit-down restaurant, ask questions about cooking methods: "Is it fried? Breaded? Batter-dipped and fried?" If so, avoid it. Opt for fish that is baked, broiled, steamed or grilled, without oil or butter. Watch out for condiments and sauces such as drawn butter, cream sauce and cheese sauce.

In fast-food restaurants, make smarter choices. A serving of Flavorbaked Fish at Long John Silver's, for instance, has just 3 grams of fat, while Wendy's Fish Filet Sandwich will set you back 27 fat-grams.

BECOME LABEL-LITERATE

If you live in the real world and buy processed foods, it's necessary to know what's in them. And that means reading food labels. Take for example a sandwich ham advertised as "95% fat-free." What the claim actually means is that fat makes up just 5% of the ham's *weight*.

PASTA, RICE AND POTATOES:
IT'S WHAT'S ON TOP THAT COUNTS

One cup of enriched pasta provides vitamins, minerals, about 10% of the USRDA for protein and less than one gram of fat—all for just over 200 calories. But even the healthiest pasta turns into a high-fat, high-calorie dish when it's drenched in Alfredo sauce or served with a pound of sausage. One cup of pasta with a quarter-cup of marinara or red clam sauce and a tablespoon of grated Parmesan cheese has only about 275 calories, or about the same as a cup of low-fat yogurt sweetened with fruit preserves. Also, don't overlook Asian noodles such as soba (buckwheat), udon and saifun (cellophane), which are particularly good in chicken broth with vegetables.

The same principle applies to rice, a low-fat, nutrient-rich food that makes for excellent side and main dishes, particularly when it's whole-grain brown rice. Instead of topping it with butter, butter sauce or gravy, serve it as a side dish with a few drops of sodium-reduced soy sauce or as a main dish covered with beans or stir-fried chicken and vegetables. Watch out for packaged rice dishes that contain added fat; most of them don't need to be made with the butter or oil as suggested in the cooking instructions. And don't be fooled into thinking that a packaged rice dish is fat-free because the Nutrition Facts list fat content as zero. Some manufacturers give nutritional information "as packaged," so that the fat called for in cooking is not reflected.

The best toppings for a low-fat baked potato include nonfat sour cream, low-fat or nonfat yogurt, salsa and fresh herbs such as chopped dill, parsley and chives.

It has nothing to do with the true measurement, the *calories* that come from fat. About 40% to 60% of calories in sandwich ham come from fat, which is a long way from the low-fat claim.

Most food labels have a section called Nutrition Facts (see the example on the facing page). This is where you'll find an accurate description of fat in grams, not percentages, as well as calories and other elements contained in the food.

In particular, take note of the following information:

■ *Serving size*. Pay attention to the number of servings in the container. If you buy a bag of chips that contains four servings and you eat half the bag, you'll have to double the calories and fat on the label since you've eaten two servings.

■ *Calories*. Watch out for "fat-free" foods. While they contain no fat, they still have calories. And from a weight-control standpoint, all calories count! The label will tell you if the food is too calorically dense for your dietary goals.

■ *Fat-grams*. Once you know your fat budget, it's relatively easy to decide whether any particular food "fits."

■ *Saturated fat*. If you want to avoid high total and LDL cholesterol levels, buy foods with a low saturated fat value.

■ *Fiber*. There's a big difference between two slices of French bread (1.5 grams of fiber) and the same amount of pumpernickel bread (4 grams of fiber)—particularly if you're trying to reach the recommended level of 20 to 35 grams of fiber a day.

TRANS FATS

Not yet listed in Nutrition Facts, trans fats may be worse for your arteries than saturated fat. If the ingredients list includes heavily hydrogenated oils, you can be sure trans fat is in the food.

■ *Sugars*. Remember, 4 grams of sugar equals one teaspoon. Quaker Cap'n Crunch, for instance, lists 12 grams of sugar per serving. Think of it as three teaspoons.

■ *Sodium*. Your goal is to consume 2,400 milligrams or less of sodium a day—or approximately one teaspoon of salt. To give you an idea, a cup of Newman's Own Pasta Sauce, for instance, has 1,400 milligrams of sodium.

■ *Dietary cholesterol*. Remember the guideline of no more than 300 milligrams a day.

Nutrition Facts

Serving Size ½ cup (114 g)
Servings Per Container 4

Amount Per Serving

Calories 90   Calories from Fat 30

% Daily Value*

Total Fat 3 g **5%**

Saturated Fat 0 g **0%**

Cholesterol 0 g **0%**

Sodium 300 mg **13%**

Total Carbohydrate 13 g **4%**

Dietary Fiber 3 g **12%**

Sugars 3 g

Protein 3 g

| Vitamin A | 80% | * | Vitamin C | 60% |
| Calcium | 4% | * | Iron | 4% |

* Percent Daily Values are based on a 2,000-calorie diet. Your daily values may be higher or lower depending on your calorie needs:

	Calories	2,000	2,500
Total Fat	Less than	65 g	80 g
Sat Fat	Less than	20 g	25 g
Cholesterol	Less than	300 mg	300 mg
Sodium	Less than	2,400 mg	2,400 mg
Total Carbohydrate		300 g	375 g
Fiber		25 g	30 g

Calories per gram:
Fat 9   Carbohydrate 4   Protein 4

In addition to Nutrition Facts, food labels also contain advertising and descriptive terms. In the past, terms like "light" and "low-fat" could be used virtually any way the packager wished. The FDA now requires such eye-catching nutrition terms to meet specific definitions. Believe us—they make for fascinating reading!

OLD TERMS, NEW MEANINGS

WHAT THE NEW LABEL SAYS	WHAT THE NEW LABEL MEANS
FREE	The product contains no or only negligible amounts of calories, cholesterol, fat, sodium or sugar.
Calorie-free	Less than 5 calories per serving.
Cholesterol-free	Less than 2 milligrams cholesterol and 2 grams or less saturated fat per serving.
Fat-free	Less than 0.5 grams fat per serving.
Sodium-free	Less than 5 milligrams sodium per serving.
Sugar-free	Less than 0.5 grams sugar per serving.
LOW	May be used on foods that can be eaten frequently without exceeding the dietary guidelines for fat, saturated fat, cholesterol, sodium, sugar and/or calories.
Low calorie	40 calories or less per serving. *(When it comes to meals and main-dish items like frozen dinners and entrées, this guideline translates into about 120 calories or less in 3.5 ounces of food.)*
Low cholesterol	20 milligrams or less cholesterol and 2 grams or less saturated fat per typical serving. *(A main dish or meal labeled "low cholesterol" has about 60 milligrams of cholesterol per 10 ounces.)*
Low fat	3 grams or less fat per100 calories. *(Watch out for milk products, which have been exempted from the "low fat" regulation. So, "2% milk" will be termed "low fat" even though it contains 5 grams of fat per serving.)*
Low saturated fat	1 gram or less saturated fat per serving. *(A main dish can usually make this claim if less than 10% of its calories come from saturated fat.)*
Low sodium	140 milligrams or less sodium per serving. *(This translates into about 400 milligrams of sodium in a typical 10-ounce main dish, or 600 milligrams in a 16-ounce meal.)*
Very low sodium	35 milligrams or less sodium per serving.

OLD TERMS, NEW MEANINGS (*continued*)

WHAT THE NEW LABEL SAYS	WHAT THE NEW LABEL MEANS
HIGH	means the food must contain 20% or more of the Daily Value for a particular nutrient. "Rich in" or "excellent source" may be used instead of "high."
GOOD SOURCE	means that a serving of the food supplies 10% to 19% of the Daily Value for a particular nutrient.
LIGHT or *LITE*	can mean a number of different things: • If a food contains 50% or more of its calories from fat to begin with, such as sausage or cheese, "light" means that at least half its fat has been removed. • If a food is less than 50% fat to begin with, it can be called "light" if *either* the fat content has been cut in half *or* the calories have been reduced by a third. • For a main dish or meal, "light" means that the dish meets the definition of either "low calorie" or "low fat." • "Light" can also mean that the sodium content of a low-calorie, low-fat food has been reduced by at least 50%. However, if the sodium is reduced by 50% in a food that is not low in fat and calories, the label must state "light in sodium." • "Light" can also refer to color or texture, but the label must say so clearly. It can be also be used without explanation when "light" has traditionally been part of the food's name, e.g., brown sugar or cream.
REDUCED	means that a product contains 25% less of a nutrient (such as fat) or of calories than the regular product.
MORE	tells you that a serving of food contains 10% more of the Daily Value for a nutrient than the regular food. The label on the calcium-fortified orange juice, for example, could specify that the product supplies "more calcium" than regular juice.

OLD TERMS, NEW MEANINGS (*continued*)

WHAT THE NEW LABEL SAYS	WHAT THE NEW LABEL MEANS
LEAN and *EXTRA-LEAN*	describe the fat content of certain meats, poultry, seafood and game meats.
Lean	Less than 10 grams of fat, 4 grams of saturated fat and 95 milligrams of cholesterol per serving. *(With the exception of many main dishes and entrées, a "lean" food generally has more fat than a "low fat" food and more saturated fat than a "low in saturated fat" food.)*
Extra-lean	Less than 5 grams of fat, 2 grams of saturated fat and 95 milligrams of cholesterol per serving. *(With the exception of many main dishes and entrées, an "extra-lean" food generally has more fat than a "low fat" food and more saturated fat than a "low in saturated fat" food.)*
PERCENT FAT-FREE	must now be used only on foods that meet the "low fat" or "fat-free" definitions. However, it may still be misleading as it describes the percentage of fat by weight, not the percentage of calories from fat.

87 GO LEAN

We get about one-third of our daily fats from animal foods, and this is hardly a healthy situation. "Our excessive intake of meat is killing us," says the *American Journal of Cardiology*'s Dr. William C. Roberts. "We fatten our cows and pigs, kill them, eat them, and then they kill us."

The trick is to modify the meat in our diet, not to eliminate it altogether. Meat is a good supplier of protein, iron and B vitamins; it's particularly effective in repairing muscle tissue broken down by regular exercise. And not all meat is high in fat and calories; ounce for ounce, a slice of apple pie has more than double the amount of fat contained in lean meat.

But not all cuts of meat are the same. Some favorite meats—T-bone steak, prime rib, New York strip, rib eye, rib roast, brisket, pork spare ribs and lamb roast, for example—can have 20 to 30 grams of fat per 3.5-ounce serving. And few people limit themselves to such small servings.

Fortunately, modern breeding and trimming methods have made leaner cuts available, many containing just 6 to 9 grams of fat and under 200 calories per 3.5-ounce serving. For beef, choose "Select" grade over "Choice" and "Prime." Look for cuts labeled *round* or *loin*, or any of these: tenderloin, London broil, flank steak, club steak, and round, eye of round and sirloin tips.

THE SKINNY SIX

CUT OF BEEF (3.5 oz.)	CALORIES	GRAMS OF FAT	GRAMS OF SATURATED FAT
Top round, broiled	179	4.9	1.6
Eye of round, roasted	166	4.9	1.8
Round tip, roasted	183	6.9	2.3
Top sirloin, broiled	192	7.1	2.8
Top loin, broiled	205	9.3	3.5
Tenderloin, broiled	208	9.9	3.7

For pork, lamb and veal, the leanest cuts are labeled *loin* or *leg*. Some smart choices include extra-lean canned ham, pork tenderloin, Canadian bacon, pork center loin, fresh ham, lamb loin chop, lamb leg, veal leg and veal loin. Also, most cuts of game, such as buffalo, elk and deer, are lower in fat than either beef or chicken.

If you're a meat-aholic, try some of these ideas:

■ *Cut down on frequency.* If you're among the many Americans who still eat bacon for breakfast, bologna for lunch and pork chops for dinner, switch to having meat at just one meal each day. Also reduce the number of red meat days to perhaps three a week, if you can. Look for opportunities to use more poultry, fish, beans, grains and vegetables. When you do include meat in a meal, go for the best. Why use up your fat budget on a greasy burger when you could enjoy roasted pork tenderloin?

■ *Read labels.* Some deli meats can have 12 grams of fat per ounce, and meat entrées are typically among the fattest of frozen meals since many of them come in "he man" portions, smothered in fatty sauces and gravies, and surrounded by other high-fat foods. A good rule of thumb to follow is no more than 3 grams of total fat per 100 calories.

■ *Use healthy cooking methods.* Roasting, broiling, grilling, baking and stewing allow fat to drip off, whereas frying seals fat in. In general, the longer meat cooks, the more fat it loses, so medium and well-done are preferable to rare.

■ *Watch portion size.* A three-to-four-ounce serving of lean meat often contains fewer than 200 calories, but many people simply eat too much, even when a lower-fat cut is chosen. Portion control seems to be particularly difficult for men, who list red meat (especially steak, hamburgers and pizza with meat topping) as a favorite food. So, what constitutes an appropriate serving of about 3.5 ounces? It's the size of a woman's palm, or an audiocassette (not a video!) or a standard deck of cards.

■ *Order smart.* In a sit-down restaurant, ask for meat entrées to be lean, well-trimmed and cooked in a low-fat manner. Order a small piece of London broil, veal or sirloin done to "medium" or "well done," and ask that no butter or oil be used in the preparation.

HOW TO STRETCH MEAT

If you use meat in chili, casseroles and stir-fries, you can use a lot less. This works particularly well if you substitute grains and beans for part of the meat in many recipes. As an example, you can cook one thinly sliced steak in a stir-fry with crisp vegetables. It will feed four people as deliciously as four steaks but with a reasonable amount of fat and calories.

Skip fatty sauces. If you order beef, ask for the "petite," "queen" or "8-ounce" cut rather than the "king" or "16-ounce" portion. Ordering smart in fast-food restaurants and delicatessens is also key. A hamburger at Jack in the Box at 280 calories and 11 grams of fat is a far cry from their Ultimate Cheeseburger at 1,030 calories and 79 grams of fat.

WATCH OUT FOR GROUND BEEF 88

The best way to minimize the fat content is to buy the leanest ground beef available. And that means reading food labels.

In the past, descriptions like "lean" or "extra-lean" were used, but new labeling laws have banned such terms. Instead, ground beef must be described in lean-to-fat ratios by weight. Look for meat with a high lean-to-fat ratio. The figures in the chart below refer to four-ounce, medium-broiled servings of ground beef:

% LEAN/% FAT BY WEIGHT	CALORIES	FAT-GRAMS
73% lean/27% fat	291	21
80% lean/20% fat	268	18
85% lean/15% fat	240	14
90% lean/10% fat	199	11
95% lean/5% fat	155	6

ADD SOY TO YOUR DIET 89

Americans tend to think of soy foods as, well, not too good—either a gelatinous goo or dry and tasteless. We need to think again. Today the choices and varieties of soy foods are plentiful, and that's important because significant cardiac benefits come from these foods. It's not actually that hard, since you can find soy in soybeans, soy milk (available in fortified versions and in several flavors), tofu (soybean curd which comes in different consistencies: firm, soft and silken), sports bars that contain soy, tempeh (a chewy, soft soybean cake), soy nuts (peanut-like), veggie burgers, textured vegetable protein (TVP, a good substitute for ground beef), breakfast cereals fortified with soy, isolated soy protein powder (for adding to shakes and baked products) and soy flour. Grams of protein for common soy foods are listed below.

FOOD	PROTEIN (Grams)
Soy milk, 8 oz.	6.0
Tofu, 3 oz.	
Firm	8.5
Silken	6.0
Tofu yogurt, 8 oz.	8.0
Miso, 1 tbsp.	2.0
Soybeans, cooked/canned, ½ cup	13.0
Soybean sprouts, 1 oz.	4.0
Soybean burgers, 3.5 oz.	10.0
Soy crumbles, ground, ½ cup	9.0
Soy flour, ¼ cup	8.0
Soy nuts, ¼ cup	12.0

SPEAKING FROM EXPERIENCE

It's hard to get the recommended 25 grams of soy protein a day on the American diet, and most days I don't reach it. But I'm trying to do a few things regularly that will help. I'm using soy milk in cocoa and on cereal—I can pick up about 5 grams there. And I'm eating cereals fortified with soy. A ¾-cup serving provides 5 to 8 grams of protein. But the easiest way to reach my goal is to eat Japanese soybeans, edamame, as a snack food. These blanched soybeans come in little pods about the size of baby lima beans and have a sweet, nutty taste. You can use them in salads or stir-fries, but I eat them the Japanese way: just squeeze the pods with your fingers and pop the beans into your mouth. A half-cup serving contains about 16 grams of protein. —*J.P.*

Keep your intake balanced: 25 grams of soy protein and 30 milli-grams of isoflavones daily are deemed cardioprotective, but soy is not a "magic bullet." It should be eaten as part of a balanced diet, not in lieu of it. And bear in mind that soy foods are most effective for heart health when they are substituted for meat and other products containing animal protein.

GET AN OIL CHANGE

Most of us eat too much fat. But what's more to the point is that we eat the wrong *type* of fat, choosing the ones that raise cholesterol over those that lower it.

To go over the basics: all vegetable oils contain 120 calories and about 14 grams of total fat per tablespoon. They differ primarily in the types of fatty acids in their makeup: saturated, polyunsaturated and monounsaturated. While we tend to catalog an oil as one of the three types, in reality no fat is made up exclusively of one type of fatty acid. See below for an idea of how many fat-grams are contained in a table-spoon of the most common oils.

TYPE OF OIL	MONO-UNSATURATED	POLY-UNSATURATED	SATURATED
Monounsaturated			
Almond	10	2	1
Canola	8	4	1
Olive	10	1	2
Peanut	6	5	2
Polyunsaturated			
Corn	3	8	2
Cottonseed	2	7	4
Safflower	2	10	1
Sesame	5	6	2
Soybean	3	8	2
Sunflower	3	9	1
Walnut	3	9	1
Saturated			
Coconut	1	0	12
Palm	5	1	7
Palm kernel	2	0	11

Monounsaturated vegetable oils are the best choice for your heart. All of them are beneficial, but in the world of cardiac health olive oil rules. It reduces the risk of clot formation within coronary arteries while lowering "bad" LDL cholesterol when substituted for saturated fats.

In the past, monounsaturated oils were viewed as being essentially neutral with respect to cholesterol—not harmful, but not particularly healthful, either. The science changed radically, however, when Dr. Scott Grundy of the University of Texas Southwestern Medical Center published his landmark study on the effectiveness of monounsaturated fats in lowering cholesterol levels. "This may explain why populations using olive oil—Italians, Greeks, Cretans— have fewer heart attacks than do other populations," says Dr. Grundy. Investigation in this area also indicates that canola oil can be instrumental in reducing the risk of coronary heart disease. As Dr. Grundy has observed, "While olive oil may explain the low incidence of heart problems among Mediterranean populations, canola oil may explain it for Asian populations. In both cases, the monounsaturated oils are used as replacements for saturated fats."

The next healthiest choice is *polyunsaturated oils*. According to Dr. Margo Denke, a lipids expert at the University of Texas Southwestern Medical Center, polyunsaturated oils reduce LDL cholesterol levels when substituted for saturated fats, but this benefit is somewhat blunted by the fact that they also lower levels of beneficial HDL. And when they're hardened into solid fats—for instance, in stick margerine—polyunsaturated oils increase cholesterol-raising trans fats.

Saturated fats are the worst choice for cardiac health because they cause cholesterol, particularly LDL cholesterol, to rise significantly. In addition to animal foods, sources of saturated fats include palm oil, palm kernel oil and coconut oil.

See the following tips on how to avoid saturated fats and choose more monounsaturated fats.

■ *Reduce animal foods.* Instead of a small salad, a half-cup of rice and a giant steak, switch to a large salad, a full cup of rice, two vegetables and half a chicken breast.

■ *Read labels.* Avoid products in which oils have been hydrogenated and foods made with tropical oils. Beware of terms like "all-vegetable oil" and "made with 100% vegetable oil," since they do not identify the oil used. Another favorite advertising term is "made with one or more of the following oils—soybean, cottonseed, palm and/or coconut oil." When you can't tell which oil a food contains, stay away.

■ *Use high-quality oils.* Because virgin or extra virgin olive oil is so flavorful, you may be able to use less and still produce the desired taste with fewer calories.

■ *Try flaxseed.* Since the oil in flaxseed contains high levels of cardioprotective omega-3 fatty acids, many experts recommend adding about two tablespoons of ground flaxseed to your daily diet.

TOO MUCH OF A GOOD THING?

Healthy oils are most effective when they *replace* unhealthy fats. But some people apparently think that if a little olive oil is good, a lot of it must be even better. The rule is all fats in moderation, even the healthy ones.

If you're used to making sandwiches with butter on two pieces of bread and switch to soft corn oil margarine to replace the butter, that isn't much of a change. But if you use margarine on one piece of bread and mustard on the other piece, that *is* a change. Not only have you shifted to a healthier fat, but you're taking in less total fat. Remember, too high an intake of fat, even the healthy kind, can contribute to overweight and increase cancer risk. There is no need to consume large amounts of any fat, whether it comes from a steer or from olives.

Sprinkle it on yogurt, cereal or salads, mix it with juice or add it to baked goods and soups. Keep ground flaxseed refrigerated. Ready-made flaxseed breads, muffins, cereals and breakfast bars can be found in many stores.

■ *Remember that healthy oils are not magic elixirs.* Despite all their benefits, they do not offset poor dietary choices, smoking and a sedentary lifestyle.

91 BE PICKY ABOUT POULTRY

With the exception of duck and goose, poultry is an excellent substitute for red meat: lower in fat, lower in calories and really tasty. Chicken breasts pan-fried in a nonstick pan are as easy to cook as minute steaks. Roasted and broiled chicken take no more work than a pork roast. Roasted turkey breast is a great alternative to roast beef. And ground chicken and turkey breast can be used as a substitute for ground beef in many recipes, including tacos, chili and spaghetti. But don't be fooled into thinking that all poultry is created equal. One example: half a rotisserie chicken (the kind usually found in the deli department of a grocery store) has 41 grams of fat and 665 calories.

Below are a few principles that will keep you from making high-fat/high-calorie mistakes.

■ *Select the leanest cuts.* A simple rule will lead you to the leanest cuts of chicken and turkey: *choose a skinless white breast.* Unlike red meat, poultry is not marbled with fat; instead, the fat is concentrated just beneath the skin. If you remove the skin before cooking, you'll save about five grams of fat per piece of chicken. If you prefer to cook poultry with the skin on, be sure to remove it before serving. In addition, white meat has about one-third less fat than dark.

The table on the facing page will help you see the differences in 3.5-ounce portions of roast chicken and turkey.

POULTRY MEAT	GRAMS CALORIES	GRAMS OF OF FAT	SATURATED FAT
Chicken			
Light meat, skinless	165	3.5	0.9
Light meat, w/ skin	195	7.7	2.1
Dark meat, skinless	205	9.6	2.6
Dark meat, w/ skin	250	15.6	3.5
Turkey			
Light meat, skinless	155	3.2	1.1
Light meat, w/ skin	195	8.2	2.3
Dark meat, skinless	185	7.1	2.4
Dark meat, w/ skin	220	11.4	3.5

■ *Use healthy cooking methods.* Frying a chicken breast in oil, lard, vegetable shortening or grease will offset any low-fat benefit, as will smothering it in fatty gravy. Use cooking methods that allow fat to drip off, such as roasting, broiling, barbecuing, baking, steaming and stewing. If you do fry, use a nonstick pan with cooking spray, flavored vinegar, defatted broth or wine.

■ *Watch out for ground turkey.* Processed poultry products like chicken hot dogs, turkey bacon and turkey bologna often contain dark meat, skin and fat. Consequently, they can be as fat as—or fatter than—their beef and pork counterparts. One of the worst offenders is ground turkey. Some brands contain 13 to 16 grams of fat in a four-ounce serving. Be sure you're buying "ground turkey breast," not just "ground turkey." Made from skinless white meat, ground turkey breast has just 3 to 4 grams of fat per serving.

■ *Read food labels.* While Healthy Choice Chicken Oriental with 2 grams of fat would fit your budget, there is little chance that Swanson Hungry-Man Chicken Pot Pie with 41 grams of fat would work. Look for frozen chicken meals with no more than 3 grams of fat per 100 calories.

■ *Use portion control.* "People have been heavily blitzed with the message to eat less fat," says Dr. Walter Willett, chief of nutrition at Harvard's School of Public Health. "But replacing a 12-ounce steak with the same amount of poultry doesn't make sense. Instead, servings of poultry—or any animal food—should be three or four ounces, surrounded by grains, beans, vegetables, fruit and other foods rich in complex carbohydrates and fiber."

■ *Order smart.* In a sit-down restaurant, order baked, broiled, roasted or barbecued poultry without skin and with any sauces served on the side. In fast-food restaurants, avoid fried chicken, wings or nuggets. (Wendy's Grilled Chicken Sandwich at 290 calories and 7 grams of fat is quite different from its Chicken Club Sandwich at 500 calories and 23 grams of fat.) At a delicatessen, a turkey sandwich is a great choice as long as you don't ask for it to be larded with mayonnaise, bacon and cheese; instead, order it with mustard, lettuce and tomato.

DON'T PASS THE SALT

The key to cutting down the amount of sodium you eat is being conscious of how much of it you actually eat. It's easy enough to be careful about table salt and obviously salty foods like pickles, bacon and potato chips. (Salt is sodium chloride. It's the sodium in salt that is a health issue.) But it's much harder when the sodium is a hidden ingredient. And it *is* hidden—in foods like cheese, peanut butter, bread, cereals and commercial salad dressings and spaghetti sauce. One ounce of corn flakes has nearly twice the sodium found in an ounce of salted peanuts, and two slices of white bread contain more sodium than 14 potato chips.

Here are some ways to steer clear of salt:

■ *Eat more fresh foods* and fewer processed foods. A medium potato contains just 5 milligrams of sodium; processed into potato chips, it has 1,560 milligrams. Fresh peas contain .9 milligrams of sodium per one-fourth cup; the same amount of canned peas, 230 milligrams. A 3-ounce portion of steak has 55 milligrams of sodium; a frozen meat loaf dinner, about 1,300.

■ *Hide the salt shaker.* If you need additional seasoning on your food, use non- or low-sodium spices such as black pepper, garlic or garlic powder, tarragon, chili flakes, chili powder, lemon juice or combinations of homemade or commercial dried herbs and seasonings (such as Mrs. Dash and Spike). Avoid soy sauce and similar sodium-rich seasonings. If you're a salt diehard, consider using a one-hole shaker.

■ *Reduce salt in cooking.* Question when salt is called for in a recipe. Sometimes less salt or no salt will do. If you determine that salt is truly needed, reduce the amount called for by at least a fourth. After a few weeks, reduce the amount by another fourth. Use lemon juice, flavored vinegars, herbs and spices to bring out natural flavors.

■ *Read food labels* and familiarize yourself with the most commonly used advertising descriptions:

> *Low sodium* means 140 milligrams or less per serving.
>
> *Very low sodium* means 35 milligrams or less per serving.
>
> *Sodium-free* means less than 5 milligrams per serving.
>
> *Reduced sodium* means at least a 25% reduction from the regular food.
>
> *Unsalted* means no salt added, but not necessarily no sodium added.

■ *Learn other names for sodium.* In addition to salt, these include baking soda, baking powder, celery salt, garlic salt, onion salt, kosher salt, rock salt, seasoned salt, sea salt, sodium ascorbate, sodium benzoate, sodium caseinate, sodium citrate, sodium erythorbate, sodium nitrate, monosodium glutamate (MSG), sodium bicarbonate, sodium propionate, sodium saccharin and sodium phosphate.

■ *Order smart.* In a sit-down restaurant, ask that your food be prepared without added salt, garlic salt, sea salt or MSG. At a fast-food restaurant, ask to see the nutritional breakdown of the various dishes. There's a big difference between a Jack in the Box Ultimate Cheeseburger with 1,176 milligrams of sodium and an Arby's Regular Roast Beef Sandwich at 588 milligrams. And to be on the safe side, make sure your at-home meals are lighter in sodium on days when you eat a meal in a restaurant.

93 MAKE YOUR MUSTACHE FAT-FREE

Milk is rich in vitamins, minerals, protein and calcium, but some types of milk also come with unwanted baggage—too much heavily saturated fat. The challenge is to choose milk products that are tasty, nutritious and not loaded with excess fat. Here's what you can do:

■ *Make the best milk choice*: fat-free (also called nonfat and skim). Only 2% of its calories come from fat, yet it has all the calcium and protein benefits of whole milk. Fat-free buttermilk and 1% "light" milk are also good choices. See the breakdown for different types of milk on the facing page.

SPEAKING FROM EXPERIENCE

When we started to change our family diet, my daughter Anne was six years old and my son Joe was four. They both said there was no way they would drink "blue milk." What we did was mix the 2% milk that they were drinking with nonfat milk, which we wanted them to drink. Over time we increased the nonfat portion and decreased the 2% portion, until finally they were drinking 100% nonfat milk.

The only problem was, we served it to them in a 2% container, and one day at breakfast Anne asked me, "Dad, is this milk any good?" "It tastes fine to me," I said. "Why do you ask?" "Because the container says it's a year old," she replied.

At that point I told her that she and Joe were drinking nonfat milk. They wanted to go back to 2% milk (on principle, I think), but their taste buds had changed. They now actually *liked* nonfat milk.

The secret is to take small steps. Move from whole milk to 2%, then to 1%, and finally to fat-free milk over a period of about four to six weeks.   —*J.P.*

TYPE OF MILK (8 fl. oz.)	CALORIES	GRAMS OF FAT	GRAMS OF SATURATED FAT
Whole milk	150	8.1	5.1
Whole chocolate milk	210	8.5	5.3
2% reduced-fat milk	125	4.7	2.9
2% reduced-fat chocolate milk	180	5.0	3.1
1% low-fat milk	100	2.6	1.6
Fat-free milk	85	0.4	0.3

Replacing a cup of whole milk with the same amount of fat-free milk saves 8 grams of fat—the same as two pats of butter! At three cups daily, that's a yearly calorie saving equal to 22 pounds of body fat.

■ *Be moderate in your consumption,* even if you're concerned about osteoporosis. How much calcium do you actually need each day? The National Institutes of Health recommends the following guidelines:

AGE	MILLIGRAMS OF CALCIUM
1 to 5	800
6 to 10	800 to 1,200
11 to 24	1,200 to 1,500
Women 25 to 50	1,000
Women 50 to 65 taking estrogen	1,000
Women 50 to 65 not taking estrogen	1,500
Men 25 to 65	1,000
Men or women over 65	1,500
Pregnant or lactating women	1,200 to 1,500

At about 300 milligrams of calcium per cup, fat-free milk is a calcium powerhouse. But remember, other foods can also be good calcium sources: fat-free and low-fat yogurt and cheese, calcium-fortified orange juice and cereals, collard greens, sardines, salmon, kale and soybeans.

GET YOUR B'S

Foods rich in folate, vitamin B_6 and vitamin B_{12} reduce high levels of homocysteine in the blood, an emerging marker for coronary artery disease, heart attack and stroke. Here are some ways to make sure you're getting enough:

■ *Choose complex carbohydrates.* Leafy green vegetables like asparagus and spinach are rich in folate, as are tomatoes, oranges and other citrus fruits, as well as oatmeal. But pound for pound, it's hard to beat legumes, beans and peas. Pintos, garbanzos, baby limas, blacks, navies and small white beans have 250 micrograms or more of folate, while cranberry beans and black-eyed peas have 350 micrograms.

■ *Choose fortified cereals.* Many cereals and grains are fortified with B vitamins. Some have 400 micrograms of folate in one cup.

■ *Use healthy cooking methods.* According to Dr. Mary Frances Picciano, professor of nutrition at Pennsylvania State University, "Folate is a surprisingly delicate vitamin, and the more a food is processed or cooked, the less folate it's likely to contain." So even if you're eating more than one serving a day of vegetables, if that serving is fried, overcooked, or processed beyond recognition, it's probably not doing much for your folate levels.

The recommendation is for 400 micrograms of folate daily. For B_6, the USRDA is 1.3 milligrams daily for women and 1.7 milligrams for men. For B_{12}, it's 2.4 micrograms daily.

FOLATE

FOOD	MICROGRAMS
Black-eyed peas, 1 cup	350
Cranberry beans, 1 cup	350
Cooked asparagus, 1 cup	262
Cooked spinach, 1 cup	262
Cooked lentils, 1 cup	258
Oatmeal, 1 cup	199
Orange juice, 1 cup	109
Cooked broccoli, 1 cup	80

VITAMIN B$_6$

FOOD	MILLIGRAMS
Banana, 1 medium	.48
Avocado, ½ medium	.42
Hamburger, 3 oz.	.39
Chicken, 3 oz.	.34
Fish, 3 oz.	.29
Potato, 1 medium	.20
Cooked spinach, ½ cup	.16
Rice, brown, ½ cup	.16

VITAMIN B$_{12}$

FOOD	MICROGRAMS
Liver, beef, 3 oz.	68
Clams, canned, ½ cup	19
Oysters, canned, 3.5 oz.	18
Tuna, 3 oz.	2
Yogurt, 1 cup	1
Milk, nonfat, 1 cup	.9
Halibut, 3 oz.	.8
Egg, 1 large	.8
Chicken, 3 oz.	.4
Cheese, cheddar, 1 oz.	.2

MOVE THE CHEESE

Americans are gaga for cheese—to the tune of 30 pounds or so a year for each and every one of us. According to the Stanford Center for Research in Disease Prevention, cheese is the hardest food for us to trim from our diet, particularly for women, who rank it much higher than meat as a "favorite and frequently consumed food," right behind chocolate and ice cream.

The problem is that, while cheese is a good source of protein and calcium, it can also be a concentrated source of fat, saturated fat and calories. Most regular cheese is about 60% to 80% fat, two-thirds of which is saturated. This means that a typical 1.5-ounce serving, about one and half slices of American cheese, contains as much fat as three and a half pats of butter, or about 14 grams of fat. The key is balance.

■ *Know what you're eating*. Fat content fluctuates greatly with different types of cheese:

TYPE (1 oz.)	GRAMS OF TOTAL FAT	GRAMS OF SATURATED FAT
Regular, or full-fat	9 to 11	6 to 7
Reduced-fat, or part-skim	5 to 7	3 to 5
Light	2 to 4	1 to 3
Fat-free	Less than 0.5	Trace

■ *Read food labels*. This is the only way to know how fatty a cheese really is. (Just because the label says a cheese is "part-skim," "low-fat" or "semi-soft" doesn't necessarily mean it's low in fat.) And pay attention to serving size as well. Most labels for cheese use a one-ounce serving size—a pitifully small amount for a cheese lover.

■ *Grate it*. "Stretch" cheese by grating it, then use teaspoons—not cups—to flavor vegetables, salads, soups and pasta. A sprinkle of sharp cheese such as Parmesan, Romano or feta, added at the last moment, will zip up your meals without much added fat.

■ *Try fat-free and low-fat varieties*. Using a fat-free cheese on a sandwich, say, will save you 10 grams of fat and 70 calories. Low-fat is also good, but be careful of cheeses that are "lower in fat." A reduced-fat cheddar, for instance, may have 5 grams of fat per ounce—less than regular, but still a lot.

■ *Make taste an issue*. If you don't like the cheese, you won't eat it, no matter how much fat and calories it saves you. If you can't find a fat-free or reduced-fat cheese that satisfies you, stick with regular cheese—as long as it fits into your fat budget.

HIDE THE SUGAR BOWL

Commonly used in coffee and tea, in homemade baked goods and on cereal and fruit, table sugar contributes about 30% of our total sugar intake. Consider using less or no sugar in drinks or using a sugar substitute. Use fresh or dried fruit on cereal. And when cooking from a recipe, reduce the amount of sugar called for by one-third; normally, there is no change in taste. Apple juice and applesauce are good sugar substitutes in baking.

Here are some other ways to cut back:

■ *Limit processed foods.* These foods provide about 70% of the sugar we eat. Some sources are obvious because they taste sweet: examples include breakfast cereals, soft drinks, canned fruit, ice cream, gumdrops and jam. But many processed foods, such as peanut butter, tomato sauce and canned soups, have hidden sugar. Even ketchup has sugar!

■ *Read labels.* Remember that 4 grams of sugar equals one teaspoon. So, if the label states that your breakfast cereal has 12 grams of sugar, take a moment to visualize the three teaspoons of sugar you're about to eat.

■ *Don't be misled by the names given to ingredients.* When you read the list of ingredients on a food label, watch for sucrose, maltose, dextrose, lactose, fructose, malt, corn solids, corn syrup, honey, molasses, invert sugar, raw sugar, maple sugar, corn sweetener, malted barley, date sugar and turbinado. Also, it's advisable to avoid any product whose label lists sugar, under any name, among the first three ingredients.

■ *Switch to fresh fruit.* Americans eat almost 21 pounds of candy each year. And when we're not snacking on Snickers, we're often indulging in other sugar-rich desserts. But keep this in mind: a four-ounce serving of iced chocolate cake contains about 10 teaspoons of sugar. A much better way to satisfy your sweet tooth is with the natural sugar found in a ripe peach, a crisp apple or an ice-cold watermelon wedge.

LIQUID CALORIES

Most people who drink soft drinks aren't aware of the incredible amount of sugar—and calories—that can be crammed into a can or bottle.

SOFT DRINK (12 oz.)	CALORIES	TEASPOONS OF SUGAR	% OF CALORIES FROM SUGAR
Coca-Cola	144	9.3	100
Mountain Dew	178	11.0	100
Pepsi-Cola	158	10.0	100
Shasta Orange	172	11.8	100
Sprite	142	19.0	100

In addition, liquid calories don't fill us up. A study at Purdue University had participants eat 450 calories worth of jelly beans every day for four weeks and 450 calories worth of soda every day for another four weeks. On the days they ate jelly beans, the participants ate about 450 fewer calories of other foods. But on the days that they drank soda, they ended up eating 450 calories more than normal. "Liquid calories don't trip our satisfaction mechanisms," says Dr. Richard Mattes, author of the study.

Other studies show that girls who drink the most cola have five times the risk of broken bones. According to Dr. Grace Wyshak of Harvard School of Public Health, sodas tend to replace milk, so girls who consume too much of them may be taking in less calcium. And colas in particular contain phosphoric acid, which may spur calcium loss from bone.

Whenever possible, skip soft drinks in favor of water. Keep a large pitcher of water in your refrigerator. Or, if you prefer, rely on bottled water. Many people like a mixture of one-third orange juice and two-thirds carbonated water—it tastes like a soft drink but has fewer sugar calories.

■ *Stay away from fat-free baked goods.* These items are generally loaded with sugar to boost their flavor. "If you don't have a weight problem when you start eating low-fat muffins, you may have one afterward," says Netty Levine, R.D., at Cedars-Sinai Medical Center in Los Angeles. "They may take out some fat, but they add more sugar, which jacks up calories. And watch out for the portions. That calorie figure on the label is for one serving, but a big muffin may be three or more servings. That could make it a 450-calorie muffin!"

■ *Be smart about sugar substitutes.* Even though the FDA condones moderate use of sugar substitutes, we should still be wary of them. Studies show that they encourage us to maintain a taste for very sweet foods, which can lead to overindulgence and weight gain. Also, some people have trouble understanding that a diet cola does not offset the calories in a pepperoni pizza.

DRINK BLACK TEA

Tea has long had a reputation as a cure for frazzled nerves or blue moods, and green tea is associated with a decrease in cancer risk. Now studies suggest that drinking at least one cup of black tea daily could cut your risk of heart attack and stroke significantly.

The benefit may be due to powerful plant chemicals known as flavonoids. Found naturally in black tea, flavonoids are powerful antioxidants that may protect blood vessel linings from injury and inflammation. In addition, they have the same anticoagulant property that aspirin has, reducing the ability of blood platelets to stick together.

The latest findings are fairly dramatic. A 1999 study headed by Dr. Michael Gaziano, a heart specialist at Brigham and Women's Hospital, selected 340 men and women who had suffered heart attacks and matched them by age, gender and neighborhood with people who had never had heart attacks. The study then investigated their coffee- and tea-drinking habits for one year. Of great importance was the adjustment of the study for factors that could have skewed the results, such as smoking, exercise, alcohol intake and family history of heart disease, which allowed the researchers to zero in on beverage consumption. Few of the subjects drank one beverage exclusively, so they were categorized by their strongest preferences. Dr. Gaziano found that those who drank one or more cups of black tea every day slashed their heart attack risk by a

SPEAKING FROM EXPERIENCE

Whole grains are a nutritional bonanza—low in fat, rich in nutrients such as protein, B vitamins and vitamin E, good sources of fiber and low in calories. They're also central to reducing the risk of heart disease. But it can be difficult to incorporate them into your meals throughout the day.

For starters you can think of whole grains as side dishes rather than just breakfast foods. One cup on average provides 3 to 10 grams of fiber but only about 200 calories. Of course, you may have to wean your family from the more processed versions. One mother told me that her son loved white rice but hated brown rice. She simply mixed them—one-half white, one-half brown—until her son's taste buds adjusted and the family progressed to *all* brown rice.

In addition, most of us eat only rice, wheat or corn, so I recommend experimenting with other grains such as whole or pearled barley, bulgur and whole-wheat couscous.

Dietitian Bev Utt suggests trying different whole grains in one-dish meals. You might start with couscous, for example, then layer on sautéed peppers, green onions and other vegetables, garbanzo or black beans, and even a small amount of chicken or meat. One-dish meals are a great way to maximize whole grains in your diet.   —*J.P.*

staggering 44%, compared with those who did not drink tea.

The same result was found in a study of 805 Dutch men who consumed a diet rich in black tea, apples and onions, all of which contain large quantities of flavonoids. Not only was heart attack risk reduced substantially, but those who drank more than four cups of tea a day cut their risk of stroke by

PLANT PROTECTION
Don't depend on tea for all your flavonoids. Fruits and vegetables are also very good sources. So is red wine.

69% over those who drank less tea. And finally, a Boston University study found that tea may work directly on blood vessels that have lost their elasticity by restoring the vessels' ability to dilate when pulse rate quickens.

Such a positive result from the research translates into a strong lifestyle recommendation to drink more black tea. But let's put it in perspective:

■ *Don't imagine that drinking tea will offset an unhealthy lifestyle.* If you really want to maximize the effect of tea, add it to healthy habits. It won't work if you're smoking, sitting on a couch and eating junk foods.

■ *Don't drink green or herbal tea* if you want the benefit of flavonoids.

■ *Don't worry about condiments, temperature or form.* Milk, sugar and lemon do not diminish the effect of flavonoids. Neither does drinking your tea hot or cold. (Some people make a day's supply with three tea bags in 20 ounces of water, cool it in the refrigerator, transfer to a container and sip all day long.) And there is no difference between tea prepared with loose tea leaves, tea bags or granulated crystals.

■ *Don't go crazy.* The amount of tea needed to provide a cardioprotective effect is still under debate. Until we know the "threshold" dosage (whether it's one or six cups a day), remember your grandmother's advice: "Moderation in all things."

■ *Don't stop worrying about caffeine*, which can stimulate the heart, produce extra heartbeats, increase heart rate and raise blood pressure. Pound for pound, tea contains more caffeine than coffee. One way to minimize caffeine is by brewing full-leaf tea. Since the smaller the leaf, the stronger the concentration of caffeine, a tea bag made from cut-leaf tea or "dust" will release nearly twice as much caffeine per cup as full-leaf tea. Another way is to shorten the brewing time. A four-minute infusion of black tea will provide 40 to 100 milligrams of caffeine, while a three-minute infusion will provide only 20 to 40 milligrams.

GET YOUR ANTIOXIDANTS FROM FOOD

According to the American Heart Association, "As a general rule, it is always preferable to get vitamins and minerals such as beta-carotene, vitamin C and vitamin E in a nutritious diet rather than through supplements. We continue to recommend that Americans eat a variety of foods daily from all the basic food groups."

Beta-carotene is concentrated in very dark green and deep yellow fruits and vegetables. It has no USRDA, but many experts recommend a range of 5 to 30 milligrams daily.

FOODS HIGH IN BETA-CAROTENE

FOOD	MILLIGRAMS OF BETA-CAROTENE
1 cup carrot juice	38
½ cup cooked sweet potato	17
½ cup cooked canned pumpkin	16
½ cup cooked carrots	11
½ medium cantaloupe	8
½ cup raw carrots	5
1 medium mango	5
½ cup cooked spinach	4

Vitamin C is readily found in a variety of fruits and vegetables. The USRDA is 60 milligrams daily; however, research suggests that the optimal level of vitamin C for cardiovascular protection may be 500 to 1,000 milligrams per day.

FOODS HIGH IN VITAMIN C

FOOD	MILLIGRAMS OF VITAMIN C
½ medium cantaloupe	195
1 medium grapefruit	100
½ cup raw red pepper	95
1 cup honeydew melon	92
1 cup papaya	87
1 cup strawberries	84
1 kiwi	75
1 medium orange	70
½ cup orange juice	60
½ cup cooked broccoli	58
½ cup cooked brussels sprouts	49
½ cup raw green pepper	45
1 cup raw tomato	34
½ cup cooked sweet potato	32
1 cup raspberries	31

Vitamin E is the toughest of the antioxidants to get through diet alone. Many sources of vitamin E, such as nuts and seeds, vegetable oils and peanut butter, are rich in fat, so it can be a challenge to balance an adequate intake of vitamin E against the potential for breaking your fat budget.

Although the USRDA for vitamin E is 20 milligrams (30 International Units), experts suggest that a cardioprotective level is 133 to 533 milligrams (100 to 800 International Units).

FOODS HIGH IN VITAMIN E

FOOD	MILLIGRAMS OF VITAMIN E
1 cup Total cereal	20
3 tbsp. sunflower seeds, dry roasted	14
½ cup granola	8
1 oz. almonds	7
¼ cup wheat germ	5
2 tsp. peanut butter	3
1 tbsp. olive oil	2

KNOW YOUR MARGARINES

The dairy section is full of margarine options—so many that it's sometimes hard to know what to buy. Here are two rules to keep in mind:

■ *Avoid stick margarine.* When an oil is hardened to produce a food product, as corn oil or safflower oil is to produce stick margarine, the hydrogenation process increases trans fatty acids. The harder the margarine, the more trans fat it contains. And, remember, trans fats increase blood cholesterol.

■ *Choose soft margarine.* Because neither liquid and tub margarines are heavily hydrogenated, they are more heart-healthy than stick margarine. Be sure, however, to choose a soft margarine made with a polyunsaturated oil such as safflower oil or corn oil.

■ *Choose cholesterol-lowering margarine.* In a recent study from the University of Texas Southwestern Medical Center, 23 families ate butter while another 23 families used cholesterol-lowering margarine. After five weeks the adults on the "margarine diet" experienced an 11% drop in LDL cholesterol.

Dropping total and LDL cholesterol by double digits simply by eating those margarines is indeed remarkable. There are, however, a few things to consider:

■ Study participants who got the best cholesterol-lowering results used plant stanol margarine in place of—not in addition to—other spreads.

THE NEW MARGARINES

Both Benecol and Take Control contain plant stanol esters, which have somewhat the same cholesterol-lowering effect as oat bran. Benecol is used as a spread as well as in cooking, baking and frying. Clinical trials conducted in Finland and the United States showed it to be effective in reducing total cholesterol and LDL cholesterol levels by an average of 10% and 14%, respectively. Take Control is used as a spread but not in baking or frying. Trials indicate that the use of this plant stanol margarine may lower LDL cholesterol by 7% to 10%.

■ Be aware of fat and calories. A pat of Benecol contains 5 grams of fat and 45 calories. At the recommended amount of three pats per day, that's 15 grams of fat and 135 calories. A pat of Take Control contains 6 grams of fat and 50 calories. At the recommended two pats per day, that's 12 grams of fat and 100 calories. If you're restricting dietary fat for purposes of weight loss and cardiac health, be certain that two or three pats of margarine a day will fit into your fat budget.

■ And finally, plant stanol margarine is not a cure-all. Don't eat a poor diet and then try to offset it with cholesterol-lowering margarine. There is no offsetting mechanism when you spread Benecol or Take Control on a croissant.

The bottom line is to keep your perspective. When you choose to eat fat, make the healthiest choice you can, be it olive oil, canola oil or plant stanol ester margarine. Then remember that healthy fats are still fat.

HAVE A DRINK

In moderation, alcohol is associated with a reduced risk of heart attack and stroke. But heavy drinking can cause cirrhosis, cancer, birth defects, brain damage and fatal accidents, and can contribute to overweight, obesity and Syndrome X. An excessive intake of alcohol can also impair the pumping capacity of the heart. And recent

EAT TO BEAT STRESS

When we feel stressed, we tend to seek out sweet, fatty food that raises our mood but unfortunately also raises our weight. But we don't have to resort to chocolate (the "edible tranquilizer"), ice cream, cookies and cake to boost our serotonin levels. Complex carbohydrates can have the same effect. Dr. Leigh Gibson at University College in London recommends the following foods to fight emotional eating:

- Fresh fruit or fruit canned in its own juice
- Whole-wheat toast with jam
- Multi-grain waffle with light syrup
- Tomato soup
- Sweet potato, or baked potato with light sour cream and chives
- Oatmeal
- Lightly sweetened whole-grain cereals such as Multi-Grain Cheerios

research shows that it can raise levels of C-reactive protein, a harbinger of coronary inflammation.

In other words, if you drink alcohol, be smart about it:

- *If you don't drink, don't start* simply because of the potential health benefits of alcohol. Exercising regularly, eating right and not smoking all have major health benefits and no downside.

- *If you do drink, do so in moderation*—which means no more than one to two drinks a day for men, one for women. This does not mean averaging a drink a day by abstaining on weekdays and binge-drinking on weekends. That pattern is clearly harmful to health.

- *Understand what constitutes a drink*: 12 grams (one-half ounce) of pure alcohol. This is the amount in 12 ounces of beer, 1.5 ounces of 80-proof liquor or 5 ounces of wine.

- *If you have a condition that could be aggravated by alcohol*, such as high blood pressure, elevated triglycerides, obesity, cardiomyopathy (a weakened heart) or atrial fibrillation, or if you're taking prescription medications, talk with you doctor about whether or not drinking is safe for you.

■ *Understand that alcohol is not a magic cure-all* for poor lifestyle habits. Not smoking, eating a diet low in saturated and trans fats, and exercising regularly—these should be first and foremost among your lifestyle habits

■ *Strive for a balanced diet.* While it may be good news to learn that beer contains a potent antioxidant (xanthohumol), the bad news is that you would have to drink 117 gallons of beer a day to obtain its maximum health benefits. Be sure you're getting sufficient antioxidants from multiple food sources.

■ *Determine if you can afford the extra calories* that come in alcoholic beverages, particularly if you're trying to lose weight. Ounce for ounce, alcohol has almost as many calories as fat has.

BEVERAGE	CALORIES
Scotch, whiskey, gin, vodka (1.5 oz.)	
80-proof	97
86-proof	105
90-proof	110
94-proof	116
100-proof	125
Brandy, cognac (1 oz.)	65
Liqueurs (1 oz.)	75 to 100
Dry wine (3.5 oz.)	87
Sweet wine (3.5 oz.)	142
Beer, ale (12 oz.)	140 to 165
Light beer (12 oz.)	95 to 105

REWRITE YOUR FAVORITE RECIPES 101

A trip to the bookstore is often the first step for many people trying to change their diets. They buy a low-fat cookbook, shop for hard-to-get ingredients with unpronounceable names, spend hours in the kitchen and are then disappointed when the family refuses to eat the great new dish they've prepared.

Here's why. We like our own food, our own favorite recipes, better than we like the recipes of other people. *The fact is that most American families prepare 12 recipes 80% of the time.* So instead of worrying about how to create a hundred new low-fat meals, it's more effective to reduce fat and calories in those recipes that already have your family's stamp of approval.

Let's say your family likes to have French toast on Sunday mornings. The traditional recipe calls for mixing whole milk and four whole eggs, dipping bread in the mixture and frying it in bacon fat. How can this recipe be lightened without losing taste? First, you can use nonfat milk instead of whole milk; Egg Beaters, or one whole egg and three egg whites, instead of four whole eggs. Next, instead of bacon grease, use a nonstick pan or griddle with a little cooking spray. Now you can afford to top the French toast with fresh fruit and yogurt, fruit compote, or even a small dollop of soft margarine and a little maple syrup. It will be fantastic.

 EAT YOUR BEANS

Beans and legumes are great sources of complex carbohydrates, fiber, folate, protein, phytochemicals and other nutrients, yet contain little or no fat and no cholesterol. In particular, they contain *soluble* fiber, which is effective in lowering blood cholesterol.

A good way to include beans, peas and lentils—the most common types of legumes—in your diet is to mix them with other foods. Examples are black beans and rice, white bean and tuna salad, pasta and beans, bean tacos and falafel. Dietitian Bev Utt suggests one-dish meals: "A Tex-Mex salad, for instance, uses greens as a base. Then add black beans, canned corn, green onions and sautéed chicken. I use a light ranch dressing and serve with a warm tortilla."

Add lentils, split peas, black beans or white beans to soups and stews. Use pinto beans with ground beef or textured vegetable protein in tacos and burritos. And add navy, kidney and garbanzo beans to salads. Be adventurous.

EASY ON THE MAYO

Regular mayonnaise is a fat disaster, with about 12 grams of fat and 2 grams of saturated fat per tablespoon—ounce for ounce, more fat than spareribs. But there are options. "Light" or "calorie-reduced" mayonnaise usually contains half the fat and saturated fat of regular mayonnaise. Examples with 3 to 5 grams of fat per tablespoon include Hellmann's/Best Foods Reduced Fat, Miracle Whip Light, Kraft Light and Weight Watchers Light. "Fat-free" mayonnaise has less than one-half gram of fat and only a trace of saturated fat per tablespoon. Some good examples are Kraft Free, Miracle Whip Free and Smart Beat Fat Free.

But here's a case where you should let your taste buds guide you. Some people like "fat-free" mayonnaise on a sandwich, particularly when a spicy mustard is used, but prefer "light" mayonnaise when it comes to tuna salad. Also, remember that just because you use reduced-fat mayonnaise, it doesn't mean you can use twice as much.

HOLD THE BUTTER

Few foods are so rich in fat that they fall outside the prescription for low-fat eating, but butter is one. Not only is butter rich in fat—a single pat contains 4 grams of fat, a tablespoon almost 11 grams of fat—but over 50% of the fat content is saturated. Ounce for ounce, butter is fatter than prime rib. It's also insidious. A pat here, a spread there—it adds up all too quickly. If you're concerned about calories and cholesterol, the best advice is to avoid butter altogether.

1 teaspoon of butter	=	1 teaspoon of regular mayonnaise
	=	2 teaspoons of French or Italian salad dressing
	=	3 teaspoons of mayonnaise-type salad dressing
	=	3 teaspoons of cream cheese
	=	4 teaspoons of table cream
	=	5 teaspoons of sour cream

BE SMART ABOUT SNACKS

Americans love to snack. On average, we eat snack foods over 200 times a year, and we're eating more all the time. Annual candy consumption, for instance, recently jumped from 19 to 25 pounds per person.

There is actually nothing wrong with snacking, provided you make smart choices. Indeed, it may be healthier (in terms of reduced weight and cholesterol) to eat small meals throughout the day rather than two or three large ones. The problem for most people is what they choose to eat rather than how often they eat.

Most popular snacks are excessive in fat, sodium, sugar and calories. Potato chips, the all-American favorite, get 50% to 60% of their calories from fat. Eating eight ounces of chips is tantamount to adding 12 to 20 teaspoons of oil to a baked potato!

Here are some ways to be smart about snacks:

■ *Restock your cupboard and refrigerator.* The first step should be to replace cookies, chips and other high-calorie munchies with healthier, nutrient-packed snacks.

■ *Eat more fruit.* Sweet, tart, chewy or crunchy, fresh fruits are one of the best deals around. One hundred calories will get you any of the following:

> an apple * 5 apricots * a banana * half a cantaloupe *
> 20 cherries * one grapefruit * 29 grapes * 1 or 2 oranges
> * a nectarine * 2 peaches * a pear * 3 plums * a cup of
> raspberries * 2 cups of strawberries * 2 or 3 tangerines *
> 10 ounces of watermelon * ⅕ of a honeydew melon

Try fruits in different forms. Frozen grapes, for instance, are a refreshing alternative to fatty snacks. And dried fruits, while higher in calories, are a valuable source of fiber and nutrients.

■ *Fill up, not out.* Choose watery vegetables like cucumbers, radishes, celery, zucchini, red and green peppers, cauliflower, mushrooms and broccoli: all are under 10 calories per ounce.

■ *Eat nuts in moderation.* First, let's look at the bad news—the fat and calories—in nuts. The figures in the table below apply to dry-roasted, one-ounce portions:

TYPE	CALORIES	GRAMS OF FAT	GRAMS OF SATURATED FAT
Almonds	167	14.8	1.4
Brazil nuts	186	18.8	4.6
Cashews	163	13.2	2.6
Filberts/hazelnuts	191	19.1	1.4
Peanuts	160	14.0	2.0
Pecans	190	20.0	2.0

On the other hand, let's remember that nuts are artery-friendly: rich in unsaturated fats, vitamin E, omega-3 fatty acids, fiber and B vitamins. Several studies have found that including nuts in the diet may reduce LDL cholesterol. In the Nurses' Health Study, women who ate more than five ounces of nuts a week had a 35% reduction in their heart attack risk compared with women who ate one ounce of nuts a week or none at all.

So, should nuts be part of a heart-healthy diet? By all means, yes, especially if they take the place of chips or a candy bar. Just don't pick up a whole jar of peanuts and sit down in front of the TV.

■ *Look for alternatives.* A regular-size Baby Ruth gets its 300 calories from 3 teaspoons of fat and 10 teaspoons of sugar: a nutritional disaster. So what do you do when the craving hits? Try sweet and smooth snacks like fruit sorbet, frozen grapes, low-fat and nonfat yogurt, ice milk, angel food cake, sherbet, juice and applesauce. If nothing but chocolate will do, go small and eat a mini-bar. You can also cut up a favorite candy bar into bite-size pieces you pop in the freezer. When a craving

BUY LESS, EAT LESS

Research suggests that buying packaged foods in giant economy sizes can increase consumption by as much as 43%. A smarter strategy: buy big, then repackage contents into smaller sizes at home.

RECOMMENDED SNACKS

CARBO-RICH

Low-fat popcorn

Chex mix

Whole-grain crackers

Cracker sandwiches (low-fat cheese, fruit spread)

Fruit dipped in fat-free caramel

Frozen bananas, grapes, berries, mango

Veggies and dip (low-fat yogurt, black bean, salsa)

Fruit juice popsicles

Cereal by the handful

Rice pudding

Twice-baked potatoes

Raisins

Caramel-covered rice cakes

Cracker Jack

Pretzels

Dried fruits

CALCIUM-RICH

Frozen yogurt

Vanilla pudding

Light ice cream

Tapioca

Yogurt

Hot chocolate made w/ fat-free or 1% milk

Flavored low-fat milks (chocolate, strawberry)

Veggies w/ fat-free cream cheese

English muffin w/ low-fat or fat-free cheese

PROTEIN-RICH

Turkey jerky

Bean dip on tortilla chips

Lean meat roll-ups

Peanut butter on: veggies, crackers, apples, English muffins, bagels, cracker bread

Sliced turkey breast

O.K. ONCE IN A WHILE

Sponge cake

Fruit rollups

Cookies

Cupcakes

---

hits, eat one piece. By the time the candy thaws in your mouth, which can take several minutes, your craving may be satisfied.

Don't be fooled by many of the so-called "energy bars." The "energy" in most bars is simply calories. Many have the same profile as candy bars. Be sure to read the label.

Traditional potato chips can be among the worst of snacks, with 8 to 10 grams of fat—and about 1 gram of saturated fat—per ounce. Some varieties are available with reduced fat and calories. One ounce of Pringles Original Potato Chips (about 17 chips) contains 160 calories and 11 grams of fat, while the same amount of Pringles Light Crisps has 130 calories and 6 grams of fat. But if you "can't eat just one" (ounce, that is), it's best not to start.

Cookies, crackers, bagels, pretzels and muffins come in low-fat varieties; however, they may not be low in calories. An oversize bagel may easily contain 300 calories. A Dunkin' Donuts banana muffin may be low in fat at just 1.5 grams, but it still contains 240 calories. A single SnackWell's Devil's Food cookie has 50 calories. Be sure to read labels whenever possible. And be realistic about the size, amount and calories of such snacks.

Popcorn is as American as apple pie and can be a whole lot leaner. A four-cup serving of plain air-popped popcorn has only one gram of fat. Many brands of microwave popcorn have a richer taste than air-popped, yet are genuinely lower in fat. Watch out for ready-to-eat popcorn, such as that found in movie theaters. A study by the Center for Science in the Public Interest found that a medium-size bucket of movie popcorn could contain as much as 43 grams of fat and almost 650 calories. Hit it with "butter" topping and it climbs to 71 grams of fat and 910 calories. That puts it in triple-cheeseburger country. Moreover, much of the fat used in this kind of popcorn is saturated.

■ *Drink water.* Research shows that five to eight glasses a day will help to curb snacking tendencies.

DRESS SALADS LIGHTLY

Which has more fat and calories: a tablespoon of salad dressing or a tablespoon of hot fudge? You're wrong if you picked the hot fudge. Commercial salad dressings are about 90% fat, or about nine grams of fat per tablespoon. To put this in perspective, a single packet of Thousand Island dressing at McDonald's contains more fat than one cup of Ben & Jerry's premium chocolate ice cream!

A better way to dress a salad is with balsamic vinegar or balsamic vinegar mixed with a bit of olive oil. If you use commercial dressings, be sure to try one of the many "nonfat" (also called "no-oil") and "light" (also called "calorie-reduced") versions. "Light" dressings will save, on average, about seven grams of fat per tablespoon. However, fat-grams and calories can add up rapidly even from

"FAT-FREE" WARNING

In the past five years, Americans have embraced fat-free foods with a vengeance (more than 5,900 new items are introduced each year), but the average adult has gained eight pounds over this period! "People perceive fat-free food as good and think they can eat as much as they want," says Cathy Nonas, director of the Van Itallie Center for Nutrition and Weight Management at St. Luke's–Roosevelt Hospital in New York City. "But snacking all day can rack up as many calories as eating a meal, without providing any of a meal's nutritional benefits."

When first introduced, many fat-free foods were tasteless and bland (think rice cakes). Food manufacturers then decided to offset flavor loss by increasing the amount of refined sugar. As a result, many fat-free foods now have calories comparable to—and some-times higher than—their full-fat versions. In addition, when health experts called for a reduction of dietary fat to reduce the risk of heart disease, cancer and obesity, no one expected that an aggres-sive food industry would grab onto the message with such single-mindedness. "We said nothing about calories, and neither did the food industry," says Nancy Ernst, nutrition coordinator of the National Cholesterol Education Program. "So what's being promoted is high-sugar, no-fat products that do not help weight maintenance and in some cases translate into weight gain."

To make matters worse, people simply eat too many fat-free foods. According to Dr. Chris Rosenbloom of Georgia State University, "Research shows that if people are told the food is fat-free or lower in fat, they tend to eat three to five times as much as they normally would if the food contained fat. If I put out a plate of Toll House chocolate-chip cookies, you might eat one or two, maybe 100 or 120 calories. But if I put out a box of fat-free cookies, chances are you'll eat 8 or 10."

"light" dressing if you use it too freely. "Nonfat" dressings can be a better choice, although they differ greatly in taste. Experiment.

If you do eat regular or "light" dressing, a good tip is to serve it on the side. Dip your fork into the dressing, then eat the salad. You'll get all the flavor of the dressing while minimizing your fat and calorie intake.

FIGURE OUT FAST FOOD

Quick, cheap and tasty, fast food is almost irresistible. Unfortunately, most of it is laden with excessive fat, sodium, sugar and calories. And it's getting worse. Not too long ago, a McDonald's Quarter Pounder with 430 calories and 21 grams of fat was pretty much king of the hamburgers. Today, it looks positively lean next to the Double Western Bacon Cheeseburger at Carl's Jr. with 794 calories and 46 grams of fat, or Jack in the Box's Ultimate Cheeseburger with 1,050 calories and 78 grams of fat. Even Taco Bell's Taco Salad in the Shell— a salad!—has 850 calories and 52 grams of fat.

In a perfect world, no one would eat this kind of fast food. But this isn't a perfect world, and sometimes we don't want to cook, or we're running late, or we just want the stuff. The best way to handle this reality is to make smart food choices within a fast-food environment:

FAST FOOD	CONTENT
McDonald's Hotcakes (w/o margarine)	340 calories, 8 grams of fat, 1.5 grams of saturated fat
Subway 6" ham sandwich (w/o cheese and mayo)	261 calories, 4.5 grams of fat, 1.5 grams of saturated fat
Arby's Light Roast Chicken Deluxe sandwich (w/o cheese and dressing)	260 calories, 5 grams of fat, 1 gram of saturated fat
Wendy's Grilled Chicken Sandwich (w/o cheese and dressing)	300 calories, 7 grams of fat, 1.5 grams of saturated fat
Jack in the Box Chicken Teriyaki Rice Bowl	550 calories, 3 grams of fat, 0.5 grams of saturated fat

Arby's, Burger King, Wendy's, McDonald's and other fast-food places offer salads with nonfat salad dressing.

Now all you need to do is put all this knowledge into practice. Suppose you're in the mood for a hamburger, and you order the following at McDonald's:

MEAL #1

ITEM	CALORIES	GRAMS OF FAT	GRAMS OF SATURATED FAT
Quarter Pounder with Cheese	530	30.0	13.0
French fries, large	540	26.0	4.5
Strawberry shake	560	16.0	11.0
Apple pie	260	13.0	3.5
Total	1,890	85.0	32.0

Meal #1 has a lot of fat, saturated fat and calories for the amount of food eaten. But what if you ordered smarter?

MEAL #2

ITEM	CALORIES	GRAMS OF FAT	GRAMS SATURATED FAT
Hamburger	280	10.0	4.0
French fries, small	210	10.0	2.3
1% milk	100	2.5	1.5
Total	590	22.5	7.8

Here are some things to watch:

■ *Serving size.* As the number of hamburger patties increases, so does fat. Single hamburgers have about 2 ounces of meat; quarter-pounders, about 3 ounces; triple burgers, 4 or more ounces. Many deli sandwiches are large enough to feed two people.

■ *Add-ons.* Cheese, bacon, mayonnaise or mayo-based "special sauces" often come on hamburgers. Instead, opt for lettuce, tomato, onion, ketchup or mustard. Avoid fatty gravies and sauces on chicken and fish.

■ *Side orders.* A large order of French fries can contain more fat and calories than a quarter-pound hamburger. Coleslaw, onion rings and potato salad are also high in fat and calories.

■ *Chicken and chicken nuggets.* Battered and fried, often with skin on, these items can be high-fat disasters.

■ *Extra cheese.* Two slices of Domino's 14-inch Hand Tossed Pizza with sausage, pepperoni and extra cheese have 760 calories, 36 grams of fat and 16 grams of saturated fat. Instead, order a cheese pizza with half the cheese, extra tomato sauce, and load up on vegetables instead of meat. You'll have a pizza your heart can live with.

DON'T GO MENU-MAD

Over half of all meals eaten in the United States—or 40% of our average food budget—are eaten in restaurants. We obviously find the experience pleasurable. But dining out can pose a serious problem for cardiac health. Restaurant foods generally contain liberal amounts of fat in the form of oil, butter, cream, lard, meat drippings, fatty meat, cheese and cheese sauce. In addition, many items are fried, deep-fried, pan-fried and sautéed. As a result, restaurant meals can be high in fat, calories and saturated fat, as well as salt and sugar. So what can you do to enjoy restaurant food without penalizing your health? Here are a few tips:

■ *Choose to eat healthy.* The operative word is "choose." Make a mental decision to combine good taste and good health.

■ *Know fat content.* Your budget represents the maximum amount of fat-grams you can have in a day and still be on a lean, balanced diet. Once you know how much fat comes in an average serving of your favorite restaurant foods, you'll be able to determine if the foods fit your budget.

For example, let's suppose your fat budget is 40 grams of fat and you'd like to go out for dinner at an Italian restaurant. If you know ahead of time that pasta in a marinara sauce, linguine in red clam sauce and even spaghetti with two small meatballs all have under

20 grams of fat, you can budget your eating throughout the day to make any of these selections. But without that knowledge you can make mistakes. Pasta in a white, pesto or Alfredo sauce can contain 50 to 90 grams of fat.

■ *Don't set yourself up to overeat.* If you skip meals all day long to "save calories" for a restaurant meal, you can be so famished by dinnertime that you succumb to your appetite and overeat. A better plan is to eat breakfast and lunch, but make them lean. This will allow for more calories and fat at dinner, but it will keep you from feeling famished. Be sure to stay hydrated throughout the day so that you'll be a little full when you order. Watch out for alcohol as it can increase your hunger. Be aware of portion sizes. If you order beef, ask for the "petite," "queen" or "8-ounce" cut rather than the "king" or "16-ounce" portion. Avoid buffets and "all-you-can-eat" restaurants. Share desserts. And resist any urge to join the "clean plate club."

■ *Be inquisitive.* Ask questions about how each dish is prepared. Is it made with butter, margarine, cream, oil or animal fat? Is it fried or deep-fried? Is salt or sugar added? Restaurant personnel can be very helpful with regard to meal content and preparation. Also, look for key words on the menu. Avoid foods described as buttery, sautéed, fried, pan-fried, crispy, creamed, au gratin, scalloped, au lait, à la mode, au fromage, marinated, basted or prime. Stay away from béarnaise, beurre blanc and hollandaise, butter sauce, cream sauce, aioli, pesto, or anything served in its own gravy or cheese sauce. Better choices are: steamed, in broth, in its own juice, poached, garden-fresh, roasted, broiled, stir-fried and lean.

PORTION PATROL

Be conscious of how much you're eating. In a study at Pennsylvania State University, researchers found that when they served men 2.5 cups of macaroni and cheese, the men ate 1.9 cups. But when they were served a 5-cup portion, they ate 2.5 cups. After the meals, participants rated their fullness the same, regardless of how much they had eaten.

■ *Choose your restaurant carefully.* Know where you can get food that tastes great yet won't hurt your nutritional goals. It's harder to order smart in a prime rib restaurant that specializes in oversize portions.

■ *Be aware of portion distortion.* Oversize servings are turning Americans into oversize people. Share an entrée. Push half to the side and ask for a doggy bag. Or order from the appetizer menu.

LIMIT CAFFEINE 108

Americans consume about 33 million gallons of coffee a day, equal to 30 seconds of full flow at Niagara Falls. Chocolate ranks number one for women on surveys of "favorite and most frequently eaten" foods. And soft drinks, cola in particular, have replaced water as America's drink of choice. One of the reasons for the popularity of coffee, chocolate and soft drinks is a common component: caffeine. In a society that never rests, it keeps us alert, awake and energized.

CAFFEINE CONTENT

ITEM	MILLIGRAMS OF CAFFEINE
Coffee, 8 oz.	
Drip	150
Brewed	135
Instant	95
Decaffeinated	5
Espresso (1.5 to 2 oz.)	100
Tea, 8 oz.	
Black	50
Green	30
Instant	15
Decaffeinated	2
Chocolate	
Milk chocolate candy, 1 oz.	6
Cocoa, water mix, 8 oz.	14
Soft drinks, 12 oz.	
Coca-Cola	45
Pepsi-Cola	37
Diet Pepsi	35
Dr Pepper	40
Mountain Dew	55

But too much caffeine has a negative impact on cardiac health. It stimulates the heart, forcing it to work harder and in some instances producing extra heartbeats. Caffeine can also increase heart rate and blood pressure and, according to some studies, the amount of fatty acids in the bloodstream. A Johns Hopkins University study of over 1,000 men found that those who drank five cups of coffee a day had nearly three times the risk of heart disease as those who drank no coffee.

Research to date has not conclusively linked heart disease to moderate consumption of coffee, but it seems reasonable that those concerned with cardiac health should avoid overstimulation of the heart by caffeine. That advice also holds true for people desiring weight control. Caffeine can cause blood sugar to drop, producing feelings of hunger that can sabotage good dietary intentions. And finally, too much caffeine may cause insomnia, nervousness and stomach upset.

Should you avoid caffeine altogether? Probably not. But if you drink coffee all day long, eat chocolate frequently or drink soft drinks regularly, it may be prudent for you to examine your dietary habits and consider changes to reduce caffeine intake.

FLOSS AND BRUSH YOUR TEETH

Okay, so this one isn't exactly about eating, but it does have something to do with cardiac health. A number of studies show a link between periodontal (gum) disease and an increased risk of heart attack. In fact, it's estimated that a person with periodontal disease is two to three times more likely to have a heart attack than one without periodontal disease.

Here's the theory. Plaque that builds up on the teeth produces chronic inflammation of the gums, causing irritation, redness, swelling and bleeding when you brush. If the plaque isn't removed, the gums separate from the teeth, leaving pockets that fill with bacteria. The most common strain found in these pockets is *Streptococcus sanguis*. When it enters the bloodstream, this bacteria may be a significant causative factor in heart attacks and strokes.

Dental bacteria seem to undermine cardiovascular health in three ways. First, infections from dental plaque can cause injury to coronary artery walls. Second, people with gum disease are more likely to produce an inflammatory response that may place them at elevated risk of suffering a heart attack. And finally, gum disease can initiate blood clotting. While cholesterol buildup may narrow the artery opening, a blood clot is what seals the opening, choking off blood flow in narrowed heart or neck arteries, triggering heart attacks or strokes. Researchers at the University of Minnesota, led by Drs. Mark Herzberg and Maurice Meyer, found that *Streptococcus sanguis* produces a protein called PAAP (platelet aggregation associated protein), which forms on the bacteria's outer cell walls. Blood platelets then stick to the protein and begin to clot, blocking arteries and, if severe enough, potentially inducing heart attacks.

Not everyone agrees that gum infections are a risk for heart disease, but it seems prudent to:

■ *Brush your teeth* at least twice a day. Electric toothbrushes, rinses and toothpaste help to prevent periodontal disease.

■ *Floss* at least once a day.

■ *See your dentist* for cleaning regularly. People who are genetically predisposed to dental plaque buildup have a 20% chance of developing periodontal disease. If this concerns you, talk to your dentist about a test that can identify people at risk.

■ *Be sure your diet includes* plenty of complex carbohydrates, especially fruits and vegetables. Reduce sugar and highly refined carbohydrate foods such as baked goods.

■ *Consider bone implants* to replace dental bone lost from periodontal disease.

■ *Consider aspirin therapy* to ease inflammation and damage to the arteries and to promote anticoagulation. Be sure to talk to your doctor.

■ *Chew sugarless gum* to help fight dental decay. Gum containing xylitol, a sweetener made from birch bark, has been shown to partially suppress the growth of cavity-promoting bacteria in the mouth.

Epilogue

WHEN WE WERE WRITING THIS BOOK, we sometimes found ourselves overwhelmed by the staggering incidence of heart disease in this country. We wanted to help the millions of people afflicted to help themselves. At those moments we remembered this inspirational story from *Chicken Soup for the Soul* by Jack Canfield and Mark V. Hansen.

ONE AT A TIME

A friend of ours was walking down a deserted Mexican beach at sunset. As he walked along, he began to see another man in the distance. As he grew nearer, he noticed that the local native kept leaning down, picking something up and throwing it out into the water. Time and again he kept hurling things out into the ocean.

As our friend approached even closer, he noticed that the man was picking up starfish that had been washed up on the beach and, one at a time, he was throwing them back into the water.

Our friend was puzzled. He approached the man and said, "Good evening, friend. I was wondering what you are doing."

"I'm throwing these starfish back into the ocean. You see, it's low tide right now and all of these starfish have been washed up onto the shore. If I don't throw them back into the sea, they'll die up here from lack of oxygen."

"I understand," my friend replied, "but there must be thousands of starfish on this beach. You can't possibly get to all of them. There are simply too many. And don't you realize this is probably happening on hundreds of beaches all up and down this coast? Can't you see that you can't possibly make a difference?"

The local native smiled, bent down and picked up yet another starfish, and as he threw it back into the sea, he replied, "Made a difference to that one!"

Appendix I
Prescriptions, Procedures and Programs

1. DRUG THERAPY

Sometimes managing stress, exercising more and watching your diet—the front line in cardiac risk reduction—are just not enough. You may need drugs as an adjunctive therapy to better control certain markers. Of course, the information in this section does not replace consultations with your doctor, but it will give you a better understanding of your options and the right questions to ask.

Aspirin Therapy

As noted earlier, the risk of a heart attack increases with the blood's propensity to clot and seal off a coronary artery. Clotting can also stop blood flow to the brain, causing a stroke. It is important, then, to reduce any tendency toward dangerous coagulation.

A recent study, published in the *New England Journal of Medicine*, suggests that taking aspirin regularly is one of the best ways to reduce clotting risk. Aspirin's anticoagulant ability prevents platelets from sticking together, thereby lessening the chance of clots forming and blocking narrowed coronary arteries. As one researcher described it, "Aspirin is like the lumberjack who prevents logjams."

Three other major health benefits can be derived from aspirin therapy:

- Regular aspirin use may ease the severity of new heart problems. According to one report, hospitalized patients with chest pain were far less likely to have experienced a heart attack if they were on aspirin therapy at the time.

SEE YOUR DOCTOR

It's important to talk to your doctor *before* taking any drug. But it's equally important to *keep* talking. Science changes; new drugs are developed; old drugs are made more powerful; and combinations of some drugs and/or food supplements may be dangerous. It's crucial to keep up.

CARRY UNCOATED ASPIRIN WITH YOU

Many doctors recommend carrying regular aspirin tablets with you to be used in a cardiac emergency. A study of over 17,000 patients found a 23% reduction in the death rate and a 49% reduction in new or recurrent heart attacks when aspirin was taken within 24 hours of experiencing heart attack symptoms. As a result, doctors now advise that people who think they're having a heart attack should chew and swallow one regular *uncoated* adult aspirin (325 mg). It's estimated that this recommendation, if widely adopted, would save an additional 5,000 to 10,000 lives in the United States each year.

- Aspirin can help to minimize damage at the onset of a heart attack. Studies show that when taken during or immediately following a heart attack, aspirin reduces the risk of death immediately and during the first five weeks after the attack.
- Aspirin decreases coronary artery inflammation.

Both the FDA and the American Heart Association strongly recommend aspirin for "secondary" prevention. Clearly, an aspirin regimen can be beneficial for people who have suffered a heart attack or stroke, who have undergone coronary bypass surgery or balloon angioplasty or who have stable angina. The research results are unequivocal: aspirin therapy can prevent heart attacks in people with a history of heart disease. Indeed, aspirin could reduce new heart problems by about 25% in patients with known cardiovascular disease.

In one study of 6,174 adults with heart disease, Dr. Patricia Gum and her colleagues at the Cleveland Clinic found that regular aspirin users experienced a 33% lower mortality rate during a follow-up period of three years as compared with patients who didn't take aspirin.

Should everyone with heart disease be on aspirin? Absolutely not. For people with certain heart rhythm irregularities (such as atrial fibrillation), other anticlotting medications may be more effective. Very rarely, aspirin has been linked to problems with nasal polyps and asthma; moreover, some diabetics shouldn't use it. Combining aspirin with some medications like Coumadin or anti-inflammatory drugs such as ibuprofen can lead to severe bleeding problems. There may also be other serious interactions between aspirin and other drugs a person may be taking.

However, for the vast majority of patients with heart disease, the benefits of aspirin therapy clearly outweigh the risks. Talk with your doctor to determine if aspirin therapy could be of benefit to you. "Doctors usually recommend one of two courses," says Dr. William Castelli. "You can take a baby aspirin, about 81 milligrams, daily; however, it's recommended that you supplement with a 325-milligram booster on the first and 15th day of the month. Or you can take a 325-milligram tablet every other day." According to Dr. Edward Giovannucci, a researcher on the Nurses' Health Study, "Four to six regular-size aspirin tablets a week seem to provide the maximum benefit. Gobbling more tablets or higher doses will not help to further reduce risk and may increase side effects."

ASPIRIN ALONE?

A just-published study of heart attack patients at 78 VA medical centers came to a surprising conclusion: giving heart attack survivors a combined low dose of the more expensive anticoagulant drug warfarin (Coumadin) with low-dose aspirin did not prevent heart attacks or strokes better than aspirin alone. Patients began therapy within two weeks of suffering a heart attack and were followed for an average of nearly three years. Mortality rates, recurrent heart attacks, and strokes were virtually identical in the combined therapy and aspirin-only groups. "We had hoped the combined regimen might double the effectiveness of the drugs, but it didn't," said Dr. Louis Fiore, one of the principal researchers.

Cholesterol-Lowering Drugs

Elevated cholesterol is a predictive marker for heart disease and heart attack, so it needs to be managed carefully to reduce cardiovascular risk. Most people can lower their cholesterol by 10% to 20% by adopting a low-fat diet, exercising and losing weight. But for some people, lifestyle changes alone are not strong enough to combat "bad genes." That's why more than 10 million Americans use drug therapy to reach their cholesterol goals.

A number of effective drugs are available to help control total cholesterol, LDL, HDL and triglycerides. Talk to your doctor to determine if drug therapy is appropriate for you.

Statin Drugs

Introduced in the late 1980s, statins are most doctors' drug of choice for lowering total and LDL cholesterol. Statins block cholesterol production in the liver; the body, which needs a certain amount of cholesterol to function, compensates by drawing on cholesterol found in the blood. This reduces the amount of cholesterol that could damage arteries. Depending on the drug and dosage, statins typically decrease total cholesterol by 22% to 42%, lower LDL cholesterol by 18% to 55%, increase HDL cholesterol by 5% to 15% and reduce triglycerides by 7% to 30%.

Taken in capsule form, statin drugs are the only lipid-lowering drugs that have been proven to reduce the risk of death from cardiovascular disease. They also have been shown to reduce the risk of first and second heart attacks. Commonly prescribed statins include:

DRUG	BRAND NAME
Pravastatin	Pravachol
Lovastatin	Mevacor
Simvastatin	Zocor
Atorvastatin	Lipitor
Fluvastatin	Lescol

BEFORE YOU START . . .

Before you take a statin drug, be sure to discuss with your doctor whether or not you meet the indications for therapy. A study of 29,000 primary-care patients drawn from Boston's Brigham and Women's Hospital found that fewer than one in three taking statin drugs to prevent heart disease met National Cholesterol Education Program guidelines for who should take the drugs. According to Dr. Susan Abookire, the study leader, a number of factors explain the results. "Doctors may not follow the guidelines or keep up with current research on statins. To be on the safe side, some physicians may prescribe more medication rather than less; and finally, doctors are influenced by what their patients want, which is driven by advertising."

Statin drugs are generally recommended for people whose LDL is 190 milligrams per deciliter (mg/dl) or higher; those whose LDL is 160 mg/dl or higher and have at least two other risk factors for heart disease; or those whose LDL is 130 mg/dl or higher and who have known cardiovascular disease.

Statin drugs are so effective that doctors are increasingly using them for people who have "normal" or only slightly elevated cholesterol levels. One study published in the *British Medical Journal* concluded that statins could reduce the risk of dying from a heart attack by 30% even among those with normal cholesterol levels and no sign of cardiovascular disease. That's because the non-cholesterol effects of statins, such as controlling clotting and inflammation, may be as important as the cholesterol effects. In the Air Force/Texas Coronary Atherosclerosis Study, researchers found that statin drugs also reduced levels of C-reactive protein. "Statins are turning out to be a real two-for-one," says Dr. Paul Ridker of the Brigham and Women's Hospital. "They certainly reduce cholesterol. But they also reduce C-reactive protein, an independent predictor of heart disease."

In addition, recent tests suggest that statins may help to ward off

Alzheimer's disease, osteoporosis and, in combination with aspirin, colon cancer. The efficacy of statins is reflected in the most current National Cholesterol Education Program Guidelines, which suggest that about 36 million Americans could benefit from drug therapy, up from a previous estimate of 15 million Americans. Says Dr. Antonio Gotto, former president of the American Heart Association, "I'm not recommending putting statins in the drinking water, but millions more people could benefit from their use."

So, what's the downside? First, statins are costly. Next, you presumably have to be on these drugs for the rest of your life, but to date the effects of such long-term use are virtually undocumented. More significantly, in rare cases statins can cause elevations in some liver enzymes that could ultimately result in liver damage, so people using these drugs need regular blood testing. In addition, statins have been linked to very rare reports of a muscle weakness called rhabdomyolysis, a potentially life-threatening condition in which muscle cells are destroyed and released into the bloodstream. It can cause severe muscle pain, mainly in the calves and lower back, and may result in kidney failure. Patients on statins should report any unusual muscle tenderness or fatigue to their physician.

> ### NIX THE GRAPEFRUIT
>
> Unlike other citrus fruits, grapefruit contains substances that disable certain enzymes in your body, sometimes for many hours. Without these enzymes, some statin drugs end up in the bloodstream at higher concentrations, which can put you at risk for serious muscle aches or weakness. Although an *occasional* small glass of grapefruit juice may be fine, experts recommend not drinking it at the same time you take the medication.

Resins

Also called bile acid sequestrants, these drugs—considered the safest of the lipid-altering drugs—have been used successfully for over 20 years to reduce LDL cholesterol. Usually taken as a sandlike powder mixed with juice or water, resins bind with bile salts in the intestines and flush them out of the system. To replenish the bile acid pool, the liver then draws cholesterol from the bloodstream, thereby reducing the blood's LDL concentration. In addition, resins promote cholesterol elimination in stools.

Resins are especially effective for people with high cholesterol who cannot tolerate statins. They're also less expensive than statins and have fewer potentially serious side effects. However, unless taken in huge amounts, resins usually do not produce the dramatic drop in cholesterol that statin drugs do. In addition, it's more of a hassle to take them, particularly when you're away from home. Furthermore, resins can raise the triglyceride level and have only very modest effects on raising HDL cholesterol.

Some of the most prevalent resins include cholestyramine (Questran), colestipol (Colestid) and colesevelam (WelChol). Questran and Colestid cannot be taken in combination with other medications, including statins; they may bind to and remove such drugs. WelChol, a newer drug, does not have these drawbacks, which is why it's believed to be especially effective as adjunctive therapy for people already on statin drugs who need further cholesterol reduction.

Niacin

Also called nicotinic acid or vitamin B_3, niacin is an old standby for cholesterol control. Inexpensive and effective, it decreases total and LDL cholesterol, the latter by 5% to 25%. However, it does something that most other cholesterol drugs do not: niacin lowers triglycerides by 20% to 50% and increases HDL by 15% to 35%. Accordingly, niacin is the best HDL cholesterol raiser of the lipid-altering agents. In some cases, niacin is prescribed along with a statin drug to maximize the therapy.

Niacin is effective only in massive doses, usually one to three grams (1,000 to 3,000 milligrams) per day, or 50 to 100 times the USRDA. Unfortunately, large doses of niacin can have bothersome side effects—including flushing, hyperglycemia, hot flashes, itching, nausea, blurred vision and headache. Usually side effects disappear as tolerance is gained. Sustained-release versions of niacin, taken once a day (instead of two or three times as with vitamin B_3), seem to help.

Since a rare but more serious side effect is liver damage, you should never take massive doses of niacin—even though you can buy it over the counter—without first consulting your physician. Then, be sure to have your blood test checked for liver function. If you have liver disease, diabetes, gout, peptic ulcers or glaucoma, or if you're on a blood thinner, your doctor may not recommend niacin therapy for you.

Some of the most common brands of niacin include B_3-50, B_3-500-GR, Niacin SR, Niacor, Niaspan ER, Nico-400, Nicolar, Nicobid and Slo-Niacin.

Be Wary of Over-the-Counter Cholesterol Fighters

A number of over-the-counter products claim to lower cholesterol, but once again, some of these claims are hollow. Here's a quick rundown:

■ *Soluble fiber* in capsules and powders, often found in health food stores, is not effective in reducing cholesterol. Stick with foods that are rich in soluble fiber—oatmeal, oat bran, apples, oranges, beans and corn.

■ The jury is still out on soy protein powder, whereas foods such as soy milk, tofu and soybeans are effective.

■ There is little evidence that garlic oil, garlic powder, or garlic supplements lower cholesterol.

■ Fish oil capsules do not lower cholesterol levels, although they can help to reduce triglycerides.

■ Stay away from a dietary supplement of red yeast extract called Cholestin. It may be less of a supplement and more of an unapproved drug.

The bottom line: don't self-medicate.

Fibrates

These drugs, notably gemfibrozil (Lopid) and fenofibrate (Tricor), are mainly used to decrease triglycerides, usually from 20% to 50%. An additional benefit is that they can increase protective HDL by 10% to 20% and decrease harmful LDL by 5% to 20%. Gemfibrozil lowers the triglyceride level as well as or more effectively than any of the other lipid-lowering drugs, but it has only modest effects on LDL cholesterol levels. Also, it sometimes raises rather than lowers LDL cholesterol.

Side effects of these drugs include digestive problems, gallstones and muscle weakness.

Hormone Replacement Therapy

Since the risk of heart disease increases markedly as women pass menopause, many scientists and doctors have thought that estrogen exerts a cardioprotective effect and that hormone replacement therapy (HRT) could reduce the rate of postmenopausal cardiac events. Surprisingly, however, the Heart and Estrogen/Progestin Replacement Study (HERS), the first large-scale randomized clinical trial to test this hypothesis, found that treatment with oral estrogen plus progestin did *not* reduce the overall rate of new heart attacks in postmenopausal women with known coronary disease. Several theories have been proposed to explain these disappointing results, including an inadequate follow-up duration (4.1 years). Yet two just-published reports in the *Journal of the American Medical Association*, involving an extended follow-up (6.8 years) of the HERS subjects, came to a similar conclusion.

Recently, the results of the Women's Health Initiative trial, the largest study ever conducted in the United States of women's mid-life health issues, reported an increased overall health risk in healthy postmenopausal women taking combined HRT as compared with women who were given a placebo. Between 1993 and 1998, 16,608 women aged 50 to 79 who had not had a hysterectomy were randomly assigned to two groups: one took Prempro (estrogen and progestin), the other a sugar pill. Although it was scheduled to run until 2005, the study was stopped prematurely because the women taking Prempro demonstrated a higher incidence of heart attack, stroke, breast cancer and blood clots.

Prompted by these new studies, the American Heart Association has now updated its recommendations, suggesting that HRT should not be used for the purpose of preventing a second heart attack or death among women with established heart disease. It also advises against starting or continuing combined HRT for the prevention of coronary heart disease. On the other hand, the AHA has emphasized that further results from the Women's Health Initiative trial will be needed in order to assess the risks and benefits for women taking estrogen alone.

In summary, combined estrogen and progestin—a treatment used by millions of women for relief of menopause symptoms as well as the prevention of other serious health problems—should not be taken long-term. Talk to your doctor about HRT in light of these new findings and your personal and family health history. "The message is not that all women should stop hormones," says Dr. Margery Gass of the University of Cincinnati. "It's that each woman should consider why she's on HRT—and how she might accomplish her health goals another way."

ACE Inhibitors

Angiotensin-converting enzyme inhibitors, or ACE inhibitors, belong to a class of cardiac drugs called antihypertensives, normally administered to patients with high blood pressure but also used to treat congestive heart failure or after major heart attacks where considerable heart damage has occurred. ACE inhibitors may be referred to either by their generic names, which commonly end in "il"—such as benazepril, captopril, enalapril, lisinopril, and ramipril—or by their brand names: Lotensin, Capoten, Vasotec, Zestril or Prinivil, and Altace. These medications are believed to block an enzyme that produces a substance that causes blood vessels to constrict. By relaxing or dilating blood vessels, they end up reducing blood pressure and increasing the supply of blood and oxygen to the heart muscle.

The Survival and Ventricular Enlargement (SAVE) Trial enrolled over 2,200 major heart attack survivors and randomly assigned them to either a placebo or treatment with an ACE inhibitor. Patients were then followed for an average of three and a half years. Drug therapy reduced the risk of death by about 20%, recurrent hospitalizations by 22% and recurrent heart attacks by 25%, as well as reducing the need for coronary bypass surgery or balloon angioplasty.

The Studies of Left Ventricular Dysfunction (SOLVD) Trials also assessed the effects of ACE inhibitor therapy in patients with a his-

SPEAKING FROM EXPERIENCE

Doctors today have an impressive array of pharmaceutical weapons to use in the fight against heart disease, but I sometimes worry about the downside. Many people think drugs are magic cures that will solve their cardiovascular problems without any lifestyle effort on their part. They forget that drugs are *adjunctive therapies*, meaning that they are used in addition to, not instead of, healthy lifestyle changes.

Take statins, for instance. These drugs are very effective in lowering LDL cholesterol, but that does *not* mean a person taking them can eat a high-fat diet. That's why drugs come after healthy lifestyle changes in the Piscatella Protocol.   —*J.P.*

tory of heart failure and residual cardiac impairment. Follow-up averaged slightly more than three years. Overall, drug therapy reduced cardiovascular mortality, new heart attacks and recurrent anginal pain by about 20% each.

Although the results of these well-designed follow-up studies have consistently demonstrated fewer subsequent cardiovascular complications in patients assigned to ACE inhibitor therapy, it remained unclear whether a broader population of heart patients (those without major heart damage) would also benefit from such therapy. Recently, this question was resolved when the Heart Outcomes Prevention Evaluation (HOPE) study was stopped before its scheduled conclusion because of overwhelming evidence that ramipril reduced the overall number of cardiovascular problems by a remarkable 22%. Moreover, investigators also found that drug-treated patients developed heart failure and diabetes less frequently and had fewer interventional procedures, such as coronary bypass surgery and balloon angioplasty.

Beta-Blockers

Formally called beta-adrenergic blocking agents, these drugs are used to treat high blood pressure, relieve angina, abolish heart rhythm irregularities and prevent recurrent heart attacks. Referred to by either their generic names, which commonly end in "ol" (as in atenolol, metoprolol, nadolol, propranolol and timolol), or their brand names (Tenormin, Lopressor or Toprol, Corgard, Inderal and Blocadren), they work by affecting the response to certain nerve impulses throughout the body. Consequently, they decrease the heart's blood and oxygen requirements by reducing its workload while helping it to maintain a normal rhythm.

Long-term administration of beta-blockers after a heart attack has been unequivocally shown to improve survival rate. In the Beta-Blocker in Heart Attack Trial (BHAT), nearly 4,000 heart attack survivors were followed for an average of 25 months. The first year, mortality for patients who were randomly assigned to receive beta-blocker therapy was reduced by 39% as compared with mortality for their counterparts, who received a placebo. However, among one-year survivors, benefit from continued treatment appeared to be largely restricted to those at the highest risk of new or recurrent heart attacks.

Another analysis of 16 major trials, involving more than 18,000 heart attack patients, demonstrated convincingly the therapeutic benefit of starting treatment soon after the cardiac event. Beta-blocker therapy reduced the risk of death by 20% and of recurrent heart attacks by 25%. These percentages were based on all patients, regardless of whether they faithfully adhered to their prescribed drug regimen. Accordingly, the benefits may be even greater for compliant and high-risk patients.

Several mechanisms may explain the reduced cardiovascular mortality with long-term beta-blocker therapy after a heart attack. A chief effect of beta-blockers in numerous studies appears to be a reduction in sudden cardiac death, supporting the belief that these drugs combat potentially lethal heart rhythms. Others suggest that the lowering of heart rate and blood pressure may be especially important in reducing the potential for cardiac ischemia (lack of blood to the heart), which has been linked to threatening heart rhythms. Beta-blockers may also lessen the workload of the heart muscle, which may decrease the size of a heart attack if administered before or soon after the onset of symptoms, and reduce the potential for blood clotting.

In summary, beta-blocker therapy can be useful for preventing subsequent heart attacks and potentially fatal rhythm disturbances in heart attack survivors. Patients who may also benefit from these medications include the elderly, individuals with heart failure or lung disease and heart attack survivors who have not undergone coronary bypass surgery or balloon angioplasty.

2. TESTING FOR CORONARY HEART DISEASE

If angina or other symptoms have you worried about coronary heart disease, it makes sense to schedule a physical exam that will evaluate the condition of your heart and arteries. Your doctor will take your family history, listen to your heart, check your blood pressure and pulse, and probably assess your weight and body-fat distribution. You should also have a blood test for total cholesterol, LDL, HDL, triglycerides and glucose.

In addition, because of the latest research, many physicians are now evaluating levels of homocysteine and C-reactive protein (indicators of arterial inflammation) and fibrinogen (a marker for the propensity of blood to clot).

In the event that heart disease is suspected, a variety of diagnostic tests may be employed to help analyze your situation. Given the fact that sudden cardiac death is the first sign of heart disease for thousands of people each year, diagnostic tests are becoming increasingly important. Such tests are administered on a progressive basis and can usually be grouped into three levels of sophistication: basic, intermediate and advanced. Promising new tests are also in the works.

Basic Tests

One of the most common diagnostic tests is the *chest X ray*. By examining photographs of the chest's interior, the doctor can assess the size of the heart (which could be enlarged due to heart failure), discover certain structural abnormalities and detect fluid in the lungs.

An *electrocardiogram* (ECG) is part of most annual physicals and is recorded while the patient's heart is "at rest." Electrodes attached to the arms, legs and chest allow the doctor to evaluate the electronic impulses given off by the heart and look for evidence of rhythm irregularities, chamber enlargement, ischemia (insufficient blood supply via the coronary arteries) and heart attack. Sometimes ECG readings are taken continuously over a 24-hour period using a Holter monitor hooked up to chest electrodes. Readings over a period of time can show heart rhythm irregularities and, to a lesser extent, evidence of insufficient blood supply to the heart.

Unfortunately, a resting ECG will not generally disclose a blockage until it completely obstructs the artery channel. When the heart is not under a heavy workload, the ECG results may be "normal" even when the channel is severely blocked, as long as the muscle is getting enough blood to meet its resting oxygen requirements. Only when an artery is severely obstructed and blood flow is impeded to the point where the heart has an insufficient oxygen supply does the ECG show an abnormality. A few years ago, for instance, a prominent mayor of Chicago died of a heart attack as he was leaving his cardiologist's office after an examination in which his resting ECG was normal.

"PENILE STRESS TEST"

For some men, impotence may indicate impending heart disease. In a recent study, 50 men were referred to a medical center because the cause of their erectile dysfunction could not be determined. Although none of the men had symptoms, 20 of them had significant coronary artery blockages. Researchers may eventually categorize impotence as a "penile stress test" that can warn of serious heart problems.

A simple test called the *ankle/brachial blood pressure index* (ABI) measures blood pressure in the upper arm and in the ankle. If a pressure reading in the ankle is significantly lower than that in the arm, an increased risk of peripheral vascular disease (atherosclerosis of the lower extremities) may be indicated, particularly in people over age 50. This condition is frequently observed in people with coronary heart disease.

Intermediate Tests

If the basic tests show a problem, or if the doctors need more information, one of the intermediate tests will likely be used. These may include an exercise stress test or a diagnostic technique called echocardiography.

Exercise Stress Tests

Basically an ECG performed during exercise, usually on a treadmill or stationary bike, the standard exercise stress test evaluates the heart when it is beating more rapidly than when it's at rest. The intensity of the exercise increases as the test progresses, and blood pressure readings are taken at intervals to assess the heart's pumping power when the workload is increased. Often used to evaluate symptoms such as shortness of breath or chest pain, an exercise stress test is successful in detecting coronary heart disease in about 70% of people with the disease.

When a person is at rest, significant blockage of the coronary arteries (generally considered to be 75% or more) may not be severe enough to result in an insufficient delivery of oxygen to the heart muscle. During exercise, however, an impaired blood supply to the heart may cause anginal chest pain, a change in the ECG pattern (called ST-segment depression), or both.

This test provides a very good diagnostic and prognostic tool, particularly for middle-aged men. Doctors have even found it to be effective in identifying men with silent cardiac ischemia, in which coronary arteries are narrowed and blood flow is diminished but no angina or other symptoms are present. Studies have found that men who have silent ischemia and other risk factors (such as high cholesterol, high blood pressure and smoking) have four to six times the risk of heart attack. By identifying the increased likelihood of disease with an exercise stress test, additional diagnostic studies (such as thallium or cardiolite stress testing and/or cardiac catheterization) can be used to clarify the location and the extent of the coronary blockages, so that preventive action can be taken.

There is one note of caution, however. Exercise stress tests are not always predictive, especially for young men and women or for middle-aged women. Sometimes these tests fail to detect slight blockages and thus produce false-negative results. More often, they suggest coronary heart disease when it does not exist; this is called a false-positive result and is associated with young women in particular. Nonetheless, these tests provide an enormously powerful prognostic tool, especially when taking fitness and non-ECG measures into account.

An exercise stress test with *myocardial perfusion imaging* permits doctors to observe the manner in which blood moves through the vessels and is taken up by the heart. A small amount of thallium or cardiolite is injected intravenously while the patient is near maximal exercise on a treadmill and the heart is being "stressed." Immediately after the test an X-ray scan is taken and compared with another scan taken while the heart is at rest. This test can reveal inactive scar tissue (the result of a previous heart attack) and areas deprived of oxygen due to reduced blood flow. By examining these

RECOVERY HEART RATE: A NEW PROGNOSTIC INDICATOR

An exercise stress test is also a good way to give doctors a look at their patients' heart recovery rate, or how much the heartbeat slows after they have exercised to exhaustion and then recovered.

Normally the maximal heart rate drops between 15 and 25 beats soon after exhaustive exercise, but researchers discovered that for people whose heart rate falls 12 beats or less at one minute after exercising, the risk of dying within six years is four times greater.

images, doctors can pinpoint potential sites of coronary artery blockages.

Patients who are limited in their ability to exercise may benefit from *pharmacologic stress testing*, which uses medication such as dobutamine to increase heart rate or persantine to dilate coronary arteries. This form of testing is associated with an accuracy of 85% to 90% in detecting significant coronary blockages.

Radionuclide ventriculography traces a nuclear isotope that has been injected into the patient's bloodstream. During exercise, the patient pedals a stationary bike in the supine, upright or semi-upright position while X-ray pictures are taken to determine how much of the isotope is being pumped out of the heart's ventricles during each beat. Taken at varied angles, the pictures can also measure chamber volume and identify wall motion abnormalities. An advantage of this noninvasive technique is that it is highly accurate in detecting the presence of coronary artery disease. Moreover, it can be used serially to evaluate the effects of medication, balloon angioplasty and bypass surgery.

Echocardiography

Used more and more these days to provide additional diagnostic information, echocardiography relies on a recording sensor to bounce ultrasound waves off the heart to create an image of the muscle at work. Echocardiography can show areas of the heart that have been damaged by a heart attack. It can also be combined with a stress test to reveal wall motion abnormalities, which can indicate areas of the heart that are not receiving enough blood.

In addition, according to Dr. Daniel O'Leary of the Tufts–New England Medical Center, ultrasound can detect cumulative damage to blood vessels before any symptoms are experienced. Dr. O'Leary's recent study shows that ultrasound can identify thickening of the carotid artery walls in the neck, a powerful predictor of heart attack or stroke in elderly people.

Advanced Testing

Coronary angiography, also known as cardiac catheterization, is the definitive "gold standard" test for coronary heart disease. First, a thin plastic tube called a catheter is inserted into an artery in the leg or arm and threaded into the heart. Then a dye is injected into the catheter. As the dye flows through the coronary arteries, each of which is only about the size of a strand of cooked spaghetti, the doctor can identify and assess narrow spots and blockages via X-ray imaging.

Its ability to show specific sites of narrowing makes angiography a key diagnostic technique when evaluating the need for balloon angioplasty or bypass surgery.

SPEAKING FROM EXPERIENCE

I was apprehensive going in for my angiogram—after all, this was an invasive procedure—but the medical team explained what was happening step by step and that relaxed me. I was awake and alert the whole time. I expected some pain when the catheter was inserted, but all I felt was a slight pressure.

I really couldn't feel any of the catheter's movement as it was threaded into my heart. There was a feeling of sudden heat, like a hot flash, when the dye was released, but it lasted only a moment or two. What kept my mind off the physical aspects of the procedure was the fact that I could watch what was happening on a monitor. I could identify the arteries, see when the dye was released and, unfortunately, pinpoint the place where the artery narrowed and I had a problem. It was this test that convinced me to have bypass surgery. —*J.P.*

Promising New Diagnostic Tests

Computed tomography (CT) is now being used to find early coronary heart disease by detecting calcium in the coronary arteries. Calcium deposits, believed to be by-products of inflammation and precursors of artery blockages, are considered predictors of increased risk of heart disease and stroke. One study showed that patients whose calcium buildup increased 20% or more each year had an 18-fold greater chance of suffering a heart attack than those with less calcium in the heart. Thus if the CT scan shows a large amount of calcium, a narrowing of the coronary artery is suggested. People with calcium deposits tend to be smokers with high cholesterol levels and high blood pressure.

The newest tomographic test, called *electron-beam computed tomography* (EBCT), is 10 times faster than the standard CT scan and therefore capable of producing a rapid evaluation of calcium deposits in the coronary arteries. The theory is that EBCT is simply better than cholesterol screening at identifying high-risk patients. In a study by Dr. Harvey Hecht, published in the *Journal of the American College of Cardiology*, 304 women underwent both cholesterol testing and EBCT scans. The results showed that cholesterol screening failed to identify nearly half the women over age 55 who exhibited signs of heart disease; in women under 55, cholesterol screening failed about 40% of the time.

Recently, Dr. Paolo Raggi and associates studied 632 symptom-free patients with coronary risk factors who were screened by EBCT and followed for an average of 32 months for the development of cardiac events (heart attack or sudden cardiac death). Their results showed that calcium scores of 0 were associated with an event rate of 0.1% per year; in contrast, the annualized event rate was 2.1% for scores of 1 to 99, 4.1% for scores of 100 to 400 and 4.8% for scores over 400. Interestingly, calcification scores above 100 were associated with cardiac event rates that were higher than those of patients

CARDIAC CALCIFICATION SCORE

10-Year Event Rate (%)

50 — 40 — 30 — 20 — 10 — 0 —

Zero   1 to 99   100 to 400   Over 400

with known coronary heart disease. The investigators concluded that the risk of subsequent cardiac problems is greatly increased in the presence of coronary artery calcification.

While CT and EBCT scans are reliable, most experts believe they are not for everyone. "Because calcium deposits do not automatically lead to heart disease in all cases, it is too soon to recommend widespread screening," says Dr. Carlos Iribarren, a researcher at Kaiser Permanente in Oakland, California. Other authorities emphasize that coronary plaque with calcium is generally mature, more stable and not prone to rupture. In addition, coronary calcification is found in virtually all men older than 60 and women over 70 years of age. If you have two or more cardiac risk factors but no symptoms, the test may be useful in evaluating your condition. However, the benefit of routine screening for heart disease with EBCT remains unproven.

Finally, *intravascular ultrasound* (IVUS) has great promise in detecting unstable coronary lesions, those most likely to rupture and clot. IVUS is similar to a cardiac catheterization in that it uses a long, thin tube threaded into the coronary arteries. However, the tube carries an ultrasound probe at its tip to take sonar pictures from the inside of the artery. The images show the amount of plaque, its shape and composition, and to what extent it has infiltrated the channel opening as well as the artery wall.

3. REVASCULARIZATION TREATMENTS FOR CORONARY HEART DISEASE

If heart disease is diagnosed, your doctor may recommend a number of options including medications (such as nitroglycerin to reduce angina, statin drugs to lower cholesterol or aspirin therapy), a low-fat diet, an exercise program, stress management techniques and smoking cessation. In addition, depending on your symptoms and/or the severity of the disease, you may be a candidate for coronary revascularization.

Balloon Angioplasty

The most common revascularization procedure is balloon angioplasty (600,000 to 700,000 are done each year), also called percutaneous transluminal coronary angioplasty (PTCA). In this procedure, a small, flexible catheter is inserted into an artery in the leg or arm and then threaded through the arterial system into the coronary arteries. Using X rays as a guide, the cardiologist can move the catheter into the narrowed spot.

Next, a second catheter with a tiny balloon on its tip goes through the first catheter. When the second catheter reaches the clogged artery, its balloon is inflated. The balloon gently pushes the fatty plaque against the wall of the artery, thus opening the artery so blood can flow more easily. At this point, the balloon and catheters are taken out. Angioplasty takes an hour or two and is done under local anesthesia. Not everyone is a candidate for this procedure; in some cases, blockages are so tortuous or severe that it cannot be performed.

In stretching the walls of the coronary arteries, the balloon catheter may cause slight arterial injuries. Unfortunately, such

---

REPEAT REVASCULARIZATIONS

In early March 2001, as Vice President Dick Cheney recuperated after doctors once again unblocked a coronary artery, questions resurfaced about high-tech treatments and their effectiveness. Cheney has had four heart attacks (the first 24 years ago), a quadruple bypass operation and two balloon angioplasties, yet his cardiac history is not that unusual. About 700,000 angioplasties are performed each year. Bypass surgery is done about 500,000 times annually. Many are repeats.

These numbers teach us a sobering lesson: the vessels used to bypass blocked coronary arteries may close, other coronary arteries can become clogged or scar tissue may form at a metal stent implanted to reopen an artery—as was the case with the vice president. Each of these can jeopardize the heart, causing symptoms or new events to occur.

Fortunately, aggressive medical treatment in combination with lifestyle changes can slow, halt and sometimes even reverse the progression of heart disease.

---

injuries can promote the formation of blood clots. In 4% to 12% of procedures, clot-related complications occur. To reduce this likelihood, anticoagulant drugs such as aspirin, heparin and clopidogrel (Plavix) are used during and after balloon angioplasty.

Early on, this procedure had a high failure rate and often had to be repeated. But in 1994 the Food and Drug Administration approved the use of the Palmaz-Schatz stent, a tiny, flexible cylinder designed to prevent the collapse of a vessel that has been opened. Made of stainless steel, the mesh-like stents provide support and serve as a kind of scaffolding to keep the artery open. Although stents are now the workhorse in this cardiac procedure, scar tissue forms at the sites of up to 30% of these stents, and the blood vessel clogs or narrows again, a condition known as restenosis.

Researchers such as Dr. Gregory Chapman at the University of Alabama at Birmingham believe that this Achilles' heel of angioplasty may be overcome by coating stents with sirolimus, a drug that prevents thickening of the inner walls of blood vessels. Initial results of trials are very positive. In one study of 30 patients, tests after a period of four months revealed no restenosis; after eight months, none of the patients had suffered a heart attack or stroke and none needed a second angioplasty. Stents are now even being used in emergency situations to open up blocked coronary arteries during heart attacks.

Recent studies show that acute heart attack patients fare better with angioplasty, especially when it's preceded and followed by selected anticlotting drugs (clopidogrel and aspirin), than with clot-busting drugs known as thrombolytic therapy.

Bypass Surgery

For multiple blockages, typical in people suffering from severe coronary heart disease, coronary artery bypass graft (CABG, pronounced "cabbage") may be recommended. Although bypass surgery is performed about a half-million times a year, it remains a major, expensive operation and is not without potential complications such as heart attack and stroke. Surgeons cut open the breastbone, pry apart the rib cage and stop the exposed heart as they reconfigure the blood vessels to reroute blood flow to the heart.

Bypass surgery is used to redirect blood vessels around the blocked areas. The operation typically takes three to six hours. The surgeon harvests a vein from the leg or an artery from the chest and attaches one end of the blood vessel to the aorta. The other end is attached to the coronary artery below the point where it is clogged. This creates a new arterial channel that will allow blood to flow freely to the heart. Literally "bypassing" the blocked area, the procedure has a high long-term success rate, especially when the chest artery is used.

Minimally invasive direct coronary artery bypass surgery is a newer, gentler technique that allows for a less invasive approach to bypassing blocked coronary arteries. Instead of opening the chest and working on a heart that is stopped, the surgeon operates with

SPEAKING FROM EXPERIENCE

Bypass surgery probably saved my life, but people considering this procedure should be aware of four things. To start with, it's designed to take away the pain of restricted blood flow, yet it does not take away the underlying cause—coronary heart disease— even though it may put you in a better position to bring about the lifestyle changes that are needed to stabilize and potentially reverse the disease.

Second, a bypass doesn't necessarily last forever. If you don't take care of it by adopting a healthy lifestyle, you might get just a few years out of it. Third, the physical recovery can be daunting. I had some complications, so it took me about six months to regain my strength and stamina. Others have done it sooner.

Finally, you have to be prepared for mental changes. According to a study at Duke University, about 42% of bypass patients experience a subtle change in personality and suffer an impairment of memory and cognitive abilities five years after surgery. At my seminars, I've had wives of bypass patients tell me, "This is not the man I married. His personality is different." Further studies are needed to determine the importance of such changes to real-world behavior. However, many physicians hypothesize that these results are more often found in patients who have undergone bypass surgery while on the heart-lung machine, particularly if the operation takes over four hours.   —*J.P.*

fiber-optic scopes through small incisions between the ribs to work directly on the beating heart.

For this reason, the procedure is sometimes called "keyhole surgery." No heart-lung machine is used. This procedure avoids the massive chest damage inflicted by open-heart surgery and reduces pain, recovery time and expense.

Emerging
Interventional Techniques

A number of innovative procedures are being used on a limited basis. Although much more experience needs to be gained in the use of these techniques before they become as common as angioplasty and bypass surgery, many doctors believe them to be the wave of the future.

Radiation therapy is a new technique used to complement angioplasty. One of the ongoing problems in coronary revascularization is that in a significant number of patients who undergo balloon angioplasty, the arteries close up again within six months after the procedure. Although the use of stents has helped, about 30% of stented vessels are closed due to restenosis at the six-month mark. Many doctors feel that radiation therapy as an enhancement to angioplasty may be the answer. That's because radiation inhibits cell growth (as it does with cancer).

In this procedure, tiny radioactive pellets are sent through a catheter to the blockage in the artery and then held in place for several minutes to deliver a dose of radiation before being retrieved. The radiation inhibits scar tissue that could result in subsequent restenosis. A study involving 24 patients showed almost no narrowing of blood vessels six months after angioplasty. Broader studies are planned before the technology will be approved on a large scale in the United States.

Off-pump coronary artery bypass (OPCAB) is another new surgical technique. In conventional open-heart bypass surgery, doctors work on a heart that has been stopped. The job of circulating oxygen-rich blood throughout the body is performed by the heart-lung machine, which slightly raises the risk of complications such as mental impairment. Using OPCAB, surgeons open the chest as in normal bypass surgery but operate on the beating heart without the use of the heart-lung machine. A special tool restrains the section of the heart being worked on. While potential complications may be minimized, OPCAB is more difficult to perform than conventional surgery and is not yet widely used.

Angiogenesis is a process in which new arteries can be made to grow in the walls of the heart. While still in the experimental stage (it does sound a lot like something out of science fiction!), several clinical trials are under way to assess its potential. The process involves implanting tiny "growth factor" capsules in the walls of the heart to spur the growth of new blood vessels. It could be particularly important for people with arteries so diseased that angioplasty and bypass surgery have been ruled out. "We *can* grow new vessels," says Dr. Michael Simons, director of the Angiogenesis Research Center at Beth Israel Deaconess Medical Center in Boston. "But at this stage we're still groping our way through, trying to figure out the biology."

One of the newest and most controversial options is *percutaneous myocardial revascularization* (PMR). In this procedure, doctors thread a laser-tipped catheter to a part of the heart that is not receiving sufficient blood. Quick blasts from the laser punch 30 or more tiny holes in the heart. In clinical trials this has caused an increase in blood flow and has relieved angina. One problem is that no one is certain why this procedure works. Some doctors believe it to be a beneficial treatment in last-ditch cases; others feel that a placebo effect, not PMR, is responsible for any positive results in patients. More testing is planned.

4. CARDIAC
REHABILITATION PROGRAMS

Whether you're working to prevent heart disease or facing treatment after a heart attack, bypass surgery or angioplasty, the approach is very similar. Both instances call for addressing the underlying causes of heart disease: hypertension, cigarette smoking, high-fat diets, obesity, unbridled stress and a sedentary lifestyle. Current thinking holds that multifactorial risk-factor modification using diet, drugs and exercise may slow, halt or even reverse the progression of heart disease.

Such modification is often fairly simple to achieve before a cardiac event takes place. There is no great pressure for immediate change, so you can gradually ease into an exercise program or trade your double burger for a healthier chicken sandwich. But it's not the same for those who have experienced a heart attack or who have been diagnosed with coronary heart disease. Making lifestyle changes is often very difficult. In addition to confusion over what to do and how to do it, and fear about future health, there often is an added burden: the belief that total change must take place immediately. This can produce such mental stress that the heart patient becomes immobilized and accomplishes nothing.

Cardiac rehabilitation programs can help. Designed to provide a mix of education and action in a supportive environment, they make it easier for patients to take charge of their lifestyle habits and achieve a better quality of life. Moreover, rehab staff provide doctors with valuable ongoing surveillance data (e.g., unusual shortness of breath, heart rhythm irregularities and the development of new anginal symptoms), enabling them to better monitor their patients. Most programs define themselves as being in the business of "helping patients to help themselves."

The objectives of cardiac rehabilitation are to increase physical fitness, decrease symptoms, stop cigarette smoking, modify cholesterol and other lipids, decrease body weight and body fat, reduce blood pressure and generally improve psychosocial well-being. To those ends, contemporary programs offer a menu of services to meet individual needs. And in order to accomplish their objectives, structured programs are generally staffed by a mix of health professionals: doctors, cardiac nurse specialists, exercise physiologists, dietitians and behavior therapists. However, health professional–guided, home-based rehabilitation has been shown to be an effective alternative to formal programs.

Cardiac rehabilitation programs are generally based on three to four phases:

■ *Phase I*, called the inpatient phase, takes place while the patient is still hospitalized following a heart attack or surgery and includes low-level walking, self-care activities and intermittent sitting or standing. Risk factors, post-hospital medical care, medications and limitations are discussed with the patient and his or her family as they receive support and insight into what the future holds for them.

■ *Phase II* is the beginning of outpatient cardiac rehabilitation, usually lasting from 4 to 12 weeks. During this time the patient starts

SPEAKING FROM EXPERIENCE

When I had my surgery in 1977, I didn't go to rehab. It wasn't available at the time, so I just went home and tried to make the best of it. My questions about which exercise I should do, how hard I should exercise, how to change my diet or manage stress went unanswered—until I started investigating these topics on my own.

Cardiac patients and their families should not be in that situation. I tell patients to be proactive with their doctors about getting into a cardiac rehab program, where they'll receive information, instruction, exercise therapy, ongoing medical surveillance and support. —*J.P* a formal, ECG-monitored rehabilitation program under the direction of the cardiac rehabilitation medical team. Exercise conducted during this phase (usually on a treadmill or an exercise bike) not only gets the patient moving again (albeit gently) but also provides the team with information for determining the patient's clinical status and establishing guidelines for further exercise.

■ *Phase III* usually lasts three to six months. In addition to increased exercise, the patient receives counseling on risk factor modification, stress management and diet. Phase III rehabilitation normally involves the safe incremental progression of exercise together with other important lifestyle interventions. Patients usually participate in 50-to-60-minute exercise sessions up to three times a week. In addition, they are encouraged to increase physical activity in daily living.

■ *Phase IV* consists of the exercise a patient will do for the rest of his or her life, either in a medically supervised setting or on an informal (i.e., home-based) basis. Specific exercises are up to the patient: treadmill, stair climber, rowing machine, weight lifting, pool activities, aerobic dance, or less standardized routines.

Appendix II
Sources and Web Sites

1. SELECTED SOURCES

American Heart Association. *Heart Facts*, 2001.

———. "Physicians Urged to Measure Fibrinogen." January 1996.

American Medical Association. "Revised Dietary Guidelines." *Circulation* (October 2000).

Anderson, J.L., et al. "Plasma Homocysteine Predicts Mortality Independently of Traditional Risk Factors." *Circulation* (September 2000).

Anderson, J.W., et al. "Effects of Oat Bran or Bean Intake for Hypercholesterolemic Men." *American Journal of Clinical Nutrition* 40 (1984).

Andrews, T.O., et al. "Effect of Cholesterol Reduction on Myocardial Ischemia in Patients with Coronary Disease." *Circulation* (January 1997).

Armstrong, M.L., et al. "Regression of Coronary Atherosclerosis in Rhesus Monkeys." *Circulation Research* (1959).

Arruda-Olson, A.M., et al. "Cardiovascular Effects of Sildenafil During Exercise in Men with Known or Probable Coronary Artery Disease." *Journal of the American Medical Association* (February 2002).

Barefoot, J.C., et al. "Symptoms of Depression, Acute Myocardial Infarction, and Total Mortality." *Circulation* (May 1996).

Bernard, N.D., et al. "Adherence and Acceptability of a Low-Fat Vegetarian Diet Among Patients with Cardiac Disease." *Journal of Cardiopulmonary Rehabilitation* 12 (1992).

Blair, S.N., et al. "Influences of Cardiorespiratory Fitness and Other Precursors on Cardiovascular Disease and All-Cause Mortality in Men and Women." *Journal of the American Medical Association* (July 1996).

Blankenhorn, D., et al. "The Influence of Diet on the Appearance of New Lesions in Human Coronary Arteries." *Journal of the American Medical Association* (October 1990).

Bonzheim, K.A., et al. "Women and Heart Disease: Role of Exercise-Based Cardiac Rehabilitation." *American Journal of Medicine and Sports* (May/June 2000).

Boushey, C.J., et al. "A Quantitative Assessment of Plasma Homocysteine as a Risk Factor for Vascular Disease." *Journal of the American Medical Association* (October 1995).

Brown, A.G., et al. "Regression of Coronary Artery Disease as a Result of Intensive Lipid-Lowering Therapy in Men with High Levels of Apolipoprotein B." *New England Journal of Medicine* (March 1990).

Brown, L., et al. "Cholesterol-Lowering Effects of Dietary Fiber." *American Journal of Clinical Nutrition* (July 1999).

Case, R.B., et al. "Living Alone After Myocardial Infarction: Impact on Prognosis." *Journal of the American Medical Association* (January 1992).

Danesh, J., et al. "Association of Fibrinogen with Coronary Heart Disease." *Journal of the American Medical Association* (May 1998).

———— et al. "Lipoprotein(a) and Risk of Myocardial Infarction." *Circulation* (September 2000).

———— et al. "Low-Grade Inflammation and Coronary Heart Disease." *British Medical Journal* (July 2000).

Dansky, H.M., and Fisher, F.A. "High-Density Lipoprotein and Plaque Regression." *Circulation* (November 1999).

Daviglus, M.L., et al. "Fish Consumption and the 30-Year Risk of Fatal Myocardial Infarction." *New England Journal of Medicine* (April 1997).

Despres, J.P., et al. "Hyperinsulinemia as an Independent Risk Factor for Ischemic Heart Disease." *New England Journal of Medicine* (April 1996).

Dunn, A.L., et al. "Comparison of Lifestyle and Structured Interventions to Increase Physical Activity and Cardiorespiratory Fitness." *Journal of the American Medical Association* (January 1999).

Dupuis, J., et al. "Cholesterol Reduction Rapidly Improves Endothelial Function." *Circulation* (June 1999).

Enas, E.A. "Triglycerides and Small, Dense Low-Density Lipoprotein." *Journal of the American Medical Association* (December 1998).

Fletcher, G.F., et al. "Exercise Standards for Testing and Training." *Circulation* (October 2001).

Forrester, J.S., and Prediman, K.S. "Lipid Lowering Versus Revascularization." *Circulation* (August 1997).

Franklin, Barry A. "Homocysteine: A New Risk Factor for Heart Disease." *ACSM's Health and Fitness Journal* (July/August 1998).

———. "New Insights into the Value of Cholesterol Lowering." *ACSM's Health and Fitness Journal* (March/April 1999).

———. "Psychosocial Considerations in Heart Disease." *Journal of the Hong Kong College of Cardiology* (February 2001).

———. "The Downside of Our Technological Revolution? An Obesity-Conducive Environment." *American Journal of Cardiology* (May 2001).

Franklin, Barry A., et al. "Trainability of Arms Versus Legs in Men with Previous Myocardial Infarction." *Chest* (January 1994).

——— et al. "Cardiac Demands of Heavy Snow Shoveling." *Journal of the American Medical Association* (March 1995).

——— et al. "Delayed Progression or Regression of Coronary Atherosclerosis with Intensive Risk Factor Modification: Effects of Diet, Drugs, and Exercise." *Sports Medicine* (November 1996).

——— et al. "Contemporary Cardiac Rehabilitation Services." *American Journal of Cardiology* (April 1997).

——— et al. "Rehabilitation of Cardiac Patients in the 21st Century: Changing Paradigms and Perceptions." *Journal of Sports Sciences* (Special Issue, Summer 1998).

——— et al. "Avoiding Repeat Cardiac Events: The ABCDE's of Tertiary Prevention." *The Physician and Sportsmedicine* (September 2000).

———— et al. *ACSM's Guidelines for Exercise Testing and Exercise Prescription* (6th edition). Baltimore: Lippincott Williams & Wilkins, 2000.

Freemantle, N., et al. "Beta Blockade After Myocardial Infarction: Systematic Review and Meta Regression Analysis." *British Medical Journal* (June 1999).

Gotto, A.M. "Low High-Density Lipoprotein Cholesterol as a Risk Factor in Coronary Heart Disease." *Circulation* (May 2001).

Graudal, N.A., et al. "Effects of Sodium Restriction on Blood Pressure." *Journal of the American Medical Association* (May 1998).

Grodstein, F., et al. "Postmenopausal Estrogen and Progestin Use and the Risk of Cardiovascular Disease." *New England Journal of Medicine* (August 1996).

Gullette, E., et al. "Effects of Mental Stress on Myocardial Ischemia During Daily Life." *Journal of the American Medical Association* (May 1997).

Gussekloo, J., et al. "C-Reactive Protein, Stroke, and Cardiovascular Disease." *Arteriosclerosis, Thrombosis, and Vascular Biology* (April 2000).

Hambrecht, R., et al. "Various Intensities of Leisure-Time Physical Activity in Patients with Coronary Artery Disease: Effects on Cardiorespiratory Fitness and Progression of Coronary Atherosclerotic Lesions." *Journal of the American College of Cardiology* (August 1993).

———— et al. "Effect of Exercise on Coronary Endothelial Function in Patients with Coronary Artery Disease." *New England Journal of Medicine* (February 2000).

Harvard Heart Letter. "Vitamin E Supplements." Harvard University Medical School (August 1997).

Haskell, W.L., et al. "Effects of Intensive Multiple Risk Factor Reduction on Coronary Atherosclerosis and Clinical Cardiac Events in Men and Women with Coronary Artery Disease; the Stanford Coronary Risk Intervention Project (SCRIP)." *Circulation* (March 1994).

The Heart Outcomes Prevention Evaluation Study Investigators. "Effects of an Angiotensin-Converting-Enzyme Inhibitor, Ramipril, on Cardiovascular Events in High Risk Patients." *New England Journal of Medicine* (January 2000).

Heitzer, T., et al. "Antioxidant Vitamin C Has Beneficial Effect on Artery Lining." *Circulation* (July 1996).

Hennekens, C.H. "Update on Aspirin in the Treatment and Prevention of Cardiovascular Disease." *American Heart Journal* (April 1999).

Hippisley-Cox, Julia, et al. "Depression as a Risk Factor for Ischemic Heart Disease in Men." *British Medical Journal* (June 1998).

Howard, B.V., and Kritchevsky, D. "Phytochemicals and Cardiovascular Disease." *Circulation* (June 1997).

Hu, F.B., et al. "Prospective Study of Major Dietary Patterns and Risk of Coronary Heart Disease in Men." *American Journal of Clinical Nutrition* (October 2000).

Hulley, S., et al. "Randomized Trial of Estrogen Plus Progestin for Secondary Prevention of Coronary Heart Disease in Postmenopausal Women." *Journal of the American Medical Association* (August 1998).

Ironson, G., et al. "Effects of Anger on Left Ventricular Ejection Fraction in Coronary Artery Disease." *American Journal of Cardiology* (August 1992).

Jiang, E., et al. "Mental Stress-Induced Myocardial Ischemia and Cardiac Events." *Journal of the American Medical Association* (June 1996).

Knudtson, M.L., et al. "Chelation Therapy for Ischemic Heart Disease." *Journal of the American Medical Association* (January 2002).

Krantz, D.S., et al. "Effects of Mental Stress in Patients with Coronary Artery Disease." *Journal of the American Medical Association* (April 2000).

Krauss, R.M., et al. "AHA Dietary Guidelines: Revision 2000: A Statement for Healthcare Professionals from the Nutrition Committee of the American Heart Association." *Circulation* (October 2000).

Kris-Etherton, P.M., et al. "High Monounsaturated Fatty Acid Diets Lower Both Plasma Cholesterol and Triacylglycerol Concentrations." *American Journal of Clinical Nutrition* (December 1999).

Lagrand, W.K., et al. "C-Reactive Protein as a Cardiovascular Risk Factor." *Circulation* (July 1999).

Lee, C.D., et al. "Cardiorespiratory Fitness, Body Composition, and All-Cause and Cardiovascular Disease Mortality in Men." *American Journal of Clinical Nutrition* (March 1999).

Little, W.C., et al. "Can Coronary Angiography Predict the Site of a Subsequent Myocardial Infarction in Patients with Mild to Moderate Coronary Artery Disease?" *Circulation* (November 1988).

Liu, S., et al. "Fruit and Vegetable Intake and Risk of Cardiovascular Disease." *American Journal of Clinical Nutrition* (October 2000).

————— et al. "Whole-Grain Consumption and Risk of Coronary Heart Disease: Results from the Nurses' Health Study." *American Journal of Clinical Nutrition* (August 1999).

Manson, J.E., et al. "A Prospective Study of Walking as Compared with Vigorous Exercise in the Prevention of Coronary Heart Disease in Women." *New England Journal of Medicine* (August 1999).

Myers, J., et al. "Exercise Capacity and Mortality Among Men Referred for Exercise Testing." *New England Journal of Medicine* (March 2002).

Oberman, A. "Emerging Cardiovascular Risk Factors." *Clinical Reviews* (Spring 2000).

Omenn, G.S., et al. "Preventing Coronary Heart Disease: B Vitamins and Homocysteine." *Circulation* (January 1998).

Ornish, D., et al. "Effects of Stress Management Training and Dietary Changes in Treating Ischemic Heart Disease." *Journal of the American Medical Association* (January 1983).

———— et al. "Can Lifestyle Changes Reverse Coronary Heart Disease?" *Lancet* 336 (1990).

Pearson, T.A., et al. "Most Patients Do Not Achieve Target LDL Cholesterol Levels." *Archives of Internal Medicine* (February 2000).

Piscatella, Joseph C. *Don't Eat Your Heart Out*. New York: Workman Publishing, 1994.

————. *Fat-Proof Your Child*. New York: Workman Publishing, 1997.

————. *The Fat-Gram Guide to Restaurant Food*. New York: Workman Publishing, 1997.

Pitt, B., et al. "Aggressive Lipid-Lowering Therapy Compared with Angioplasty in Stable Coronary Artery Disease." *New England Journal of Medicine* (July 1999).

Pollock, M.L., et al. "The Recommended Quantity and Quality of Exercise for Developing and Maintaining Cardiorespiratory and Muscular Fitness, and Flexibility in Healthy Adults." *Medicine and Science in Sports and Exercise* (June 1998).

———— et al. "Resistance Exercise in Individuals with and Without Cardiovascular Disease: Benefits, Rationale, Safety, and Prescription." *Circulation* (February 2000).

Pope, C.A., III, et al. "Lung Cancer, Cardiopulmonary Mortality, and Long-Term Exposure to Fine Particulate Air Pollution." *Journal of the American Medical Association* (March 2002).

Rader, D.J. "Inflammatory Markers of Coronary Risk." *New England Journal of Medicine* (October 2000).

Rader, D.J., and Brewer, H.B. "Lipoprotein(a): Clinical Approach to a Unique Atherogenic Lipoprotein." *Journal of the American Medical Association* (February 1992).

Raggi, P., et al. "Identification of Patients at Increased Risk of First Unheralded Acute Myocardial Infarction by Electron-Beam Computed Tomography." *Circulation* (February 2000).

Reaven, G.M. "Insulin Resistance, Its Consequences, and Coronary Heart Disease." *Circulation* (May 1996).

Ribiero, J.P., et al. "The Effectiveness of a Low Lipid Diet and Exercise in the Management of Coronary Artery Disease." *American Heart Journal* (February 1984).

Ridker, P.M. "High-Sensitivity C-Reactive Protein." *Circulation* (April 2001).

Ridker, P.M., et al. "C-Reactive Protein and Other Markers of Inflammation in the Prediction of Cardiovascular Disease in Women." *New England Journal of Medicine* (March 2000).

———— et al. "Homocysteine and Risk of Cardiovascular Disease Among Postmenopausal Women." *Journal of the American Medical Association* (May 1999).

Rimm, E.B., et al. "Vitamin E Consumption and the Risk of Coronary Heart Disease in Men." *New England Journal of Medicine* (May 1993).

———— et al. "Vegetable, Fruit, and Cereal Fiber Intake and Risk of Coronary Heart Disease Among Men." *Journal of the American Medical Association* (February 1996).

Roberts, W.C. "Preventing and Arresting Coronary Atherosclerosis." *American Heart Journal* (September 1995).

————. "The Underused Miracle Drugs: The Statin Drugs Are to Atherosclerosis What Penicillin Was to Infectious Disease." *American Journal of Cardiology* (August 1996).

————. "Shifting from Decreasing to Actually Preventing and Arresting Atherosclerosis." *American Journal of Cardiology* (March 1999).

Rutherford, J.D., et al. "Effects of Captopril on Ischemic Events After Myocardial Infarction: Results of the Survival and Ventricular Enlargement Trial." *Circulation* (October 1994).

Sacks, F.M., et al. "Effects on Blood Pressure of Reduced Dietary Sodium and the Dietary Approaches to Stop Hypertension (DASH) Diet." *New England Journal of Medicine* (January 2001).

Sandkamp, M., et al. "Lipoprotein(a) Is an Independent Risk Factor for Myocardial Infarction at a Young Age." *Clinical Chemistry* 36 (1990).

Schuler, G., et al. "Myocardial Perfusion and Regression of Coronary Artery Disease in Patients on a Regimen of Intensive Physical Exercise and Low-Fat Diet." *Journal of the American College of Cardiology* (June 1992).

Scott, J.M. "Homocysteine and Cardiovascular Risk." *American Journal of Clinical Nutrition* (August 2000).

Sesso, H.D., et al. "Physical Activity and Coronary Heart Disease in Men: The Harvard Alumni Health Study." *Circulation* (August 2000).

Smith, S.C. "Risk Reduction Therapy: The Challenge to Change." *Circulation* (June 1996).

Smith, S.C., et al. "AHA/ACC Guidelines for Preventing Heart Attack and Death in Patients with Atherosclerotic Cardiovascular Disease: 2001 Update." *Circulation* (September 2001).

Stampfer, M.J., et al. "Primary Prevention of Coronary Disease in Women Through Diet and Lifestyle." *New England Journal of Medicine* (July 2000).

Superko, H.R. "Beyond HDL Cholesterol Reduction." *Circulation* (November 1996).

Taddei, S., et al. "Vitamin C Improves Endothelium-Dependent Vasodilation." *Circulation* (June 1998).

Third Report of the National Cholesterol Education Program (NCEP) Expert Panel on Detection, Evaluation, and Treatment of High Blood Cholesterol in Adults (Adult Treatment Panel III). National Cholesterol Education Program, National Heart, Lung and Blood Institute, National Institutes of Health, 2001.

Trevisan, M., et al. "Consumption of Olive Oil, Butter and Vegetable Oils and Coronary Heart Disease Risk Factors." *Journal of the American Medical Association* (August 1990).

Urano, H., et al. "Enhanced External Counter-Pulsation Improves Exercise Tolerance, Reduces Exercise-induced Myocardial Ischemia and Improves Left Ventricular Diastolic Filling in Patients with Coronary Artery Disease." *Journal of the American College of Cardiology* (January 2001).

Vakkailainen, J., et al. "Endothelial Dysfunction in Men with Small LDL Particles." *Circulation* (August 2000).

Vanhees, L., et al. "Prognostic Significance of Peak Exercise Capacity in Patients with Coronary Artery Disease." *Journal of the American College of Cardiology* (February 1994).

Vita, A.J., et al. "Aging, Health Risks, and Cumulative Disability." *New England Journal of Medicine* (April 1998).

Wenger, N.K., et al. *Cardiac Rehabilitation.* Clinical Practice Guideline No. 17. Rockville, Md.: U.S. Department of Health and Human Services, Public Health Service, Agency for Health Care Policy and Research and the National Heart, Lung, and Blood Institute. AHCPR Publication No. 96-0672. October 1995.

Williams, J.E., et al. "Anger Proneness Predicts Coronary Heart Disease Risk." *Circulation* (May 2000).

Williams, R.B., et al. "Prognostic Importance of Social and Economic Resources Among Medically Treated Patients with Angiographically Documented Coronary Artery Disease." *Journal of the American Medical Association* (January 1992).

2. CREDITS

Pages 34–35: Body Mass Index Table. Adapted from *Clinical Guidelines on the Identification, Evaluation and Treatment of Overweight and Obesity in Adults: The Evidence Report.*

Page 56: Duke Activity Status Report. *American Journal of Cardiology,* Vol. 64, Hlatky et al., "A Brief Self-Administered Questionnaire . . . ," pp. 651–54, 1989, with permission of Excerpta Medica Inc.

Pages 64–65: Type A Behavior Test. From *60 Second Stress Management* by Dr. Andrew Goliszek. Reprinted with permission from New Horizon Press, Far Hills, New Jersey. Copyright © 1992 by Dr. Andrew Goliszek.

Pages 71–72: Anger and Hostility Profile. Arnst Ogden Medical Center, Elmira, New York. Used with permission.

Pages 75–76: Depression Screening Test, adapted from HANDS (Harvard Department of Psychiatry/National Depression Screening Day Scale). Copyright © 1998 President and Fellows of Harvard College and Screening for Mental Health.

Pages 112–13: Life Events Scale. Reprinted from *Journal of Psychosomatic Research,* 11: 213–218, T.H. Holmes and R.H. Rahe, "The Social Readjustment Scale," 1967, with permission from Elsevier Science.

Page 135: Resiliency Test. Adapted from *The Survivor Personality* by Al Siebert, Ph.D. (Perigee Books, 1996).

Page 161: Energy Intake/Expenditure. J.O. Hill and E.L. Melanson, "Overview of the determinants of overweight and obesity," published in *Medicine and Science in Sports and Exercise,* Vol. 31, No. 11, 1999. Used with permission from Lippincott Williams & Wilkins.

Page 168: Activity Pyramid. Copyright © 2002 Park Nicollet *Health Source.* Park Nicollet Institute. Reprinted by permission.

Page 175: Borg RPE Scale. For correct usage, instruction and administration see *Borg's Perceived Exertion and Pain Scales* by Gunnar Borg, Ph.D., 1998, Human Kinetics.

Page 246: Body-Fat Percentage. Adapted, by permission, from J.H. Wilmore, 1986, *Sensible Fitness.* Human Kinetics (Champaign, Illinois), pp. 30–31.

Page 311: "One at a Time." From *Chicken Soup for the Soul* by Jack Canfield and Mark V. Hansen, pp. 22–23. 1993.

3. RECOMMENDED WEB SITES

American Association of Cardiovascular and Pulmonary Rehabilitation	www.aacvpr.org
American College of Cardiology	www.acc.org
American College of Sports Medicine	www.acsm.org
American Council on Exercise	www.acefitness.org
American Diabetes Association	www.diabetes.org
American Dietetic Association	www.eatright.org
American Heart Association	www.americanheart.org
Federal Trade Commission Consumer Line	www.ftc.gov
Institute for Fitness & Health	www.joepiscatella.com
National Academy of Sports Medicine	www.nasm.org
National Strength and Conditioning Association	www.nsca-lift.org
Nutrition Action	www.cspinet.org
Shape Up America	www.shapeup.org
Tufts Newsletter	www.healthletter.tufts.edu

Index

A

Abbott homocysteine, 24–25
Abdominal breathing, 131
Abdominal obesity, xxiv, 32–33, 61
  stress and, 109
  Syndrome X and, 48, 49
  waist circumference and, 32–33, 61, 80
Abookire, Susan, 318
Academy of General Dentistry, 140
ACE inhibitors, 323–25
Active lifestyle, 92
  see also Exercise
Activity Pyramid, 168–69
Acute alarm, 109
Addiction, 127
Adrenaline, 22, 107
Aerobic capacity or fitness, 160, 168, 197
  as cardiac marker, 4, 50–57, 82
  measurement of, 51, 54–57
  moderate, physical activities of, 52
  mortality and (graph), 53
  reclaiming of, 180
  studies on effects of, 52–54
Aerobic dancing, 204–5
Aerobic exercise, 50, 164, 168, 169–76,
    186, 187, 208
  activities for, 169–70
  biking, 162, 198–200, 203
  frequency of, 170
  intensity of, xxv, 170–75, 207
  mood disorders and, 130
  running, 159, 193–94, 198
  time factor and, 175–76
  Type A behavior and, 129
  see also Jogging; Walking
African-Americans, 5, 37, 44
Aggression, 68–69, 127
  assertiveness vs., 143
Aging:
  exercise and, xxiii–xxiv, 165–66
  reducing stiffness of, 187
Ainsworth, Barbara, 174
Air Force/Texas Coronary Atherosclerosis
    Prevention Study, 9, 318
Air pollution, xxi–xxii

Alcohol, xxxvii, 21, 115, 132, 231–32,
    293–95
  blood pressure and, 94
  caloric content of, 295
  excessive intake of, 231, 293–94
  HDL level and, 88
  inflammation and, 28, 232
  potential health benefits of, 231–32,
    293–95
Alcoholism, 105
Allen, Woody, 122
Alzheimer's disease, 10, 319
American Academy of Child and
    Adolescent Psychiatry, 105
American Academy of Family Physicians,
    105
American Cancer Association, 97
American Cancer Society, 232
American College of Cardiology, xxxv, 14
American College of Sports Medicine, 92,
    170, 176, 177, 179, 185, 187, 196,
    198, 256
American Council on Exercise, 177, 198
American Diabetes Association, 46
American diet, 5, 212–18, 228, 235, 238
  factors influencing food choices and,
    215–17
  need for changes in, 217–18
  snapshot of, 213–15
American Dietary Association, 255
American Dietetic Association, 228
American Heart Association (AHA), xviii,
    xxvi, xxxv, xxxvi, 10–11, 13, 14, 21,
    33, 42–43, 86, 97, 172, 176–77, 214,
    218, 222, 226–27, 231, 257, 290, 315,
    322
American lifestyle, 5, 30–31
  see also American diet; Sedentary
    lifestyle
American Lung Association, 57, 97
American Medical Association, 106, 220
American Psychological Association, 130
American Restaurant Association, 216
Anderson, James, 229
Androgens, 115
Aneurysms, 36

X

Y

About the Authors

JOSEPH C. PISCATELLA is the author of five books—*Don't Eat Your Heart Out Cookbook, Choices for a Healthy Heart, Controlling Your Fat Tooth, Fat-Proof Your Child* and *The Fat-Gram Guide to Restaurant Food*—all of which have been enthusiastically endorsed by health professionals. His books are used by more than 5,500 hospitals in cardiac rehabilitation, weight loss and prevention programs.

Mr. Piscatella is president of the Institute for Fitness & Health in Gig Harbor, Washington. He lectures on lifestyle management skills to a variety of clients, from Fortune 500 companies to health professionals, was the host of two PBS television specials, and is a frequent guest on network television programs. The only nonmedical member of a National Institutes of Health Cardiac Rehabilitation Expert Panel charged with developing clinical practice guidelines for physicians, he is also a member of the American Association for Cardiovascular and Pulmonary Rehabilitation.

BARRY A. FRANKLIN, who received his doctoral degree in physiology from Pennsylvania State University, is director of the Cardiac Rehabilitation Program and Exercise Laboratories at William Beaumont Hospital, Royal Oak, Michigan. He also holds adjunct faculty appointments as clinical professor of exercise science at Oakland University, professor of physiology at the Wayne State University School of Medicine and professor of family medicine at the University of Michigan. Dr. Franklin has served as president of the American Association of Cardiovascular and Pulmonary Rehabilitation as well as the American College of Sports Medicine. He is a past editor in chief of the *Journal of Cardiopulmonary Rehabilitation* and currently serves as editor for the *American Journal of Medicine and Sports*. He holds editorial positions with the *American Journal of Cardiology* and *Medicine and Science in Sports & Exercise,* and has authored or coauthored over 300 papers, abstracts, chapters and books.